Your Doctor Can't Make You HEALTHY

Evidence-based insights into protecting your health and preventing the major lifestyle killers of modern man

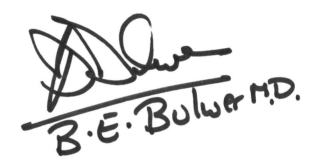

B·E·Bulwer M.D.

BERNARD E. BULWER, M.D.

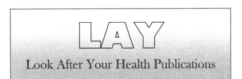

LAY
Look After Your Health Publications

www.LookAfterYourHealth.net

Boston, Massachusetts, USA

Your Doctor Can't Make You Healthy

Evidence-based insights into protecting your health and
preventing the major lifestyle killers of modern man

Published by Lay Publications, Boston, MA

Library of Congress Control Number: 2002095266

Bulwer, Bernard E. Your Doctor Can't Make You Healthy: Evidence-based insights into protecting your health and preventing the major lifestyle killers of modern man./ Bernard E. Bulwer.
    p. cm.

"A Look After Your Health Book"
Includes bibliographical references and index.
ISBN: 0-9725532-0-7

1. Nutrition.   2. Health.   3. Lifestyle.   4. Education
Cover design by Carol McLeod Design
Manufacturing: Graphic Services
403 VFW Drive, Rockland, MA 02370

Printed and bound in the United States of America

For Noor, Bertha, Elston, family, and all my teachers

To Whom It May Concern:

(Page 35)

Doctors were trained to treat diseases.
Politicians and insurance companies *promise* to look after your healthcare,
but *only you* can look after your "health."
And please …don't blame your politician, your doctor, or McDonald's.
Take a good long look at what's inside your refrigerator, your cupboard,
and at the way you spend your leisure time.
…and, take a look inside these pages
before you make up your mind.

To My Medical Colleagues:

This is not a doctor-bashing book.
We will do our patients and ourselves a favor by
letting them know that
we were trained primarily to treat their diseases.
Let them understand that good health chiefly resides with
what happens outside of the doctor's office or the hospital.

To the Politician:

There is an urgent need to shift the healthcare debate:
"More prescription drugs
and more high-technology medicine
does not mean better health."
This one calls for courage, not "political correctness."
The public needs to be told: "Good healthcare we need,
but good health is what we desperately need."
This is not a gift from politicians or doctors.
Good health follows healthy lifestyles.
It calls for greater personal responsibility mixed with a
healthy dose of politically-incorrect legislation.

The following charts (I to V) summarize the major focus of this book.

 # Prudent Cosmopolitan Diet

"The Best Diets All Under One Roof"

The Prudent Cosmopolitan Diet is a simple model of healthy eating that embraces the best of the healthiest diets in the world and places them all under one roof. It serves as a framework on which to build your personal strategy to prevent disease and optimize health *(Charts IV, V, and Chapter 8)*.

It incorporates the best of those dietary patterns that are scientifically linked to the lowest rates of nutrition- and lifestyle-related diseases. This approach addresses the urgent need to tackle the modern epidemic of obesity, cardiovascular diseases, type II diabetes, and cancer *(Chart I, II, III, and Chapter 5)*.

The **Prudent Cosmopolitan Diet** is a logical prescription for eating in modern cosmopolitan societies:

- The **foundation** is the *best of American or local foods*. The upward direction of the arrow symbolizes the need to increase the intake of these foods (Chapter 8).
- The **first pillar** is a *Mediterranean-style diet* (Chapter 8). The upward direction of the arrow (chimney) recommends increased intake of these cuisines.
- The **second pillar** is an *Asian-style diet* (Chapter 5 and Chapter 8). The upward direction of this arrow (chimney) recommends increased intake of these foods.
- The **ceiling** with the downward-pointing arrow ("chandelier") represents the advice to consume less of all foods that comprise *the Western diet* (Chapter 5 and Chapter 7).
- Hidden somewhere in the **attic** is a bottle of dietary supplements with the label marked, "*Supplements…not substitutes.*" These can play a role, but they are never substitutes for a healthy nutrition and lifestyle (Chapter 2, Chapter 6, and Chapter 8).
- Occupying the **entrance** is a human figure in running form to highlight the need for increased physical activity (Chapter 9).

Good Choices in Nutrition and Lifestyle (Chart V) summarizes the "big picture:" Your Prudent Cosmopolitan Diet, smoking cessation, and increased physical activity are the 3 key players to prevent and control a broad range of nutrition and lifestyle-related diseases: obesity, cardiovascular diseases, type II diabetes and several forms of cancer.

CHART 1

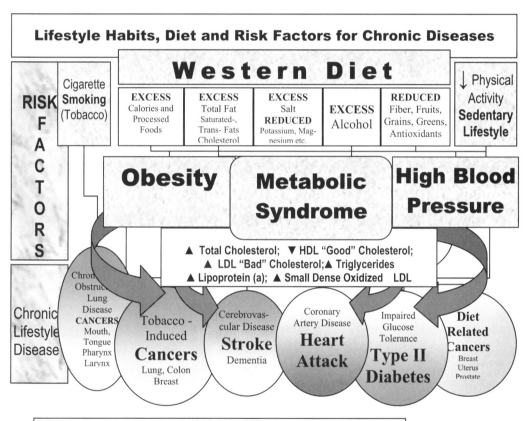

Lifestyle Habits, Diet and Risk Factors for Chronic Diseases

Western Diet

RISK FACTORS

Cigarette Smoking (Tobacco)

| EXCESS Calories and Processed Foods | EXCESS Total Fat Saturated-, Trans- Fats Cholesterol | EXCESS Salt REDUCED Potassium, Magnesium etc. | EXCESS Alcohol | REDUCED Fiber, Fruits, Grains, Greens, Antioxidants |

↓ Physical Activity Sedentary Lifestyle

Obesity

Metabolic Syndrome

High Blood Pressure

▲ Total Cholesterol; ▼ HDL "Good" Cholesterol;
▲ LDL "Bad" Cholesterol; ▲ Triglycerides
▲ Lipoprotein (a); ▲ Small Dense Oxidized LDL

Chronic Lifestyle Disease

Chronic Obstructive Lung Disease
CANCERS Mouth, Tongue Pharynx Larynx

Tobacco - Induced **Cancers** Lung, Colon Breast

Cerebrovascular Disease **Stroke** Dementia

Coronary Artery Disease **Heart Attack**

Impaired Glucose Tolerance **Type II Diabetes**

Diet Related Cancers Breast Uterus Prostate

The major behavioral risk factors increase the likelihood of developing the Metabolic Syndrome and a host of related diseases—cardiovascular diseases, diabetes, and cancer.

© B.E. Bulwer 2003

Further explanations of this chart appear in the Introduction under "Why Another Book on Nutrition and Lifestyle?" and receives extensive coverage in Chapter 5.

CHART 11

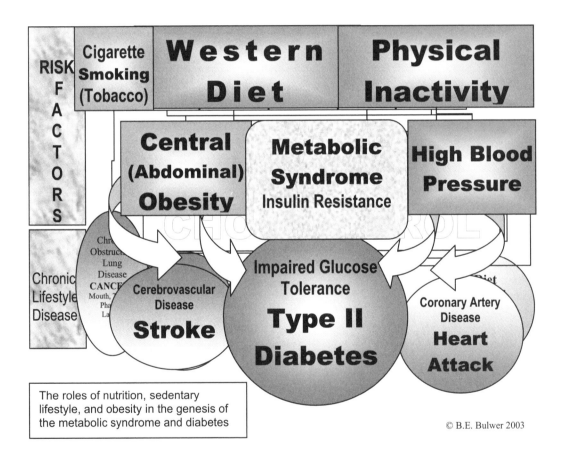

The roles of nutrition, sedentary lifestyle, and obesity in the genesis of the metabolic syndrome and diabetes

© B.E. Bulwer 2003

For further explanations of this chart, see Chapter 2 under "The Root of the Matter."

CHART 111

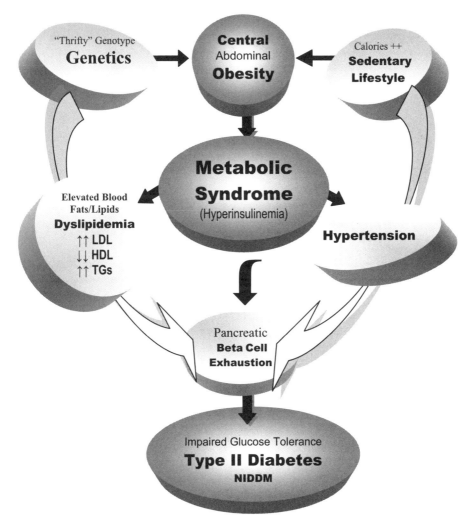

Genetics, Lifestyle, Central Obesity, and the Metabolic Syndrome

HDL—High Density Lipoprotein Cholesterol; LDL—Low Density Lipoprotein Cholesterol; Lp(a)—Lipoprotein (a); TGs—Triglycerides.

Explanations appear in Chapter 5 under "The Metabolic Syndrome—the Insulin Resistance Syndrome."

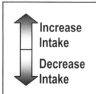

Increase
Intake

Decrease
Intake

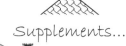

Supplements...

Not substitutes!

Worst of the

Western Diet

**High Fat, Red Meats, Highly Processed
Foods, Fast Foods, Soft Drinks
Dairy Products**

Best of

Mediterran
-ean Diets

**Vegetable Salads
Virgin Olive Oils
Wine with Meals
Fruits, Nuts, Grains**

Joie de vivre

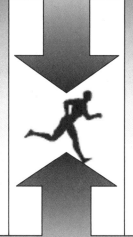

Best of

Asian Diets

**Soy Products
Green Teas
Stir frys
Greens, Fruits, Nuts,
Grains**

*High rice and noodle
intake with less meats
and fats*

Best of

American, Regional or Local Diets

**Fruits, Vegetables, Whole Grains, Nuts, Fish-especially fatty
fish, Skinless-Boneless Poultry & occasional Lean Meats**

 # Prudent Cosmopolitan Diet

"The Best Diets All Under One Roof"

Your Prudent Cosmopolitan Diet is a simple model of healthy eating that embraces the best of
the healthiest diets in the world and places them all under one roof. It serves as a framework on
which to build your personal strategy to prevent disease and optimize health.

See Chapter 8, Figure 8-3 and text "Constructing a Prudent Cosmopolitan Diet."

CHART V

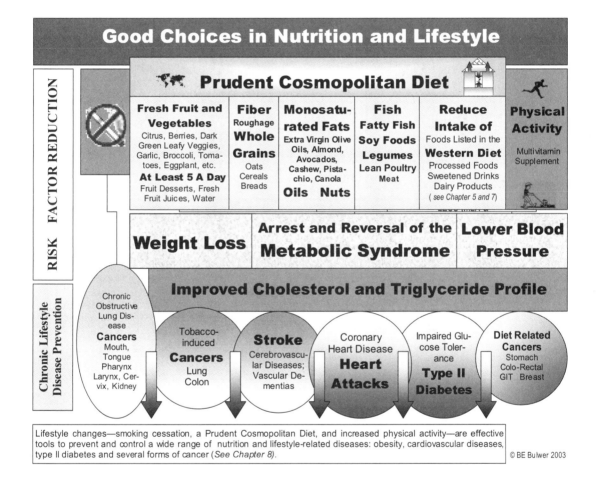

Good Choices in Nutrition and Lifestyle

RISK FACTOR REDUCTION

Chronic Lifestyle Disease Prevention

Prudent Cosmopolitan Diet

Fresh Fruit and Vegetables	Fiber	Monosatu-rated Fats	Fish	Reduce Intake of
Citrus, Berries, Dark Green Leafy Veggies, Garlic, Broccoli, Tomatoes, Eggplant, etc.	Roughage **Whole Grains**	Extra Virgin Olive Oils, Almond, Avocados, Cashew, Pistachio, Canola	Fatty Fish Soy Foods Legumes Lean Poultry Meat	Foods Listed in the **Western Diet** Processed Foods Sweetened Drinks Dairy Products
At Least 5 A Day Fruit Desserts, Fresh Fruit Juices, Water	Oats Cereals Breads	**Oils Nuts**		(*see Chapter 5 and 7*)

Physical Activity

Multivitamin Supplement

Weight Loss	Arrest and Reversal of the Metabolic Syndrome	Lower Blood Pressure

Improved Cholesterol and Triglyceride Profile

Chronic Obstructive Lung Disease **Cancers** Mouth, Tongue Pharynx Larynx, Cervix, Kidney

Tobacco-induced **Cancers** Lung Colon

Stroke Cerebrovascular Diseases; Vascular Dementias

Coronary Heart Disease **Heart Attacks**

Impaired Glucose Tolerance **Type II Diabetes**

Diet Related Cancers Stomach Colo-Rectal GIT Breast

Lifestyle changes—smoking cessation, a Prudent Cosmopolitan Diet, and increased physical activity—are effective tools to prevent and control a wide range of nutrition and lifestyle-related diseases: obesity, cardiovascular diseases, type II diabetes and several forms of cancer (*See Chapter 8*).

© BE Bulwer 2003

Summarizing the Big Picture:
Three (3) key players—
Your Prudent Cosmopolitan Diet, Smoking Cessation, and Increased Physical Activity can prevent and control the major killers of modern mankind

This chart is the main subject of Chapter 8.

A Summary of the Effects of Dietary Fats on Blood Lipids: HDL, LDL, and Triglycerides)

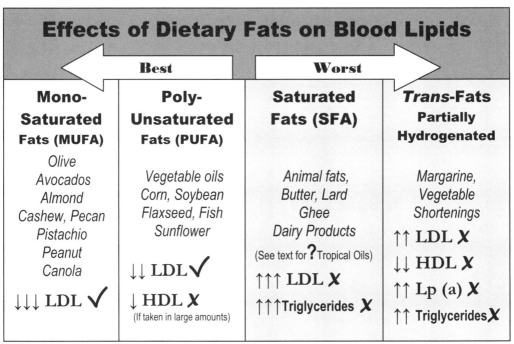

HDL—High Density Lipoprotein Cholesterol ("Good")
LDL—Low Density Lipoprotein Cholesterol ("Bad")
Lp(a)—Lipoprotein (a) Cholesterol ("Very Bad")

√--Good Effect   X--Bad Effect

This chart is discussed in Chapter 5.

About the author

Bernard Bulwer, M.D. is the editor (nutrition and diabetes studies) and director of outreach for ProCOR, a Boston-based cardiology forum dedicated to the prevention of heart disease. He was the first successful applicant for a developing world fellowship in cardiovascular diseases at the Lown Cardiovascular Center and the Brigham and Women's Hospital in Boston, Massachusetts, teaching affiliates of Harvard Medical School.

He pursued undergraduate medical training at the University of the West Indies and postgraduate studies in Nutrition at Kings College, University of London. In 1994, he was appointed clinical fellow/specialist registrar in Diabetes Medicine at the teaching hospitals of the University of Newcastle upon Tyne, England with the team of Professor Sir KGMM Alberti—president of the Royal College of Physicians and president of the International Diabetes Federation, and Professor Philip Home—chairman of the European Diabetes Federation. Dr. Bulwer served as the founding president of the Belize Diabetes Association, physician to the U.S. Embassy in Belize and the wider Belize community.

Dr. Bulwer currently holds professional memberships with the American Diabetes Association, the International Diabetes Federation, and the American Association of Clinical Endocrinologists. His experience is international, spanning congresses in the United States, United Kingdom, Cambridge University, India, and Latin America.

His major interests are nutrition, diabetes, and prevention of cardiovascular diseases.

How to use this book

This book employs several purpose-built features that make it a useful study tool. It is organized to enable the reader to easily navigate and retrieve areas of special interest. It can be read from cover to cover, but its layout will tempt most readers to browse and select their own menu (see "Who Should Read This Book" on page 35.)

📖 Useful Organizational Features

Five key charts (Chart I to Chart V) are placed at the beginning of the book to visually summarize nutrition and lifestyle and their relationships to health and disease. They appear again within the context of their appropriate chapters. A **summary of contents** is followed by a detailed **table of contents**. To gain a quick overall perspective, the reader should refer to the **overview** section on page 37. Every chapter is preceded by a **chapter outline** and a **summary** concludes each chapter. **References** (more than 1,000) for further reading and a **general index** appear at the end of the book.

📖 Shaded Texts (Insights) for Rapid Browsing

Shaded texts using larger font sizes appear within each chapter. These features serve two main purposes. First, they provide easy-to-read perspectives and insights. Secondly, they provide a way of rapidly browsing throughout the entire book. In so doing, the entire book can be quickly and comprehensively scanned.

📖 More than 100 charts, figures, and tables

This book is not stingy on charts, tables, and figures. A list of these is provided on page 29. Most consumer books offer a lot of scattered information, but fall short of providing a simple framework for grasping the essence of nutrition and lifestyle. This book deliberately fills that need by devising a series of charts that show the connections between the Western diet and lifestyles to the modern global epidemic of obesity, cardiovascular diseases, diabetes, and cancer. The Prudent Cosmopolitan Diet is a simple model to that is designed to help you navigate through the modern nutrition maze. It embraces the best of the healthiest diets in the world and places them all under one roof. They are a meaningful foundation upon which to build a healthy lifestyle plan.

⟂ Online Updates

For updates on the material covered in this book along with relevant links, please visit:

www.LookAfterYourHealth.net

CONTENTS AT A GLANCE

List of Figures and Tables 29
Acknowledgments 33
Who Should Read This Book 35
Overview 37

Part I

Introduction 43

Introduction 45

Part II

Background Issues in Health and Healthcare 59

1. Health and Healthcare: Two Very Different Things 61
2. "Pill for Every Ill" Mentality 75
3. How Much does Your Doctor Know about Nutrition? 105
4. Complementary and Alternative Medicine (CAM) 129

Part III

The Burden of Lifestyle Diseases 161

5. Common Risk Factors In Chronic Diseases: The Western Diet 163
6. Growing Older and Aging…When the Rust Steps In 209

Part IV

All That Stuff That Enters Your Mouth 249

7. Food and Choices: The "Dynamix" of Why We Eat What We Eat 251

Part V

Your Health, Charting Your Future 311

8. Nutrition Choices for Health and Disease 313
9. Lifestyle Physical Activity…Get Moving 365
10. Making Choices That Last 385

Part VI

Book Resources 397

References 399
Book Resources 445
General Index 447

TABLE OF CONTENTS

Dedication 3
Chart Summaries 5
About the Author 13
How to Use This Book 15
Contents at a Glance 17
Table of Contents 19
List of Figures and Tables 29
Acknowledgements 33
Who Should Read this Book 35
Overview 37

PART I

INTRODUCTION

INTRODUCTION

What?   Did You Say Your Doctor *Cannot*? 46
Alarming Statistics 47
Pay Now…Or Pay Much More Later 50
Perspectives of This Book 53
Why another Book on Nutrition and Lifestyle? 54
Show Me the Evidence 56
Summary 57

PART II

BACKGROUND ISSUES IN HEALTH AND HEALTHCARE

1. HEALTH AND HEALTHCARE:
Two Very Different Things

The Wrong Emphasis 63
Losing Our War on Drugs 64
Healthy Living Is Not A Killjoy 66

When Virtue Becomes a Vice 68
A Better Approach to Health..70
Less Healthcare, More Health..72
The Present and Future Challenges 73
Summary..73

2. "PILL FOR EVERY ILL" MENTALITY

A Glimpse at the Past...77
America: An Overmedicated Society 79
Direct-to-Consumer Ads and "Pester Power" 80
Programmed to Pop Pills 82
Pill-Happy Physicians 83
Looking for Quick Fixes..85
Is It Really Your Genes?..86
Is It Nature or Nurture? 87
Doomed by What Happened in the Womb?................................89
The Root of the Matter..90
How Pharmaceuticals Work..93
Placebo Effect 96
Natural vs. Synthetic; Herbs vs. Drugs......................................97
Turf War..98
Blurred Distinctions 99
"The Future Is Food" 101
Nutrition: Prompt Results, Not Quick Fixes............................101
The Problem with Doctors 102
Summary..104

3. HOW MUCH DOES YOUR DOCTOR KNOW ABOUT NUTRITION?

Introduction 107
On Automobile Mechanics and Doctors 108
What gets taught in Medical Schools 110
Postgraduate, Specialist or Residency Training 112
Important Historical Backdrop..113
The Early 1900s: Nutrition Awakened 113
The Mid 1900s: Nutrition Forsakened 114
The Years Since: Nutrition Disregarded 116
Prestige, Influence and Credibility..117
Who Dictates Research? 118

Increased Professional awareness...120
Growing Public Awareness 121
Nutrition Education in U.S. Medical Schools 122
Nutrition Education Elsewhere..125
Conclusions and Recommendations..126
The End-game..127
Summary...127

4. COMPLEMENTARY AND ALTERNATIVE MEDICINE (CAM)

The Gripe and the Hype about CAM..131
Of Egos and Attitudes 133
Why so many are turning to CAM 135
How popular is CAM? 138
Disquiet in the Mainstream Ranks 139
All those Names!...142
Definitions: CAM and Integrative Medicine...143
NIH Classification of CAM 146
    1.   Alternative Medical Systems: Chinese, Ayurveda, etc...........................146
    2.   Mind-Body Interventions: Hypnosis, Religious healing, etc....................148
    3.   Biological-Based Therapies: Herbal, Special Dietary, etc. 149
    4.   Manipulative and Body-Based Methods: Chiropractic etc...................149
    5.   Energy Therapies..150
Doctors: Mixed Reviews about CAM..150
Doctors: Concerns about CAM...152
Responsibility and Regulation of CAM 154
Conclusion and Summary...155
Addendum: Personal Perspectives 157

PART III

THE BURDEN OF LIFESTYLE DISEASES

5. COMMON RISK FACTORS IN CHRONIC DISEASES
The Western Diet and Negative Lifestyles

Observations..165
The Concept of Risk 167
Framingham Heart Study..168
Risk Factors Defined..169
The Primary Risk Factors in Lifestyle Diseases 171
    Common Risk Factors…Multiple Outcomes 171
    Tobacco Use 172
    Overweight and Obesity 173
    Sedentary Lifestyle (Physical Inactivity) 173
The Western Diet: A Closer Look 173
    Excess Food, Excess Calories 175
    Should Women Eat More During Pregnancy? 179
    Too Much Highly Processed Foods..181
    Excess Total Fats, Saturated Fat and Trans-Fats 183
    Tropical Oils: Are they as bad as some believe?................................187
    Meaty Matters 190
    Poultry..192
    Seafood 193
    Misunderstandings about Dietary Cholesterol...................................194
    Milk and Dairy Products 195
    Milk, Dairy Products, and Prostate Cancer 197
    Cured, Smoked and Charcoal-Grilled Meats.....................................198
    Excess Sodium; Reduced Potassium and Magnesium 199
    Too Much Alcohol: Weighing Risks and Benefits 200
    Reduced Fruit, Vegetables, Greens, Grains, and Fiber.......................202
Risk Charts and Tables..203
The Metabolic Syndrome—the Insulin Resistance Syndrome.......................204
Beyond Risk—Towards Maximized Health 206
Towards Aggressive Prevention 207
Summary...208

6. GROWING OLDER AND AGING:
...When the Rust Steps In

Introduction: Aging Does Not Start At 50 211
Aging: Perceptions and Misconceptions. 212
Perceptions of Youth and Aging 213
A New Paradigm on Aging 215
Definitions of Aging...215
Chronological Aging...216
An Aging Society..218
Why We Age: Theories on Aging..219
Integrated Theories..220
The Onslaughts of Free Radical Damage..220
Free Radicals and Cellular Function 221
Free Radicals and Cellular DNA 223
Free Radicals and Cell Membranes 224
Free Radicals and the Immune System 225
Free Radicals and the Cardiovascular System 226
    Blood Vessels and Cholesterol Effects 226
    The Heart, Brain, and Male Sexual Function 229
    Smoking, Free Radicals, and the Circulation 230
Free Radicals and Cancer..231
The Aging Skin: Effects of Sun, Sex, and Race................................231
    Sun Exposure 232
    Skin Aging and Race 232
    Skin Aging and Sex..233
Lifestyle Aging Accelerators...233
Stress and Modern Living: Killing Ourselves Trying To Make a Living 234
Words to the Workaholic 235
Doctors in Distress..235
Personal Reflections 235
Chronic Sleep Debt: Sleep Deprivation: 238
How to Know if You Have Not Slept Enough 239
The Medical Ravages of Sleep Deprivation 240
Never Too Late...241
Stop Smoking! It's Never Too late To Benefit..................................241
Good Nutrition Choices...242
Strengthen Those Muscles and Keep Active 243
Don't Let Your Mind Go to Waste 243
The Okinawa Formula 244
Longevity...245
Summary..247
An Ode to All Who Age 248

PART IV

ALL THAT STUFF THAT ENTERS YOUR MOUTH

7. FOOD AND CHOICES:
The "Dynamix" of Why We Eat What We Eat

Life and Choices In the Real World...253
Doctors and Governments Cannot Legislate Food Choices 255
The Complexities of Food Choices 257
Hierarchy of Food Choices 258
Socialization and Food Choices...260
Targeting the Children 262
"Ameri-sizing"...265
Economics and Food Choices...265
Politics and Food Choices 268
The USDA Food Guide Pyramid...268
The Media and Food Choices..271
Globalization and Food Choices 272
Individual Issues and Food Choices 273
Introduction to Food Processing 275
Industrial Food Processing Methods 277
Spectrum of Food Processing Methods 278
Newer Food Processing Methods 280
Processing and the Nutritional Value of Foods 280
Hidden Salt (Sodium) 283
Hidden Sugars 284
Impact of Processing on Vitamins 285
Raw or Natural Can Be Dangerous...287
Enrichment and Fortification of Foods 290
Reducing Nutrient Losses While Cooking.......................................290
Health Concerns over Some Cooking Methods 291
Food Toxins Produced during Grilling and Barbecuing..................291
Irradiated and Microwaved Foods 292
On Aluminum Pots and Alzheimer's Disease 292
Deep Fat Frying and the Reheating of Oils 293
Concerns over Technology and Agricultural Practices 294
Organic Foods; Alarm over Mad Cow Disease................................294
Organic Foods—Definitions 296

"Certified Organic" 296
Genetically Modified (GM) Foods 298
Is The American Food Supply Too Clean? 299
The Need for Balance 301
Food Labels 301
The New Food Label 303
Dissecting Food Labels 305
Deciphering "Labelese" 306
Food Labels—A Personal View 308
A Question of Balance 309
Summary 309

PART V

YOUR HEALTH...CHARTING YOUR FUTURE

8. NUTRITION CHOICES FOR HEALTH AND DISEASE

The Future is not "New" 315
Foods, Not Nutrients 316
The "Medicalization" of Nutrition 319
The Scientific Evidence for the Role of Diet in Preventing Disease 323
    Keys Seven Countries Study 323
    Framingham Heart Study 325
    Lyon Diet Heart Study 325
    Italian GISSI Prevention Trial 326
    Asian Diet Studies 326
    Dietary Approaches to Stop Hypertension (DASH) trial 327
    The Nurses' Health Study 328
    Dietary Patterns and Type II Diabetes 328
    Lifestyle Heart Trial (Ornish) 328
Constructing a Prudent Cosmopolitan Diet 329
The Prudent Cosmopolitan Diet: "The Best Diets All Under One Roof" 332
The Best of the Mediterranean Dietary Practices 332
All Olive Oils are not Created Equal 334
The Best of the Far East (Asian) Dietary Practices 338
Soy: A Great Oriental contribution 338
Milk Consumption in the Far East 339
Orientals and Greens 339
Is Rice Fattening? 340

Green Teas 340
Africa, Fiber and Whole Grains 341
Glycemic Index—Glycemic Load 342
Health Aspects of Some Fruits and Vegetables 344
Grapes, Tomatoes, Eggplant, Avocados, and Peppers 344
Citrus Fruits 345
A Wonderful Excuse for a Fruit Dessert 346
Spinach, Broccoli and Dark Leafy Greens e.g Collard, Kale, Chard....346
Blueberries, Blackberries, Strawberries, Raspberries, Cranberries.....347
Garlic, Onion, Leeks, Chives, Allium Family 347
Soft Drinks, Reconstituted Juices, Water 348
Summarizing the Prudent Cosmopolitan Diet 348
Notes on Obesity: A Growing Epidemic 350
Obesity and Quality of Life Issues 351
Obesity and Medical Handicaps 352
Overweight, Obesity, Central Obesity, Visceral Obesity 352
Successfully Tackling Obesity: Perspectives and Principles 354
Needed: "Regime Change" 355
Practical Perspectives for Successfully Tackling Obesity 356
Say "No" to Counting Calories, Special Menus, etc 357
Making Practical Choices When Shopping—Read Less Labels 358
Cooking at Home: Quick and Easy: The Way I Do It 359
When Eating Out Ask Questions (But Not Too Many) 361
Understanding Global Cuisines 362
Conclusion and Summary 363

9. LIFESTYLE PHYSICAL ACTIVITY.
...Get Moving

Victims of Our Success 367
Physical Activity Levels in America 368
Definitions 369
Increased Physical Activity: It's Role in Prevention 370
Benefits of Increased Physical Activity 370
The Evidence for Physical Activity on Health and Longevity 371
The Institutionalization of Physical Activity 372
Can Sexual Activity Qualify as Exercise? 373
It All Adds Up 374
Targeting the Children 376
Exercise Modalities and Health Benefits: A Summary 376
Why Wait Until…? 377
Potential Hazards of Exercise: Be Sensible 378
When to Check with Your Doctor 379

"On-the-Job Training"..380
The Television and Computer Age: Creative Solutions Needed.....................381
Overcoming Psychological Barriers 381
Barriers to Exercise: Foreign Considerations 382
A Good Habit is as Hard to Break as a Bad One 382
Exercise and Physical Activity—Personal Reflections....................................383
It is All about Choices..384
Summary...384

10. MAKING CHOICES THAT LAST:
From Knowledge to Action

Refuse to Be Confused 387
A Simple Perspective: Complicate it Not..388
Needed...Nutrition Education...389
People Can Change 389
On Attitudes, Perspectives, and Behavior 390
What is it That You Want? What are You Aiming For? 392
Making Choices That Last Means Going Beyond Circumstances 392
Good Changes Do Not Occur Overnight...394
Going for the Long Haul 395
People Who Succeed Are Willing To Take Responsibility..............................395
Beyond Nutrition and Lifestyle..396
Summary and Conclusion 396

PART VI

BOOK RESOURCES

References 399
Book Resources...445
Index 447

List of Figures and Tables

Figure 0-1.   Contrasting approaches to managing lifestyle-related diseases 47
Figure 0-2.   The majority of U.S. deaths are caused by negative lifestyles: 47
Figure 0-3.   Lifestyle habits, diet, and risk factors 55
Figure 1-1.   Misconceptions and negative mind-sets about healthy living 66
Figure 1-2.   Some aims and benefits of healthy living...64
Figure 2-1.   Worlds in Conflict: Some historical notions about health and disease 78
Figure 2-2.   Progressive increase in advertising spent by U.S. pharmaceutical companies 80
Figure 2-3.   Pester Power: the impact of sleek drug advertising on medical practice. 81
Figure 2-4.   Nutrition, sedentary lifestyle, obesity, the metabolic syndrome and type II diabetes .91
Figure 2-5.   Contrasting food and nutrients vs. pharmaceuticals, drugs and medicines 94
Figure 2-6.   Overlap between Food, Herbs and Drugs 100
Figure 3-1.   A Glimpse at Medical School Education 111
Figure 3-2.   Percentage of U.S. medical schools offering nutrition programs. 123
Figure 4-1.   Reasons for choosing CAM practices...137
Figure 4-2.   Percentage of CAM use in industrialized countries 138
Figure 5-1.   Global prevalence of overweight and obesity in adult populations (2001) 166
Figure 5-2.   Risk Factors for Coronary Heart Disease 171
Figure 5-3.   The three Major Behavioral Risk Factors for Cardiovascular Diseases 171
Figure 5-4.   Annual Deaths from Smoking (U.S.) 172
Figure 5-5.   The Unbalanced Western Diet 174
Figure 5-6.   Lifestyle Risk Factors and the Major Chronic Non-communicable Diseases 174
Figure 5-7.   Summary of the Effects of Dietary Fats on Blood Lipids: (HDL, LDL, and TGs). 184
Figure 5-8.   The Coronary Risk Prediction Charts 204
Figure 5-9.   Genetics, Lifestyle and Central Obesity leading to the Metabolic Syndrome...........205
Figure 6-1.   A Schema for the Progression of Disease with Aging..217
Figure 6-2.   The Spectrum of Aging and Disease 218
Figure 6-3.   Projections for an Aging Population (United States)..218
Figure 6-4.   The Elderly Population and Healthcare Resources 219
Figure 6-5.   Prevalence of Chronic Disease in the Elderly..219
Figure 6-6.   Smoking and its impact on cardiovascular system. 231
Figure 6-7.   Concerns over Physicians Stresses 237
Figure 6-8.   The Medical Ravages of Sleep Deprivation in Healthy Young Men.........................240
Figure 6-9.   The Health Benefits of Smoking Cessation 242
Figure 7-1.   Factors Influencing Food Choice and Preferences...254
Figure 7-2.   Functions of Food: Maslow's Hierarchy, as Applied to Food Habits 259
Figure 7-3.   The Acquisition of Food Habits and the Socialization process 261
Figure 7-4.   The Key Players Involved in Establishing U.S. Food Policy 269
Figure 7-5.   The popular USDA Food Guide Pyramid (Daily recommended intakes) 270
Figure 7-6.   The New Food Label, annotated. 303
Figure 8-1.   Prudent Cosmopolitan Diet—a dietary prescription for
                                            modern cosmopolitan societies................331
Figure 8-2.   Mediterranean-style Diet Pyramid..333
Figure 8-3.   Summarizing the Big Picture: The Best Diets and Healthy Lifestyles
              for Prevention and Management of the Major Killers of Modern Mankind 350

Table 0-1.   Deaths from major preventable lifestyle-related diseases (U.S.A)............................48
Table 0-2.   Costliest medical conditions, USA...49
Table 1-1.   The elements for successful outcomes in nutrition and lifestyle programs 71
Table 4-1.   Complementary and Alternative Medicine (NIH classification) 147
Table 5-1.   The Six Leading Lifestyle Diseases and their Major Risk Factors (U.S.)..................170
Table 5-2.   Comparison of the average American vs. the Japanese diets.................................177
Table 5-3.   Comparison of Daily Caloric Intake of Oriental vs. American style diet 178

Table 5-4.   Major Food Sources of Trans-Fatty Acids (TFAs) 185
Table 5-5.   Trans-fatty acid content of common foodstuffs 186
Table 5-6.   Typical Composition of Some Meats (raw) 192
Table 5-7.   Composition of Some Fish (White and Fatty Varieties) 193
Table 5-8.   Content of 3.5 oz (100 g) portions of raw shellfish 194
Table 5-9.   Composition of Milks of different species (per 100 mg) 197
Table 5-10.   Major features of the Metabolic Syndrome 206
Table 5-11.   Years You May Gain By Caring For Your Heart 207
Table 6-1.   Positive and Negative Perceptions of the Aging Process 213
Table 6-2.   Perceptions on Youth and Aging in Modern Culture 214
Table 6-3.   Changes associated with normal aging 216
Table 6-4.   Advanced Age is a Risk Factor for Several Medical Conditions 217
Table 6-5.   Theories on Aging 220
Table 6-6.   Free Radicals, Sources and Disease 222
Table 6-7.   Major Antioxidants Present in Body Fluids and Tissues 223
Table 6-8.   The Spectrum of Cardiovascular Disease 227
Table 6-9.   Five Major Aging Accelerators 234
Table 6-10.   Chief Stressors for Physicians 237
Table 6-11.   Caffeine in the Diet. 239
Table 6-12.   Simple Indicators of Sleep Deprivation 240
Table 7-1.   Important Issues Influencing Food Choices 260
Table 7-2.   Important Factors Influencing Food Choices 263
Table 7-3.   Food Choices and Socioeconomic Status in the UK 266
Table 7-4.   Understanding the Food Choices of Low Income Americans 268
Table 7-5.   Marketing Appeals in Food Advertising 272
Table 7-6.   Traditional Food Processing Methods 276
Table 7-7.   Early Industrial Food Processing Methods 277
Table 7-8.   Spectrum of Industrial Food Processing Methods (Physical Agents) 278
Table 7-9.   Spectrum of Industrial Food Processing Methods (Biological Agents) 279
Table 7-10.   Spectrum of Industrial Food Processing Methods (Chemical Agents) 279
Table 7-11.   Advantages of some food processing methods 282
Table 7-12.   Disadvantages of some food processing methods 282
Table 7-13.   Foods High in Sodium 283
Table 7-14.   Hidden Sources of Salt and Sodium 284
Table 7-15.   Some Food Sources of Hidden Sugars 285
Table 7-16.   Stability of Some Vitamins under Different Conditions 286
Table 7-17.   Vitamin C Losses during Different Methods of Processing Green Peas 287
Table 7-18.   The Effect of Storage and Cooking on Vitamin C Content 288
Table 7-19.   Heat-labile Anti-nutritional Factors 289
Table 7-20.   Reducing Nutrient Losses while Cooking 291
Table 7-21.   Health Claims Approved by Food and Drug Administration (2000) 302
Table 7-22.   The Meanings of Adjectival Descriptors Appearing on Food Labels 307
Table 8-1.   The Complex Little Soybean 317
Table 8-2.   Citrus Fruits: Composition and Related Health Benefits 318
Table 8-3.   Vitamin E (Tocopherol) Content of Some Nuts and Oils (mg/100g) 320
Table 8-4.   Vitamin E—A Complex Group of Tocopherols 320
Table 8-5.   Understanding Nutrition and Disease Relationships 324
Table 8-6.   Grades of Consumer Olive Oil 335
Table 8-7.   Summary of Health Benefits of the Mediterranean Diet 336
Table 8-8.   Varieties of Soy Foods 339
Table 8-9.   Summary of Health Benefits of Asian Diets 341
Table 8-10.   Glycemic Index and Glycemic Load of Common Foods 343
Table 8-11.   Whole Grains and their Health Benefits 344
Table 8-12.   Diseases linked to Overweight and Obesity 351
Table 8-13.   Overweight and Quality of Life 352
Table 8-14.   Degrees of Excess Body Weight and Body Mass Index (BMI) 353
Table 9-1.   Physical Inactivity / Sedentary Lifestyle Levels in U.S. Adults 368
Table 9-2.   Physical Activity Levels of U.S. Adults 369
Table 9-3.   The Benefits of Physical Activity and Exercise 371

Table 9-4.   Studies on Physical Activity and Health.. 372
Table 9-5.   Misconceptions about Physical Activity and Exercise... 375
Table 9-6.   Types of Exercises and their Health Benefits 377
Table 9-7.   Trigger Factors for Healthier Lifestyle and Physical Activity 378
Table 9-8.   Conditions that can increase the Potential Hazards of Exercise............................ 379
Table 9-9.   Conditions to Check Before Starting Exercises 380
Table 9-10.   Lifestyle Physical Activity Strategies... 381
Table 10-1.   Perspectives for Making Choices that Last.. 391

Acknowledgments

Many people have played indispensable roles in making this book a reality. I express my sincere appreciation to them all. I found out that writing a good book is a completely different ball game from giving speeches or lectures. Writing *Your Doctor Can't Make You Healthy* was like major rehabilitative surgery—with the bone surgeons doing the tough internal work followed by multiple follow-up visits to the plastic surgeons. It is still a work in progress.

I now understand why writers take sabbaticals. Working in a busy clinic with daily clinical and emergency duties and no time off or book deals certainly did not help. That I could simply dictate this book using voice-recognition software was nothing short of wishful thinking. Now I know otherwise. My sincere appreciation goes out to the many wonderful people who, in ways spoken and unspoken, up front and behind-the-scenes, contributed in sundry ways to make this effort a reality.

First, I would like to acknowledge my greatest teachers—my patients—who have been responsible for molding my thoughts on this subject. They have provided the raw material to make this book a reality.

Special Mention:

Joseph and Elston Bulwer (deceased), father, brother and great teachers; Dr. Noor Melham (UK, Iraq); Hsieh Ya Ching of Tianjin Medical University, China; David Singer, M.D., Harvard Vanguard Medical Associates, Boston, Massachusetts; Rhea Rogers, B.Sc.(St. Louis University); Le Ann Blumberg, Ph.D.(Georgetown) at the United States Department of Agriculture; the Family Medical Center Team in Belize: Ismay Bulwer, Carol Garay, Tahira Ahmad, and Janice Davis; Cedric Flowers CPA (Arkansas); John and Marta Woods and family, Belize; John Mencias, BSc. MBA(Australia), Ambrose Tillett, MSc.(UK); the Amandala Newspaper, Belize: Evan X Hyde BA(Dartmouth), Rufus X, Russell Vellos (editor); Maurice and Vivian Underwood; Mike and Martha Williams; Godwin Hulse; and Hector and Ethel Thompson; Jill McGilligin, Ph.D., King's College, University of London; Yvonne "Bunny" Staine and Ernest Staine, Attorney-at-Law; George Swift.

Those who suggested, commented, and reviewed this book especially:

Marian-Ortolf Bagley, Professor of Design Emeritus, University of Minnesota; Caroline Gentle, BA, YMCA Director, Belize; Christelle Leger of New Brunswick,

Canada, Edward Shelonka, M.D.; George Aldridge of the U.S. Embassy in Belize; Nada Hamze, teacher and poet; Jennifer Pirali-Neal, MSc.(Minnesota State University).

My teachers:

Professor Bernard Lown, M.D., Professor of Cardiology Emeritus, Brigham and Women's Hospital, Harvard School of Public Health; Shmuel Ravid, M.D., Director of the Lown Cardiovascular Center and cardiologist, Brigham and Women's Hospital and Harvard Medical School; Walter C. Willett, M.D., Dr. P.H., Chair, Department of Nutrition and Frank Stare Professor of Epidemiology and Nutrition, Harvard School of Public Health; Professor Catherine Geissler, Ph.D. and Peter Emery, Ph.D. of the Department of Nutrition, Kings College, University of London; Professor Philip Home (Newcastle upon Tyne), vice president and chairman, Clinical Guidelines Task Force, International Diabetes Federation and Professor Sir KGMM Alberti, president of the Royal College of Physicians of London and president, International Diabetes Federation; Professor Mark Walker and Dr. Martin Rutter of the University of Newcastle upon Tyne; Professor Errol Y. St. A Morrison. FRCP, FACP, Pro-Vice Chancellor, University of the West Indies, and the Medical Faculty in Mona, Jamaica and Port-of-Spain and San Fernando, Trinidad and Tobago, West Indies; Miss Sybil Reyes (late); and the Faculty of St. John's College and Queen's Square Anglican School of Belize.

For those who introduced me to international cuisine:

Sung Yu Ling and family of the Republic of China, Taiwan. Mei Su Yei of the Embassy of the Republic of China, Taiwan; the Hsieh family of Kaoshiung, Taiwan; Maria Yannakoulia, Ph.D.(UK, Athens) and Vassiliki Costarelli MSc.(UK) of Athens, Greece; Hande Mutlu, BSc.(Istanbul) and the group at the Princess Hotels International; Dr. Noor Melham (UK, Mosul); Dr. Kalvinder Bamrah, DDS (Newcastle-upon-Tyne, UK); Lystra Matura, Hassina Khan, Sellesha Khan and all those special friends too numerous to mention in Trinidad and Tobago, Jamaica, Egypt, India, Taiwan, the Sudan, Nigeria, Mexico, and Belize. They all provided me with unforgettable hospitality and a lifelong appreciation for the wonderful gift of global cuisine. To the Most High God, from whom all blessings flow and who through providence enabled me to take this task to its completion, I will always be grateful.

Who should read this book

The AIM of this book is to share with all readers a provocative, but logical way of thinking about nutrition, health, and disease.

The reader will find a spirited debate on the need to focus more on health and less on healthcare. It is offers a lengthy, but compelling argument that is bolstered by extensive research. In this pursuit, the primary focus has been to create a balanced and scientific perspective on nutrition and lifestyle, and their roles in promoting and optimizing health. **It is intended for all readers who are motivated to take more responsibility for their own health.**

It subscribes to the doctrine that "**the health of an individual is his or her primary responsibility, but the individual must first be empowered before being delegated such a task.**" In doing so however, it does not cut corners or oversimplify the issues of nutrition and lifestyle. Solid arguments cannot be based on flimsy or superficial handling of the subject matter. Though this book makes a deliberate attempt to simplify the argument, it tries not to gloss over important details upon which good nutrition and lifestyle recommendations are based.

The non-medical reader will find an abundance of information and detail, but should not be intimidated. This book is not a quickie. The subject of nutrition has left many so confused and jaded over the latest food quarrels that many people have simply tuned out. A comprehensive discussion of nutrition and lifestyle is essential for successfully navigating your way through this confusion. The information contained in this book discusses what you need to know in order to take greater responsibility for your health. This book deliberately incorporates a lot of reader-friendly features and easy-to-read guides that de-mystify important health concepts (see "How to Use This Book" on page 15).

The health and nutrition enthusiast will discover a refreshing discussion of this subject from the view of a doctor trained not just in orthodox mainstream medicine and postgraduate nutrition, but from one who is a dedicated advocate of prevention and patient empowerment. This book promises to serve as an invaluable reference and springboard from which to tackle nutrition debates of the present and the future.

This book is a must-read **for medical students and doctors**. This is not a doctor-bashing book. On the contrary, it will complement our efforts and increase our effectiveness in an area that has traditionally received little emphasis during medical training. In the current healthcare crisis that has eroded the doctor-patient relationship, patients will welcome an approach that manifests their doctors' interest in preventing as well as treating their diseases. Extensive print and electronic references are provided for those who wish to pursue further research on the subject material.

Overview

Part I. Introduction.

Introduction. This section launches a direct challenge to the status-quo—we have been treating diseases but neglecting "health." This is an unsustainable approach to tackle the modern epidemic of lifestyle-related diseases that now kill 1.7 million Americans (and 60 million people worldwide) annually. We must seriously re-think our efforts in tackling obesity and the metabolic syndrome, type II diabetes, cardiovascular diseases, and cancer. If we fail to pay the price of prevention today, we are bound to pay much more later.

Part II. Background Issues in Health and Healthcare.

Chapter 1. Health and Healthcare...Two very different things

further challenges the present emphasis on medical care and proposes a new focus—that of healthy lifestyles. Most people erroneously view healthy living as a killjoy, but a closer look nullifies this misconception. There are tremendous benefits in pursuing lifestyle prevention strategies that focus more on "health," and less on healthcare.

Chapter 2. "Pill for Every Ill Mentality" exposes the prevailing

overemphasis on drugs in a society that is racked by indiscipline, drenched in advertising, and programmed to look for quick fixes. It calls for a re-thinking of this flawed and oversimplified approach to treating lifestyle-related diseases. The dominant influence of the pharmaceutical lobby on medical education, research, and practice as well as the need to wean doctors off drug companies is highlighted. The discussion concludes with the supremacy of good nutrition and lifestyles in treating the current epidemic of chronic diseases. This approach comprehensively tackles the root causes of these diseases and provides long-term results—not quick fixes.

Chapter 3. How Much Does Your Doctor Know about

Nutrition points out that medical education neglects the teaching of nutrition in medical schools. Consequently, our doctors are generally poorly equipped to provide meaningful nutrition advice to their patients. Doctors are taught to fix health problems, not to prevent them. Therefore, the central role of nutrition in the prevention and treatment of diseases are often ignored or receive only passing mention. Fortunately, attitudes are now changing.

Chapter 4. Complementary and Alternative Medicine (CAM)

introduces this controversial subject that directly challenges medical orthodoxy and examines the reasons behind its increasing popularity and its role in preventive care. Today, most of Europe and over half the American population have adopted some form(s) of CAM practices. The major reasons behind this trend lie in dissatisfaction with the current system of healthcare, and people's desire for the pro-active and empowerment approaches that many CAM practices employ. Even though CAM therapies range from the respected and the scientific, to the ridiculous and the dangerous, there is a growing cohort of doctors who integrate the best of conventional and CAM practices.

Part III. The Burden of Lifestyle Diseases

Chapter 5. Common Risk Factors In Chronic Diseases...The

Western Diet and Negative Lifestyles lays an important foundation in understanding those risk factors that gave rise to the modern epidemic of obesity, cardiovascular diseases, type II diabetes, and cancer. Twentieth century industrialization and urbanization have been accompanied by major changes in the way people eat and live. Rising obesity rates, increasingly sedentary lifestyles, and cigarette smoking have led to major shifts in disease patterns from one of under-nutrition, to one of nutritional excesses. The Western diet and negative lifestyles are chiefly to blame.

Chapter 6. Growing Older and Aging...When the Rust Steps

In relates the journey we take every day of our lives. There are many perceptions and misconceptions about aging, and divers theories set forth on why we age. Certain lifestyle factors hasten aging and diseases; others often lead to "aging well." Insights into both are discussed. Diseases are not the inevitable consequences of aging.

Part IV. All That Stuff That Enters Your Mouth

Chapter 7. Food and Choices...The "Dynamix" of Why We Eat What We Eat presents an eye-opening look at why people choose the foods they do. The first part of this important chapter discusses in some depth the "dynamix" of food choices and the many variables that influence these choices. Insights into how socioeconomics, politics, media influences, and globalization affect food choices are provided.

The second part of this chapter introduces food processing and the impact of industrial methods on the nutritional value of processed foods. References to organic and genetically modified (GM) foods are given, and the effectiveness of the U.S. food label is questioned. The author presents the view that the food label, though it appears at first glance to be a useful tool, is riddled with loopholes that can mislead even the most seasoned professionals, much less the average consumer.

Part V. Your Health... Charting Your Future

Chapter 8. Nutrition Choices for Health and Disease is the

climactic chapter that adopts a practical and a scientifically-bolstered approach to replace the nutritional imbalances that currently characterize the Western diet. It opposes a growing trend that subtly seeks to reinvent and "medicalize" nutrition. The Prudent Cosmopolitan Diet is a simple model of healthy eating that embraces the best of the healthiest diets in the world and places them all under one roof. This approach is a departure from the popular practice of building dietary pyramids. It is a logical prescription for healthy eating in a modern cosmopolitan society. It addresses the urgent need to halt the growing epidemic of chronic diseases, along with a simple message: *There is really no need for "special diets,"e.g. special diabetic or heart disease diets. Different diets are not needed to reduce the risk of diabetes, heart disease, or cancer. Healthy nutrition and lifestyles can prevent and even reverse a host of medical conditions. The benefits include losing weight, lowering blood cholesterol and blood pressure, preventing and reversing type II diabetes, reducing the risk of heart attack, stroke, and cancer.* The chapter concludes with sound principles for tackling obesity, shopping for food, home-cooking tips, and understanding global cuisines.

Chapter 9. Physical Activity and Exercise. No discussion on healthy

lifestyle is complete without reference to this subject. This chapter is not a treatise on physical activity and exercise. However, it introduces some of the salient points needed to spur us into action. Structured exercises are good, but what will benefit most people is not special exercise outfits. Rather it is in learning practical everyday ways of increasing energy expenditure. These all add up. The author is against the "institutionalization of physical activity." This has led many to believe that physical activity demands joining fitness clubs or acquiring special exercise equipment. Increasing physical activity in modern man involves overcoming major psychological as well as physical barriers.

Chapter 10. Making Choices That Last...From Knowledge to Action.

This is the shortest and arguably one of the most important chapters. Knowledge is important...but what you do with that knowledge is far more important. Why is it that so many people *know*...yet still so many fail to *do*? Translating knowledge into action involves key strategies that can materialize into enduring lifestyle changes. These strategies may be highly personal and often go to the very core of an individual's philosophical and belief systems. It encourages individuals to set clear goals and adopt practical measures toward making the necessary changes. This chapter embodies what the author has found effective in making the transition, based on his own experience and perspectives.

Part VI. Book Resources

This last section provides a chapter-by-chapter listing of **references**, followed by a list of **book resources**, and concludes with a **general index**.

Happy reading. I trust that reading these pages will prove truly insightful.

Bernard E. Bulwer, M.D.
Editor and Director of Outreach, ProCOR
Lown Cardiovascular Center, Brookline, Massachusetts, USA
June 18, 2003

PART I

Introduction

We are at a crossroads.
Modern societies now preside over an unprecedented epidemic, full of depressing health statistics. Having arrived at this crossroads, we can choose to go down the beaten path towards more disease and more worries over healthcare. The second path is a road less traveled. It is a proven path that leads to prevention and optimal health.
The choice is ours.

Introduction

Chapter Outline

What?   Did You Say Your Doctor *Cannot*? 46
Alarming Statistics 47
Pay Now…Or Pay Much More Later 50
Perspectives of This Book 53
Why another Book on Nutrition and Lifestyle? 54
Show Me the Evidence 56
Summary 57

We have the scientific knowledge to create a world in which most cardiovascular disease could be eliminated. In such a world, preventive practices would be incorporated early in life as a matter of course; everyone would have access to positive healthy living, smoke free air, good nutrition, regular physical activity, and supportive living and working environments.[1]

Victoria Declaration on Heart Health (1992)

For the two out of three adult Americans who do not smoke and do not drink excessively, one personal choice seems to influence long-term health prospects more than any other; what we eat.[2]

1998 Surgeon General's Report on Nutrition and Health

§§§§§§§§

What? Did You Say Your Doctor *Cannot*?

> Your doctor can treat your blood pressure,
> your diabetes, or your heart disease.
> Your doctor, however, cannot make you healthy.

During the early months of pondering over a suitable title for this book, the primary goal was to present a patient-centered, rather than a doctor-centered book. It was never the intention to evoke disrespect for the medical profession or my medical colleagues.

This book sets forth a logical argument for a lifestyle-based approach to tackle the modern epidemic of obesity, cardiovascular diseases, type II diabetes, and several forms of cancer. It adopts a paradigm shift in attitudes from today's dominant hospital-based model for treating diseases, and champions instead an individual-based, prevention model for tackling these diseases (Figure 0-1).

Such a shift in attitude will not be quickly embraced by the influential medical establishment which, though slowly thawing to the need for change, remains largely frozen in a crisis-management approach to healthcare. Despite this book's stated objective to focus on prevention, it no way dismisses the superb and well-meaning efforts by the medical profession to treat those presently afflicted with these diseases. In so doing, it complements rather than substitutes, and it integrates rather than replaces the current approach to healthcare.

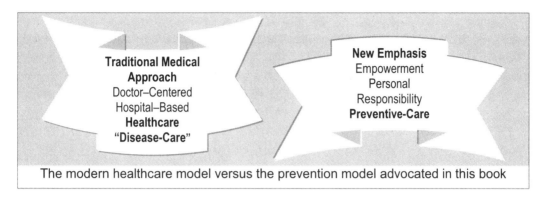

Figure 0-1. Contrasting approaches to managing lifestyle-related diseases

This book fulfils such a purpose by paying careful attention to the whole body of scientific evidence, and refrains from half-baked doctrines that are typical of many self-help books. This book is not based on the findings of single or isolated studies, which, if not placed in proper perspective, often lead to erroneous and unbalanced conclusions. We need to be careful not to miss the big picture because of fascination with marginal details. Keeping this in mind, this book does not major on the minors. In essence, a wide range of topics on preventive nutrition at the primary and secondary levels is discussed. At the primary level, the desire is to prevent lifestyle diseases. At the secondary level the challenge is to help those already affected to manage and reverse these diseases when such possibilities exist.

Alarming Statistics

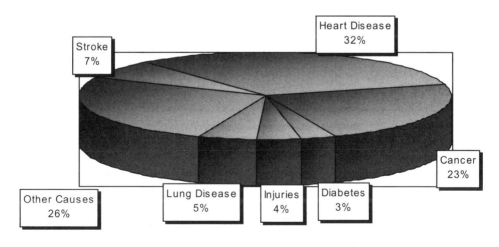

Figure 0-2. The majority of U.S. deaths are caused by negative lifestyles: smoking, unbalanced nutrition, and physical inactivity (National Center for Health Statistics, 1997).[3]

> ## Chronic non-communicable diseases account for 60 percent of the 60 million deaths worldwide, and 50 percent of the global burden of disease.
> The World Health Report 2002[4]

This book also highlights why the current system of medical care in America, despite its good and noble efforts, is being bankrupted by the rapidly rising flood of people who depend on expensive high technology healthcare. Estimates (1997) indicate that chronic diseases affect 90 million Americans and account for 75 percent of the U.S. healthcare expenditures.[5] From the early 1980s to the late 1990s, healthcare costs in the United States escalated to a whopping 1.2 trillion dollars (1998).[6]

To make matters worse, people with the least access to good healthcare suffer disproportionately more chronic diseases and have the shortest life expectancy.[7] According to mortality tables, 2.3 million Americans died in 1996 (Table 0-1).[3] The three leading causes were heart disease (733,834 deaths), cancer (539,533 deaths), and cerebrovascular diseases–mainly stroke (160,431 deaths). Diabetes ranked seventh with 61,767 deaths registered. Together these accounted for almost 70 percent of all deaths in the United States in 1996.[3] They are also the costliest diseases to treat (Table 0-2).[8]

Table 0-1. Deaths from major preventable lifestyle-related diseases (U.S.A) as a percentage of all deaths

Cause of Death	Deaths	Percent %
Major Preventable Chronic Diseases	**1,661,734**	**71.8**
Total cardiovascular diseases (heart attack, stroke, hypertension)	954, 407	41.2
All cancers	539,533	23.3
Chronic obstructive lung disease	106,027	4.6
Diabetes	61,767	2.7
Other	**652,956**	**28.2**
TOTAL	**2,314,690**	**100.00**

National Center for Health Statistics. Births and Deaths—United States, 1996. Monthly Vital Statistics Report 1997.[3]

Table 0-2. Costliest medical conditions, [8] USA

The 7 Costliest Diseases

1. Heart disease★ **$$$$$$**
2. Cancer
3. Trauma
4. Mental disorders
5. Diabetes† **$$**
6. Hypertension★
7. Cerebrovascular disease★

★ - cardiovascular disease costs   ($298bn, 2001)
† - diabetes, direct medical costs ($100bn, 1997)
$ - represents ~ 50 billion dollars

www.healthaffairs.org/1100_table_contents.php

As seen in Table 0-1 and Figure 0-2, the cardiovascular diseases (heart disease and stroke) are the most common causes of death in the United States. They account for 40 percent of all deaths annually. Today almost 1,000,000 Americans die from cardiovascular diseases every year. This translates into one person dying from these diseases every 33 seconds. The chronic diseases (Table 0-1) that cause 7 out of every 10 deaths in America account for more than more than 60 percent of the U.S. healthcare budget.[3,6]

Go beyond these death statistics and then reflect on the staggering number of Americans currently living with chronic diseases. More than 60 million Americans now live with diseases of the heart and circulation, 54 percent or 150 million are overweight. The number of new cancer cases exceeds 1.2 million annually, and for type II diabetes, 18 million Americans are now affected. Nearly 6 million hospitalizations each year are due to cardiovascular diseases. In 2001, the estimated cost of cardiovascular disease was 298 billion dollars, including loss of productivity and related costs.[9-11]

Public health authorities are also alarmed over the rise in new cases of people with type II diabetes. This was once called adult-onset diabetes, but now increasingly affects youth, principally because of rising juvenile obesity rates. Type II diabetes is fundamentally a disease of unbalanced nutrition, obesity, and physical inactivity. Diabetes affects over 150 million people worldwide. William Herman M.D. and colleagues estimated the direct medical cost (1992) in the United States for diabetes was 45 billion dollars. By 1997, costs catapulted to almost 100 billion dollars.[12,13]

Consider further the costs to the individual. Diabetes may require intensive therapy with multiple injections of insulin; this alone can exceed 4,000 dollars a year. For the diabetic who suffers visual loss or blindness, costs may total 1,900 dollars per annum for appropriate care. If kidney failure arises, the cost escalates to about 45,000 dollars for kidney replacement therapy. Lower limb amputation for infections and gangrene, a common complication of uncontrolled diabetes may cost 30,000 dollars. Coronary artery bypass surgery and balloon angioplasty to treat blocked coronary arteries (the major cause of death in people with diabetes) cost 70,000 dollars and 60,000 respectively. This is still not the complete picture. People with diabetes frequently need cholesterol-lowering drugs and treatment for erectile dysfunction (impotence) that affects up to 50 percent of diabetic men. Costs of Lipitor, Zocor, or Viagra alone can easily amount to thousands of dollars annually. Furthermore, a reduction in quality of life and productivity due to ill health escalate the costs to the individual and the nation even further. This is a glimpse of what we now face—a potential medical nightmare, full of depressing statistics.[13,14-17]

 Chronic Lifestyle Diseases:

(Obesity, Cardiovascular Diseases, Diabetes and Cancer)

Hundreds of millions of people affected ﹖﹖﹖ ﹖ ﹖ ﹖
Enormous financial burden; hundreds of billions $$$
and growing…

Pay Now! Or Pay Much More Later

People need to be told the truth: If we do not pay the price of prevention today, we are bound to pay much more later.

Given this distressing scenario, it then comes as no surprise why healthcare in America is in crisis. Indeed, healthcare worldwide is in crisis. The global projections estimate 300 million people affected with diabetes by 2025. As people live longer and as sedentary lifestyles and obesity rates escalate, the numbers of people with chronic diseases are bound to follow suit. Continued reliance on expensive drugs and new technologies will spiral the cost of healthcare further out of control.[12,18]

The healthcare crisis now occupies a central place in the American political landscape. It is destined to remain a permanent fixture of the political debates in the foreseeable future. Healthcare reform, prescription drug benefits, and the future of Medicare will remain the subjects of endless debates. While these debates heat up, the reality is that 45 million Americans are not covered by health insurance and millions more remain without adequate coverage.[19] Even when resolutions are made in the future, the overwhelming emphasis will be on "disease-care," with little effort to seriously tackle preventive behavior and personal responsibility. It must be acknowledged however, that great strides have been made in the anti-smoking crusade, as highlighted by the recent adoption of the World Anti-Smoking Treaty in May 2003.

Jessie Gruman, executive director of the Center for the Advancement of Health, challenged the folly of America's love affair with high-tech medicine. In response to a *Newsweek* report that hailed the triumph of modern medicine in successfully implanting the artificial heart, he responded with this sobering note:[20]

> Your story on health and technology was a marvel in itself—thousands of words on how to improve health, and not one of them was "behavior." If every technology advance you highlighted came to pass, more than half the population would still be at risk of premature death. Why? Because most of what kills us—heart disease, strokes, cancer, lung disease, diabetes—is controllable by what we do to prevent the illness in the first place or to manage it more wisely. When it comes to improving health, biology matters, genes matter, machines matter, but behavior really matters.

A *Time* magazine cover feature—"Drugs of the future: Amazing new medicines will be based on DNA; Find out how they will change your life"—reflects a prevalent mindset in our society today. The words of Robert Kamm provide a timely rebuke in this age of hype over wonder drugs and medical breakthroughs:[21]

> We all want to live longer and healthier lives, but to rely on the pharmaceuticals to achieve that flies in the face of experience. Taking pills to rescue us from our self-abusive lifestyle only masks real problems and ends up costing us billions of dollars a year. We ought to be investing at least as much in trying to discover why millions of us behave in ways that are not in our best interest—smoking, drinking, overworking, under-exercising and generally doing things that are bad for our health. We end up like children, crying out to the doctors, "Save us from ourselves!"

The emphasis today looks something like this: more healthcare, more research, more cures, and more money for more drugs. … Whatever became of more responsibility or more prevention? Heated debates over embryonic stem cell research and costly medical interventions may dominate the headlines, but what will dominate most people's lives is a future full of disease and disability.

Political correctness has seduced innumerable politicians to contest for what is popularly seen as the moral high ground—the more prescriptions you push, the more caring you appear. Politicians jockey for leadership of the bandwagon that peddles the message, "More prescription drugs and more high-technology medicine mean better health." This is one arena that calls for statesmanship. People need to be told the truth—healthcare we need, but "health" is what we desperately need! Good health is not a gift from politicians, or doctors, or drugs. Good health comes essentially from the choices we make. Good health follows healthy lifestyles. Political pundits consider such declarations tantamount to political suicide. It seems ironic that the Americans who treasure independence have largely swallowed the pill of excessive dependence on prescription drugs and medical interventions. As long as we pursue political expediency and play the blame game, I am afraid we are ignoring the writing on the wall. The pill of procrastination may one day become too big to swallow.[19,22]

My question is this: If the world's wealthiest nation finds it difficult (if not impossible) to provide universal and affordable healthcare at this present moment, how can we logically expect the healthcare scenario to improve when future demand is certain to escalate? If the United States, with its 20 million diabetics (and the world with 150 million more), is doing a poor job of looking after this population at the current levels of demand, what grounds are there for optimism by 2025 when the number of people with diabetes is expected to double? If we face the daunting burden of not just diabetes, but the entire host of chronic lifestyle diseases—heart disease, stroke, high blood pressure, osteoarthritis, and cancer—is there anyone who can provide reasonable grounds for optimism over the future of medical care as we know it? We are doing today's populace a disservice if we fail to highlight this. It may not deliver votes, but it will certainly deliver honesty. In case the reader construes this to be a lecture directed at the politician, it is actually directed to you. Because in the final analysis, it is you (not your politician) who will end up paying the price.[23-26]

When you consider the tangled web of politics, special interest groups, the uncertainties of future economics, and competing priorities over the healthcare dollar, the future of healthcare (as we know it) may have its days numbered. Americans have for too long been led into thinking that there will always be cures, but sooner rather than later, the reality may be a serious wake-up-call. The day that changed America and the world, September 11th 2001 (911), changes everything. Some will be for the better, but some will sadly be for the worse—at least in the short term. You do not have to have an MBA to realize this. Among its likely casualties will be the financial resources to fund healthcare programs. Homeland security, the war on terrorism, Afghanistan, Iraq, and tax cuts do not bode well for the future of health care programs. This further underscores the urgency to invest in disease prevention programs at the individual, institutional, and governmental levels.[23,27,28]

We must rethink our strategies in the war on chronic lifestyle diseases. We need a slimmer leaner approach, lest we may be left in "shock," and perhaps even "awe." If you think that we pay a high price today, just contemplate what the cost will be tomorrow. The conclusion is therefore this: pay the price of prevention today or pay dearly for our neglect and indulgences later.

Traditional Disease-Based Healthcare

Heavily influenced by politics 🏛
Emphasizes treatment, not prevention 🚑
Faces an uncertain financial future **?**

Perspectives of this Book

Most chronic diseases are the result of unhealthy lifestyles.
Doctors were trained to treat diseases.
Politicians and insurance companies promise to look after your healthcare, but *only you can* look after your health.[26]

This book reflects the author's intense desire to see individuals maximize their health and challenges the prevailing attitudes that have shifted the responsibility for personal health, from the individual, to the doctor. It provides a seasoned argument and a logical perspective on how to prevent disease and optimize health. It exposes the principal reasons behind the major killers in industrialized societies and, increasingly so, in the developing world. Getting older does not mean getting sick. Preventing disease is an achievable goal. The key to this door lies within our hands.

Why another Book on Nutrition and Lifestyle?

Many well-written books on obesity, heart disease, cancer, hypertension, aging, and nutrition are on the bookshelves. Few, however, have underscored the close interconnections that exist between these lifestyle diseases.

This book was written as a guide to address the root causes, and provide solutions to this modern epidemic of obesity, cardiovascular diseases, type II diabetes, and cancer.

Consumer books on diets and lifestyles have become quite popular over the past decade. We live in a time when many people increasingly appreciate the connection between lifestyle and health. Hardly a week goes by without a health segment on television about nutrition and lifestyle. A Harris Interactive survey (2002) titled "Cyperchondriacs continue to grow in America," revealed that 110 million Americans frequently looked for health information online.[29]

Well-written books on heart disease, cancer, overweight, hypertension, and aging fill the bookshelves. Few, however, have underscored the very close connection that exists between these many lifestyle diseases. The average book tends to focus on these as though they are completely different diseases. Modern medical practice reinforces this tradition by treating these diseases in highly specialized units. For example, people with diabetes see diabetes specialists or endocrinologists. People with heart disease are referred to the cardiologist. Textbooks and consumer books overwhelmingly reflect this separatist tradition.

The outlook of this book is considerably different. Rather than looking at these diseases as unrelated, it lumps them together as different sides of the same coin. The evidence is now clear. Cigarette smoking, unbalanced nutrition, and sedentary lifestyles lead to obesity, cardiovascular diseases, type II diabetes, and several forms of cancer. They are heavily interconnected (Figure 0-3).[30-32]

Gerald Reaven, Professor of Medicine, and colleagues at Stanford University, showed that these diseases are primarily the result of a fundamental disorder of nutrition and lifestyle. They called it the insulin resistance syndrome or the metabolic syndrome. The metabolic syndrome (as it will be referred to in this book and explained in more detail in Chapter 5) results when excess weight (especially central or abdominal obesity) leads to resistance to the action of the hormone insulin. This resistance forces the pancreas to produce more insulin (hyperinsulinemia). Over time, this triggers changes that eventually lead the development of type II diabetes, high blood pressure, and increased risk of premature death from heart attack and stroke. Other researchers have established a link between the metabolic syndrome and some forms of dementias, Alzheimer's disease, infertility (polycystic ovarian syndrome), and cancer (especially uterine cancer).[33-36]

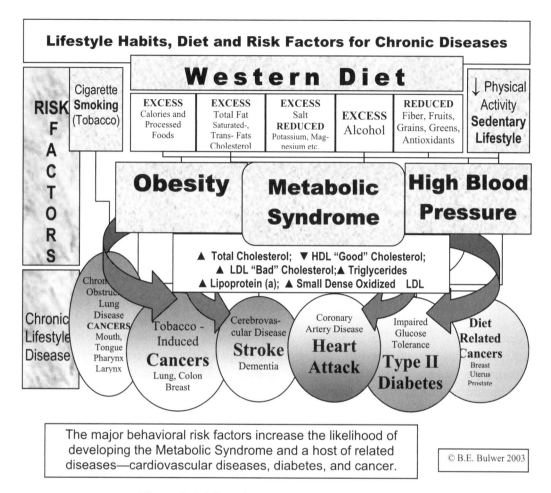

Figure 0-3. Lifestyle habits, diet and risk factors

In modern medical circles doctors get involved after these diseases are diagnosed, and then treat them according to current medical guidelines. The overwhelming bias is in favor of medical treatment—not lifestyle changes. The reasons for this are many and will be discussed in the chapters that follow. Such emphasis will do little to halt the growing global epidemic. In an article published in the *New England Journal of Medicine* (*NEJM*), Professor Reaven and colleagues advocate an approach that gets to the root of the matter:[36]

> This group of metabolic abnormalities suggests that in the treatment of hypertension, non-pharmacologic interventions that increase sensitivity to insulin, including weight reduction, low fat diet, and increased physical activity, should have a primary role.

Since the vast majority of people with type II diabetes are overweight, it seems logical that improved nutrition and physical activity (rather than better diabetes care alone), serve as the cornerstone for preventing and managing diabetes.

Your Doctor Can't Make You Healthy places the emphasis where it belongs—giving due prominence to nutrition and lifestyle in preventing disease and optimizing health. This book will provide important insights into why and how to do just that.

Show Me the Evidence

Successes have come about where people have acknowledged that the unnecessary and premature deaths that occur…are largely preventable and have empowered themselves… This epidemic can be halted—the demand for action must come from those affected. The solution is in our hands.[37]

Joint WHO/FAO Expert Report on Diet, Nutrition and the Prevention of Chronic Disease
Executive Summary, March 2, 2003

Many doctors are skeptical about lifestyle changes as a realistic alternative to medical intervention. Many contend that there is not enough "hard evidence." For them this means that unless you are referring to the gold standard of medical research—"randomized double-blind placebo-controlled studies,"—you are not referring to hard evidence, but instead to unproven therapies.[38] My response to such views is that there *are* several reliable studies to show that lifestyle changes do make a big difference. These are discussed throughout this book.

The epidemiological associations and the complex statistics involved in nutritional studies lie outside the scope of this book. For those who want to dig deeper, I will hastily recommend *Nutritional Epidemiology* by Professor Willett, M.D. of the Harvard School of Public Health. Dr. Willet and his colleagues at Harvard have been at the forefront of restoring nutrition to its rightful place in health and medical circles.[39] This issue is far too important to be seen as a turf war between medical intervention and prevention advocates. Pre-eminence must be given to find solutions to the formidable health crises that confront us. Give me the best medicine, but I still prefer the best prevention. As the old saying goes, prevention is better (and cheaper) than cure.

For those who remain dismissive of anything that seems foreign to your medical education upbringing, and who still insist on awaiting the results of gold standard medical trials, my advice is to "get real," or better yet, ponder these words on diet and cancer:[40]

> The critics' main objection that is medical advice on prevention is offered without definitive evidence… The fact is no one knows exactly which foods, in which proportions, offer the best protection against any particular malignancy. Nor does anyone know which of the myriad of chemicals in a

turnip or tomato does the most to keep our cells intact. Answering such questions will take decades of clinical study. And no matter how much we learn about nutrition, age, heredity and other unknown risk factors will still make prevention an inexact science. For now the issue is this: should we change our lives on the strength of lab studies and epidemiological associations, or should we live on cheeseburgers until the case for soy burgers is seamless? If you sift through the evidence, it is hard not to agree with Dr Gabriel Feldman, the American Cancer Society's director of prostate and colorectal cancer. "We don't need years of research," he says. "If people would implement what we know today, cancer rates would drop. It's that simple.

Follow me through this book. Nurture a questioning mind and judge for yourselves whether it all makes sense, and more importantly, whether it works.

Summary

We are at a crossroads. A global epidemic of obesity, cardiovascular diseases, type II diabetes, and cancer is upon us. These, together with a growing elderly population and rising healthcare costs serve urgent notice of a looming crisis in healthcare.

We have been led to believe that the solutions lie in providing more hi-tech medicine and more healthcare. These are noble aspirations, but with one major limitation—the numbers do not add up. With such great demand for medical services, inadequate funding for medical care, and competing priorities on the nation's financial resources, the days of healthcare (as we know it) may be numbered. These are issues over which we have little or no control.

Whether healthcare is in crisis or not, it is important to know this one thing—your doctor can help you control your diabetes, your heart disease, and make you feel better, but your doctor cannot make you healthy.

******

PART II

Background Issues in Health and Healthcare

To achieve best results in preventing nutrition-related chronic diseases, strategies and policies should fully recognize the essential role of both diet and physical activity in determining good nutrition and optimal health. Policies and programmes must address the need for change at the individual level as well as the modifications in society and the environment to make healthier choices accessible and preferable.

Joint WHO/FAO Expert Report on
Diet, Nutrition and the Prevention of Chronic Disease
Executive Summary, March 2, 2003.

Chapter 1

Health and Healthcare
...Two very different things

Chapter Outline

The Wrong Emphasis 63
Losing the War on Drugs 64
Healthy Living Is Not A Killjoy 66
When Virtue Becomes a Vice 68
A Better Approach to Health.. 70
Less Healthcare, More Health... 72
The Present and Future Challenges 73
Summary.. 73

In the year 2000, 125 million Americans, or 45% of the U.S. population, lived with at least one chronic [medical] condition. "That's 20 million more than projected 5 years ago.[1]

Dr. Gerard F. Anderson
Professor of Health Policy, Management and International Health
Johns Hopkins University's School of Public Health.

The cost of poor health is staggering and goes well beyond dollars. But the approach that offers the best solution, reduces risk, cuts demand and gets people healthy and fit is prevention. The U.S. is a nation of chronic diseases. It will get much worse, because we never deal with the causes. Individual Americans need to bring this issue to boil and keep it there until we get a health-care system premised on prevention.[2]

John J. Bagshaw

We are not going to achieve healthcare in this country unless we first recognize that there is more to healthcare than medical care…the operative word in the phrase "healthcare reform" should be "health." Yet nowhere in the proposed law is there a clear indication that the goal of this arduous reform process is to improve the health status of all Americans. Rather goals are related to medical coverage, medical care delivery, and medical costs. Sure, "health" may be the word used, but it's really a medical factor being addressed.[3]

David Smith, M.D.
Texas Commissioner of Health (1994)

§§§§§§§

The Wrong Emphasis

We waste many billions of dollars annually in diagnostic overkill for chest pain alone…Society places a much higher premium on technology than on listening or counseling…Diligent prevention invariably plays second fiddle to heroic cures.[4]

Bernard Lown, M.D., Professor Cardiology Emeritus (Harvard),
Lown Cardiovascular Center, Inventor (cardiac defibrillator), Nobel Peace-Prize Laureate,

Healthcare in America is in the "fix-it" mode. Many people have been led to believe that the answer to clogged arteries is to bypass them, or perform balloon angioplasty to re-open them. If clogging recurs or if previous medical interventions prove unsuccessful, metallic stents can be inserted to keep clogged arteries open. There is a host of amazing technologies on the horizon: novel radiation therapies, angiogenesis hormones to grow new blood vessels, and even miniature drilling devices to remove clots from arterial walls. Many see such medical breakthroughs as license for continued heart-unfriendly food habits and indulgent lifestyles.

This romance with high-tech medicine is seen by many as the solution to the epidemic of chronic lifestyle diseases. Cable television networks race to announce sensational medical breakthroughs and propagate the view that science will forever come to the rescue. Not only are such views unbalanced, but they are also unsustainable and untranslatable into affordable treatment options for the majority of patients.

Early into this administration, the Health and Human Services Secretary promoted their policy on "modernizing" Medicare along with an immediate helping hand (IHH) prescription drug proposal.[5] When Medicare was created over thirty-five years ago, there was no prescription-drug coverage. The new costs for meeting such proposals called for an increase of 153 billion dollars over a 10-year period to cover the cost of prescription drugs. Research at the National Institutes of Health to accelerate the quest for cures for Alzheimer's disease, Parkinson's disease, heart disease, and stroke, has been scheduled to receive a 3 billion-dollar raise, the largest increase in research funding to date.[6] There was virtual silence on prevention of these diseases.

There will never be enough funding for expensive medical intervention programs in the long term, and the debates over the future of Medicare and prescription-drug benefits will no doubt intensify. There is desperate need for a new approach that puts far more emphasis on prevention and personal responsibility. Ideally, this effort should start in childhood and nurtured at home, in our schools, and other institutions. But it needs to be stated that it is never too late to embark on healthy lifestyles. Simple incremental measures can make a meaningful difference at whatever stage you are in life.

Losing the War on Drugs

Current System of Medical Care

- Building more institutions and simply catering to a "drug culture" is a poor prescription.
- We have created an overmedicated society.
- We have failed to reduce the demand for prescription drugs.
- We have forgotten the lessons from the war on illegal drugs.

We are familiar with America's war on illegal drugs. This war has been fought on several fronts using a number of tactics over the past century. Billions have been spent trying to fight this scourge. Are we any closer to a solution? There is another important follow-up question: How much of a difference has it made?

On the domestic front, the United States presides over an ever increasing prison population that has, for the first time, surpassed the 2,000,000 mark. Of this number, almost 25 percent are for minor drug offences.[7] The illegal drug trade has become a major growth industry for both drug cartels and private detention corporations alike. American policy on fighting the illegal drug trade, despite many billions spent, has largely failed.

Why has this war failed? And why do millions of Americans and people around the world continue to use illegal drugs? Is it sufficient just to build more prisons and fund more law reinforcement? What about more education for inmates and potential inmates, and related measures to reduce demand? Wouldn't it be better to spend more money to rehabilitate rather than incarcerate, on prevention rather than on more policing and more prisons? The investment of resources has been unbalanced. It is futile to try to stop the illegal drug trade without reducing demand.

There is a parallel with the "legal drug trade." The major difference between this and the illegal drug trade is that we naïvely consider the use of medicinal drugs as always "good" and that of illegal drugs as "bad." Therefore, we promote more prescription drugs because we consider it a good thing. However, we need to examine closer what we are really achieving.

We certainly need the best medical facilities and the best pharmaceutical drugs for those who are really sick, but inadvertently we have birthed an overmedicated society (see Chapter 2). Medical interventions are always more costly and do not lead to long-term solutions. This is what we face; this is the reality check. … As of 2000, 125 million Americans, or 45 percent of the United States population suffered from some sort of chronic disease.[8] Americans with chronic diseases are projected to reach 157 million people or half the U.S. population by the year 2020. In terms of cost we are looking at healthcare expenses far in excess of a trillion dollars or 75 percent of U.S. healthcare expenditure. This is expected to exceed 80 percent by the year 2020.[1,9-10]

We are fighting a war that can potentially bankrupt the healthcare system. Of course this will not happen. What will happen is more of what is happening now—less people will have access to the medical care that they need. Building more institutions and catering to a "drug culture" is a poor prescription. It is time to tackle this insatiable demand at its root. This does not call for a magic wand; it simply calls for an effective prescription for healthy living.

Healthy Living Is Not a Killjoy

Most people harbor negative opinions about healthy living. Many see it as exchanging delicacies and creature comforts for horrible diets and unbearable exercises.

Contrary to popular opinion, healthy living is not a distasteful undertaking. Sadly, this is what many believe. In Western popular food culture, tastes and preferences are so deeply ingrained that there is a reflex resistance to change. This is the nature of habits. Today's food consumption patterns are a far cry from what existed 75 years ago. This has contributed to diseases that now cost a fortune to treat. To make matters worse, the physical activity front has also radically changed. Almost every mechanical invention over the past 100 years has been designed to make life easier.

Therefore, the real challenge in Western culture is how to overcome these deeply ingrained lifestyle patterns that have led to this huge burden of chronic disease. This is the question: why should people make lifestyle changes? What does it take for an individual to switch from one particular lifestyle pattern to another? The answers to these questions may vary from person to person, but the answers would be incomplete without delving into human psychology.

Human beings love their creature comforts. So much of our actions are done with this in mind. We seek pleasure and avoid pain. Fundamentally, this is how we literally survive. We avoid noxious stimuli in exchange for those that make us feel pleasant and satisfied. So much of what we now eat has been scientifically formulated to satisfy the taste buds. Embarking on healthy lifestyles in today's world can make most people uncomfortable. Most of us are not masochistic; pain does not bring us pleasure. Therefore the choices we make follow the agenda set in the world around us. This is easiest and the most natural thing to do. Anything else is met with resistance. Therefore healthy living is widely seen as a killjoy. Worse still, much of the professional advice given to us reinforces such opinions.

Erroneous Perceptions about Healthy Living

…Giving up my favorite foods!
…Unable to socialize and eat with friends anymore…
…Only for freaks and extremists.
…Such foods are tasteless, horrible, and boring foods.
…Takes all the fun and joy out of living.
☹☹☹

Figure 1-1. Misconceptions and negative mind-sets about healthy living[12,13]

Patient: "Doctor, what can I do to live longer?"

Doctor: "Don't...Don't...Stop...Don't...Give Up...."

Patient: Hmm..."So doctor, If I deny myself all my
favorites, and those things that make life
worth living...Will I live longer?"

Doctor: "No!, but it will seem that way."

Words modified from *The Lost Art of Healing* [11]

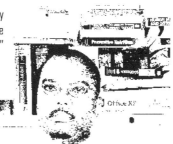

> Healthy living is not about negatives.
> It does not involve pursuing endless diets or becoming
> exercise freaks. It is not about giving up delicacies and
> pleasantries in the hope for benefits that lie decades down the
> road. Healthy living goes beyond preventing disease. It is really
> about enjoying life and optimal health.

Tastes and preferences are learned behaviors.[14] What we learn can be un-learned. For example, the taste for fatty foods is acquired, and the human body can quickly adapt to foods with less animal fats. The reason for this is not a mystery. Most people accustomed to drinking full-cream milk find the switch to full-skimmed milk initially revolting. Many complain that it is lacking in taste and texture. Interestingly, after a few weeks of adjusting to the new taste of full-skimmed milk, a return to full-cream milk can be a distasteful experience. What happened? We are creatures of habit, we had adjusted to the new taste, and reverting to a different taste, especially if it is re-enforced with negative thoughts, can be unpleasant. Think about the entire range of your personal habits. They are habits now, but a journey into the past may reveal that some of these were initially revolting. Tastes and preferences for foods and drinks are acquired. It is as simple as that.

Healthy living is an investment that pays great dividends, both now as well as the future. Too many people spend the first part of their lives unwittingly destroying their health, then end up spending the last part of their lives trying to patch things up.

Healthy living leads to genuine rewards that extend beyond preventing disease (Figure 1-2). On the social front, people who lead healthy lives generally feel better about themselves. This improved self-image filters into personal and social relationships. Maximized performance on a day-to-day basis, along with improved energy levels, is included among its many paybacks. Feeling more energetic in the morning with no need for coffee or eye-openers, or going on vacation with less worry over prescription drugs are the part of the package. It is wise to invest in your health. Our bodies were meant to last a lifetime.[15-20]

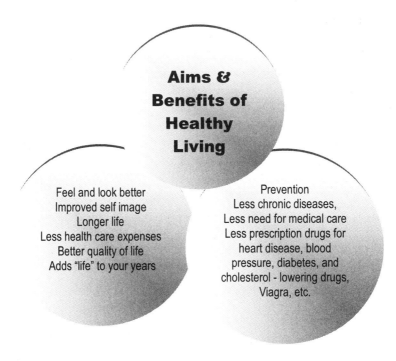

Aims & Benefits of Healthy Living

Feel and look better
Improved self image
Longer life
Less health care expenses
Better quality of life
Adds "life" to your years

Prevention
Less chronic diseases,
Less need for medical care
Less prescription drugs for
heart disease, blood
pressure, diabetes, and
cholesterol - lowering drugs,
Viagra, etc.

Figure 1-2. Some aims and benefits of healthy living.

The Sad Irony

Too many people spend the first part of their lives unwittingly destroying their health, then end up spending the last part of their lives trying to patch things up.

When Virtue Becomes A Vice

A wise man avoids all extremes. (Wisdom)

Food fulfills more than our nutritional needs. If nutrition was the only reason for eating, we would perhaps be better off getting nourishment by taking special supplements in isolated quarters. Foods satisfy our cravings, not just for food, but also for social interaction (see Chapter 7, Figure 7-1).

Social, cultural, and religious traditions serve as important backdrops for culinary delights and gastronomic indulgence in most cultures. Much of this gets lost in busy urban societies where time pressures of modern living dictate the pace of meals. In many traditional cultures, the dinner table is where families meet, social issues are discussed, and business deals are sealed. In such cultures, meals last hours … a luxury in today's time-obsessed corporate culture. The unrelenting drive towards efficiency and productivity gave birth to the fast food industry that has robbed meals of great social benefits. At the same time, it has given rise to much of the diseases that we discuss in this book.[27,28]

Knowledge is a good thing, but as a note of caution, a little knowledge can be a dangerous thing. Extremism is rampant in nutritional circles, and it has reached ridiculous extremes. Diet is important—very important, but it is not a cure-all.

Few areas have generated as much extremism as the subject of nutrition. In the weight-loss arena alone, there is a multitude of crusaders fighting their way to capture their slice of the pie in the battle of the bulge. What makes it even worse is that there is no shortage of captives willing to submit to every imaginable fad! There are those who have become through perception, real or imagined, extremely cynical about anything resembling science or modern medicine.

There is a human tendency to become fanatical after acquiring an initial injection of new knowledge. This trend, commonly seen with religious conversions, applies equally to nutrition knowledge and experiences. Communes exist where people believe that certain foods impart superiority and "special" spiritual powers over their "unenlightened brethren." Equally unfortunate are the feelings of guilt, remorse, and other psychological pressures suffered by adherents for falling short of these standards.[29,30]

If healthy equates to a never-ending pre-occupation with what to eat and what not to eat, that would be a sorry state of affairs. Something is very wrong when healthy eating starts ruining the quality of your life and dominates your social interactions. This is unhealthy! Steven Bratman, M.D.[26] coined the term "orthorexia nervosa." In his book, *Health Food Junkies: Orthorexia nervosa: Overcoming the obsession with healthful eating,* he examines an increasing problem seen in many circles in America, where well-meaning individuals go to extreme lengths to improve their nutrition. He described his personal struggles, where in his efforts to pursue healthy eating, the "poetry of his life" began to disappear:[31]

> My ability to carry on normal conversations was hindered by intrusive thoughts of food. The need to obtain meals free of meat, fat, and artificial chemicals had put nearly all social forms of eating beyond my reach. I was lonely and obsessed…For a person to eat only a handful of foods, to be isolated, to be unable to eat at restaurants or with friends, to spend the whole day thinking about what they'll eat next—those are pretty big side

effects, and quite possibly worse than the side effects of the medicine or even the sickness itself.

Healthy living is not the preserve of extremists and isolationists. It is about balance, understanding, and empowerment. It is not about making a vice out of virtue.[32,33]

A Better Approach to Health

...But the real responsibility will be that of the people themselves. The doctor will be the helper rather than the doer. Our health and longevity are in our hands.[34]

The health of an individual is his or her primary responsibility, but individuals must first be empowered before being given this important task. Nutrition education that is based on sound scientific principles can equip people to take better care of themselves. This essential tool is needed to halt the current epidemic of chronic diseases. People must understand that major limitations exist in current medical practice for treating these diseases. This is not a view coming from the fringes. There are distinguished voices that echo this call for a fundamental shift in the way we address the medical crises that confront us.

Bernard Lown, eminent Harvard cardiologist of global repute, lamented several aspects of the current system of medical care. He considers today's cardiologists to be overwhelmingly obsessed with medical interventions, with little or no interest in primary prevention. This is made worse by the clear evidence that well over 50 percent of cardiovascular diseases—diseases that cost Americans 300 billion dollars annually—are preventable. In his book, *The Lost Art of Healing, practicing compassion in medicine*, he lamented several reasons for our present predicament:[35]

> Reflecting on forty-five years of medical practice, I see that something vital appears to be vanishing. It seems to me that medicine has indulged in a Faustian bargain. A three-thousand year tradition, which bonded doctor and patient, is being traded for a new type of relationship. Healing is replaced with treating, caring is supplanted by managing, and the art of listening is overtaken by technological procedures.

Harry Hersey, a passionate advocate of prevention, declared the need for a new paradigm in our approach to promote better health over healthcare. He summed this up in his book, *New Answers to Old Questions: The Free Radical Story*:[36]

The new medicine will be different from conventional medicine. This new medicine will be practiced by health and prevention-conscious individuals, rather than by medical specialists. Progressive physicians, oriented to this new knowledge, will of course play a part: guiding their patients, providing information and advice, and occasional specific therapy. But the real responsibility will be that of the people themselves. The doctor will be the helper rather than the doer. Our health and longevity are in our hands.

In a *British Medical Journal* editorial "Towards a global definition of patient centred care," Professor Moira Stewart noted that patients prefer approaches that promote communication, partnership, and health promotion. According to her investigations, uppermost in the minds of many patients is the need for a relationship that enhances prevention and health promotion.[37] This desire by patients for a better doctor-patient relationship has led to an explosion in complementary and alternative medical practices. As frustration mounts over the current system of healthcare, an increasing number of doctors now champion an integrative or holistic approach to healthcare (Table 1-1, and Chapter 4).[4,38]

Table 1-1. The Elements for a Successful Doctor-Patient Relationship.[38]

Patient	**Doctor**
• Must see the need for change • Must feel able to make changes • Need education and empowerment • Need a simple practical strategy • Need continuity and follow-up in achieving these goals • Need the involvement of family , friends, and significant others	• Need to set achievable targets • Need to be able to translate knowledge to behavior change • Need to provide patients the tools of empowerment to achieve lifestyle changes • Must appreciate the dynamics (educational, psychological, and socioeconomic challenges) that militate against changes • Must involve patients in the decision-making process and emphasize a more patient-centered approach

Patient empowerment strengthens the doctor-patient relationship. It sends a powerful message of the doctor's interest in the patient's overall health, as much as he/she is interested in treating the patient's disease. It is an essential ingredient for meaningful relationship. The World Health Organization's document on diabetes care sums it up quite well—"A substantial part of diabetes care is patient self-care ... patients must be educated before being delegated the responsibility for daily management of their condition."[39] This is the intent of the chapters that follow. They will equip you with valuable tools to assist you to look after your health.

Less Healthcare, More Health

Current Problems with U.S. Healthcare

- Excessive reliance on high-technology care
- Excessive use of expensive pharmaceuticals
- High administrative costs
- Insurance companies and HMOs making crucial decisions on care
- Too many patients and too little time spent with doctor
- Less patient satisfaction
- Doctors under pressure "hassle factor"

Source: Adapted from J.E. Dalen, *Archives of Internal Medicine*, 2000 [38]

We live in a time when there is worldwide angst over the state of healthcare services. Aging populations, excessive reliance on high-technology, expensive medicines, and high administrative costs are chiefly to blame. James Dalen, M.D., vice president of Health Sciences at the University of Arizona Health Sciences Center, wrote his views on "Health care in America—the good, the bad, and the ugly" that appeared in the *Archives of Internal Medicine*.[38] He emphasized that Americans cannot have it both ways—"Americans want the best possible health care (now!) at the lowest possible cost." These two wishes are diametrically opposed. You get what you pay for.

Modern medicine, therefore, has found itself presiding over growing consumer discontent with healthcare, despite the unprecedented medical technological advances. Doctors themselves are not immune; they now resent being categorized as "providers" under the current system of managed care in America. Doctors are now paid less per patient seen and per procedures performed. To compensate for the financial shortfall, many doctors now spend less time with patients, leading to a predictable increase in patient dissatisfaction, as well as an increased likelihood of making mistakes.

Mistakes can easily occur during a hurried medical encounter. There is no magic in medicine. The less time you spend with a patient, the greater is the potential to make mistakes. Sending patients for more tests and costly diagnostic investigations to compensate for a hurried medical is not the way to go. Frustration levels and "hassle factors" in medical practice have risen markedly. Doctors find themselves torn between their responsibilities to patients on one hand, and the hawkish expectations of the HMO's (Health Maintenance Organizations) and insurance companies on the other. This has led some conscientious objectors to abandon their practice of medicine in this unpleasant atmosphere.

Worse still is the current medical malpractice scourge that now bedevils the practice of medicine in America. Dissatisfaction with the medical-industrial corporate culture and the virtual erosion of the doctor-patient relationship has markedly lowered the threshold for patients to sue their doctors. This has predictably driven up the cost of medical malpractice insurance and the trickle-down costs to the consumer. I am convinced that a patient is far less likely to sue a conscientious doctor who takes the time and demonstrates a genuine interest in their welfare.

The Present and Future Challenges

This continued haggling over healthcare does not bode well for the future. Prudence dictates that individuals, cognizant of the present scenario, must get involved and take more responsibility for their own health. The debates are set to continue over the future of global healthcare systems. On the financial front, views espoused by the *American Medical News*, "Surplus now, but red ink looming in Medicare forecast," questioned the financial shape of the United States Medicare program. Medicare, though reported to be in good financial condition as of the year 2000, is bound to change. Despite the fund's 36 billion dollars in surplus in 2000, a long-term crisis looms large, and is expected to come home to roost in 2010 when the baby-boomer generation retires.[39]

Explosion in medical knowledge, the rapid advances in technology, and the pressures for doctors to specialize, will continue to chip away at the time doctors spend with their patients. The medical profession pays much lip service to the need for holism. However, the reality is that patient care continues to suffer from a reductionistic approach that has reduced patients to the status of malfunctioning organs.[40] Today's time-strapped doctors who are caught in the middle, have time to do little else.

Rather than becoming depressed over future problems, we should work toward solutions. Let us stop wasting precious energy worrying over the future of Medicare and other healthcare systems. Let the politicians and the physicians sort out the best healthcare that they can deliver, but let me invite you into a sound discussion about why and how to look after your own health.

Summary

The folly in our focus is obvious. We have paid too much attention to healthcare and too little emphasis on health. It is time to recognize that better health will not come from building bigger hospitals and prescribing more drugs.

Despite common misconceptions, healthy living is not a negative pursuit. Great joys and benefits flow from healthy living. This is what we have control over—not in what happens in HMO boardrooms, or in the U.S. Congress, or in a foreign parliament—as so many have been misled to believe.

Individuals with insight will invest their time and resources into schemes that pay better dividends. Health occurs *outside* of the doctor's office. It is the product of a wise investment in a healthy lifestyle.

******

Chapter 2

"Pill for Every Ill" Mentality

Chapter Outline

A Glimpse at the Past.. 77
America: An Overmedicated Society 79
Direct-to-Consumer Ads and "Pester Power" 80
Programmed to Pop Pills 82
Pill-Happy Physicians... 83
Looking for Quick Fixes... 85
Is It Really Your Genes?... 86
Is It Nature or Nurture? 87
Doomed by What Happened in the Womb?............................ 89
The Root of the Matter... 90
How Pharmaceuticals Work... 93
Placebo Effect 96
Natural vs. Synthetic; Herbs vs. Drugs................................... 97
Turf War.. 98
Blurred Distinctions 99
"The Future Is Food" 101
Nutrition: Prompt Results, Not Quick Fixes........................ 101
The Problem with Doctors 102
Summary.. 104

We live in a culture that does not encourage self-discipline. In our advertisement-drenched society, one is encouraged to purchase answers, not to achieve them. We are taught we cannot cope by ourselves— that "the miracle of modern science has a pill for every ill." It may be good marketing, but it's not good diabetes care. Take care of yourself; there is no quick fix.[1]

                                        Peter J. Nebergall, Ph.D.

Since 1995, the rate of increase in drug expenditures has been approximately twice that of total health care expenditures, according to the Health Care Financing Administration (HCFA). The pharmaceutical industry has maintained its standing as the most profitable sector of the economy. In 1999, total health care spending reached $1.2 trillion, an increase of 5.6 percent over the previous year.[2]

            "Medicare and Prescription Drugs"-*The New England Journal of Medicine*

Then, in his final year, Dr. Dennis Burkitt exhorted us to go out there and carry the nutritional torch. ... This was a physician telling us that health comes from food, not from medicine, which was a pretty revolutionary thought."[3]

                        Canadian Medical Association Journal

§§§§§§§

A Glimpse at The Past

> Drugs and medicines are as old as man. In many ancient societies, their use was restricted to medical and religious purposes.

Mankind's love affair with drugs goes back to the dawn of civilization. The Sumerians in ancient Babylon (5000 B.C.) were versed in the uses of opium—the source of heroin and morphine. Ancient Egypt was famous for its brew. Hebrew holy men gathered special herbs for *rapha* healing, and Chinese herbalists were masters at the art of harmonizing herbal formulas to correct imbalance of *Qi*,[4] believed in Chinese tradition to cause disease. The Indian subcontinent gave us Indian hemp (cannabis), a drug that is still used by branches of Hindu Ayurvedic tradition, and increasingly today, by the mainstream medical community.

In the Western world, Judeo-Christian tradition has left its mark on modern-day attitudes towards medicinal drugs. During Mosaic theocratic rule (~1500 B.C.), Hebrew priests were the primary agents of healing. Health and disease were intertwined in a covenant relationship between the Hebrews and their God. Good health was seen as a blessing for obedience, while disease and pestilence were often curses for disobedience.[5] In many societies today, undeniable religious overtones still exist about health and disease. Rooted in the beliefs of several societies is the notion that diseases are part of the never-ending struggle between good and evil, between angels and demons, between God and the devil. This belief remains entrenched in many cultures where doctors and healers have long been regarded as intercessors between humankind and the divine.

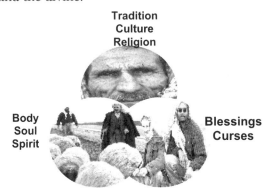

Tradition
Culture
Religion

Body   **Blessings**
Soul   **Curses**
Spirit

Figure 2-1. Worlds in Conflict: Some historical notions about health and disease

Man's preoccupation with drugs also extends to the political and legal arenas. In the history of medicine, the distinctions we use between legal and illegal drugs is a relatively recent phenomenon. In Asian and the Middle Eastern history, cannabis derivatives like hashish, Indian hemp, and amphetamine-like *catha edulis* (khat, kat, qat) were never criminalized. Alcohol, once banned during the Prohibition in the 1920's, now enjoys legal status in America and most countries in the world. In the tangled web of politics and economics, Britain fought two wars with China in the 1800s, supposedly to perpetuate the opium trade while simultaneously banning its use in Britain. Coca-Cola, the world's most recognized drink, derived part of its name from *erythroxylon coca*, the South American plant that produces cocaine. It was not until 1903 that Coke switched its formula from cocaine to caffeine.[4]

There is an interesting attitude towards disease in some Eastern traditions. People reward their physicians and healers for the promise of good health and protection from diseases. A successful outcome is recompensed in cash or kind. This was especially true, historically speaking, for promised protection from incurable diseases like leprosy that levied the ultimate social price—banishment from society. It is understandable why entire societies, faced with such stark choices, surrendered themselves to the mercy of the gods and the apothecaries. Medical knowledge as we know today did not exist.

A similar scenario exists in many parts of the world today with respect to chronic diseases. In several countries, being diagnosed with insulin-dependent diabetes is tantamount to receiving a death sentence. The lack of essential drug supplies like insulin and sterile syringes condemn many to such a fate. Renal replacement therapy for kidney failure, a major complication of diabetes, is not available in many countries of the world. Given such scenarios, it is clear why people in such settings place a high premium on health preservation. Prevention is their only option.

America: An Overmedicated Society

Modern industrial societies face a major challenge—a "culture of drugs" has taken root. Many have fallen prey to the popular belief that the best drugs and the latest therapies are the best way to tackle the modern epidemic of lifestyle-related diseases.

Despite many criticisms leveled at the modern pharmaceutical industry, few people today would prefer the days prior to Sir Alexander Fleming's discovery of penicillin in 1929, or for those days when surgery was performed using strong rum and ether as anesthesia. Undoubtedly, one of the triumphs of modern medicine has been the remarkable contribution of the modern pharmaceutical industry.

Today, drugs are everywhere. They are available over the counter or on prescription. Brand named drugs are now advertised using every conceivable media. About 150 million Americans are presently on prescription drugs. The over-the-counter drug market may be even bigger. A report appearing in the New England Journal of Medicine indicated that since 1995, total health care expenditures in the United States doubled because of increased spending on medicines. The pharmaceutical industry has today maintained its standing as the most profitable sector of the U.S. economy. [2,6]

The pharmaceutical industry is a mammoth enterprise. Almost 14 billion dollars were spent on marketing prescription drugs in 1999, and of this figure, 12 billion dollars was funneled into promoting prescription drugs to doctors (Figure 2-2). In the United States, 100 billion dollars were spent on prescription drugs in 1999. This figure rose to 132 billion dollars in 2000, an increase of almost 20 percent over the previous year. [7] Prescription drug prices have driven up the cost of retiree health expenditure to unprecedented levels. Prescription drug benefits represent 40 to 60 percent of over-65 retirees' healthcare expenses after accounting for Medicare.

Today, no American politician dares to ignore the clarion call for more prescription drugs and more drug benefits. We have inadvertently become a nation of overmedicated junkies because we have ignored the true relationship between most of these diseases and our lifestyles. In the meantime, the masses are encouraged to continue down a path that is a prescription for more of the same—more ill health, and more drug dependency. An observer once remarked, "the money is in the medicine!"

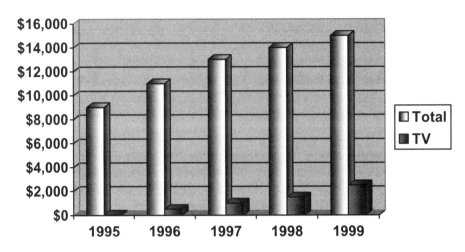

Figure 2-2. Progressive increase in advertising (in millions of dollars) spent by U.S. pharmaceutical companies (1997 to 1999)[7]

Direct-to-Consumer Ads and "Pester Power"

U.S. doctors may not have a name for it, but in England, there is a term called "pester power".
This refers to the ability of children to nag their parents into purchasing items they would otherwise not buy.[9]

You can hardly watch television without being confronted by advertisements for pharmaceutical drugs. Estimates are that more than 50 percent of consumer prescription ads currently run on television. Nexium "the new purple pill," Celebrex, Valtrex, Viagra, Lipitor, Zocor, Procrit, Allegra, Zantac, and a sizeable army of television ads have invaded the airways and the printed media. Sleek ads with before and after scenarios showing off smiling faces and handsome bodies, previously without hope, but now miraculously restored to perfect health—thanks to wonder drugs! A *British Medical Journal* article decried the dishonesty associated with the direct marketing of HIV drugs atop billboards in San Francisco's gay district. Ads that portrayed robust male models, all previously quite ill, but now wonderfully restored to perfection—climbing mountains and sailing the seven seas.

These are the images that drug companies push. The evidence is that these ads achieve their intended goals, and many consumers subsequently rush off to their doctors "demanding" these new miracle drugs.[8]

This is what increasingly confronts doctors—a growing army of patients, charging into their offices, and with singular intent—to devour the latest miracle drugs advertised on television. Patients are being increasingly seduced and many seek subtle and not-so-subtle ways of pressuring their doctors to prescribe. Verbal and non-verbal cues from patients requesting such drugs leave many doctors with little option to but to grant patients their requests (Figure 2-3).

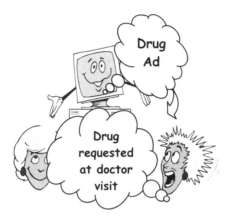

Figure 2-3. Pester Power: the impact of sleek drug advertising on medical practice.

U.S. doctors may not yet have a name for it yet, but in the United Kingdom it could be referred to as "pester power". The definition was coined in 1993 by Martin Rosenbaum, who in his article "Marketing to Schools," referred to children's ability to nag their parents into purchasing items they would otherwise not buy.[9] This clever marketing strategy to sell food and consumer items directly to children resulted in a subtle form of child-perpetrated blackmail. This needs no further explanation. We are familiar with children throwing tantrums and tirades on the supermarket aisles…that is, until they get what they want.

In a similar vein, the lives of doctors have been made more difficult since the 1997 approval of a new form of drug advertising by the U.S. Food and Drug Administration (FDA). This new advertising strategy is called direct-to-consumer (DTC) marketing. These ads peddle drugs for their respective medical uses along with anecdotal details on precautions, side effects, and advice to consult your doctor. Despite federal requirements insisting on listing the side effects, ads are delivered in such a sleek way to obscure this message. Companies that once promoted their products almost entirely to doctors, now spend about 2 billion dollars a year advertising directly to consumers—spending that has grown by almost 50 percent annually.[10]

Michael Wilkes, an assistant professor of medicine at the University of California at Los Angeles issued his verdict on the impact of the DTC marketing on his medical practice:[11]

> There's no question that this is affecting my ability to practice good medicine with my patients. I spend two-thirds of the time talking [with patients] about the ads and why they shouldn't pay any attention. That takes away from the time that I have to talk to them about potential preventions such as diet and exercise…The worst problem is that most doctors don't spend the time teaching the patients, and just prescribe the drug.

According to a report in the policy journal *Health Affairs*, marketing prescription drugs directly to consumers may be harming the quality of care. Drug ads cultivate the belief there is a pill for every ill, and contribute to the medicalization of trivial ailments. Such advertising rarely encourages lifestyle changes or non-pharmacologic interventions, a component that may be as important as any drug therapy. [11,12]

The FDA has not been oblivious to these concerns. Tom Abrams, the chief watchdog at the FDA for deceptive advertising, indicated that some ads stretch the truth, doing so with overstated claims of effectiveness and understated information about side effects. This is deception. [13] The FDA sent letters to drug companies in the year 2000 demanding changes in television commercials, magazine ads and other promotional materials. There are simply no guarantees that what you see (on television) is what you get. Indeed, the opposite is sometimes true. Consumers should view these ads with the same skepticism they would for any other advertised product.

This pressure to prescribe is a real one. The DTC marketing strategy has been successful in getting doctors to prescribe the drug in question. In fact, a number of surveys have shown that when requested to do so by patients, doctors comply with patients' requests for the advertised drug up to 80 percent of the time. [14] The direct marketing of prescription drugs to the consumer is not permitted in Europe and much of the world. This seems positive at first glance, but it is largely irrelevant in today's global village where the whole world watches U.S. television. This reality is, once it happens in America, it starts happening everywhere.

Programmed To Pop Pills

Many people have been programmed to expect medications during every doctor's visit. Many have been misled to believe that medical science has an answer to fix every ill.

Early into my medical training, it quickly became apparent that most patients expect to leave with a prescription after visiting their doctor. For many, the doctor has not done a good job if there is no prescription. Most patients have been programmed this way, you go to the doctor and it is his duty to give you something, anything. In communities where there is much poverty and illiteracy, patients are mystified by their doctor's ability to cure or to make them well. In such communities, doctors enjoy god-like status. People in more sophisticated and industrialized societies are seduced into a different sort of trap, they may sue the doctors, but many still believe that medical science has an answer to fix every ill.

There is the familiar scenario of the child suffering from the common cold. Most parents expect a prescription for antibiotics or injections for this child. They have been conditioned to believe that antibiotics will eliminate the viral infection more quickly. My pediatric colleagues confess that they frequently treat the parents as much as they treat the children. Scientific rationale is often replaced by entrenched misconceptions and fear. Generations of children have been conditioned by both doctors and parents to equate a visit to the doctor with receiving painful injections. The sick joke is that the viral attack will last seven days if left untreated, but only a week if medications are prescribed. The widespread abuse of antibiotics in such a scenario is an oft-quoted example of the injudicious use of antibiotics.

There is another example of injudicious use of prescriptions. This occurs in the treatment of the chronic lifestyle diseases. Many patients have been programmed to seek quick results from a pill. The average patient with hypertension, diabetes, or high blood cholesterol expects prescription drugs to treat these problems. This short-term, quick-fix attitude towards chronic conditions often results in costly delays in addressing the root causes of these lifestyle diseases.

Pill-Happy Physicians

Doctors find it easier to prescribe to satisfy patients' expectations. The time needed to educate and to listen to patients is in very short supply in the life of today's busy doctors.

Since doctors are so hassled in the modern medical environment, and because the doctor-patient encounter has been reduced to 10 to 15 minutes of consultation time, the quick-fix approach conveniently meshes with the current realities. As this relationship wilted, another association prospered. Doctors now enjoy a very cozy relationship with pharmaceutical companies.

Challenging this drug company-doctor relationship are consumer groups that seek to wean doctors off drug companies. Doctors are constantly showered with enticements from pharmaceutical companies delivered in the form of gifts, academic materials, and various levels or forms of sponsorships. One group opposed to this relationship publishes their list of "drug-free practitioners,"—doctors who pledge freedom from drug company influence over their clinical practice, teaching, and research. This group encourages the practice of medicine on the basis of the best available scientific evidence, and in the best interest of their patients, rather than under the influence of "advertising gimmicks and promotional ploys." [15-26]

Giving free drug samples to patients is another clever marketing tool by the pharmaceutical industry to promote their products. This is no secret. The industry counters that free samples are given to uninsured patients to reduce costs, but the real catch is that this practice influences subsequent prescription patterns of the doctor. Pharmaceutical companies gave 7.2 billion dollars in the form of free drug samples to U.S. doctors. Watchdog groups see this as a deliberate tactic to seduce patients and foster brand loyalties. The problem, however, is not just the prescription, but also the indoctrination that accompanies it. Most people believe that the way to treat all diseases is to pop a pill, and this mentality has become engrained at an early age with even wider repercussions.[27-30] In his book, *How to Raise a Healthy Child...In Spite of Your Doctor,* Robert S. Mendelssohn, M.D. addressed his disdain over this practice: [31]

> The pediatrician's wanton prescription of powerful drugs indoctrinates children from birth with the philosophy of a pill for every ill. Doctors are directly responsible for hooking millions of people on prescription drugs. They are also indirectly responsible for the plight of millions more who turn to illegal drugs because they were taught at an early age that drugs can cure anything - including psychological and emotional conditions that ail them.

Recently, the indiscriminate use of the addictive narcotic painkiller Oxycontin by some doctors sparked a nationwide controversy over physician prescribing habits. Doctors are sometimes guilty of improperly prescribing morphine and heroin. These drugs are legitimately used in intensive and coronary care units for pain and anxiety associated with heart attack, heart failure, and severe pains. Heroin (diamorphine), a more potent relative of the narcotic morphine, is preferred by British doctors because it has fewer cardiovascular side effects than morphine. Patients often receive these potent addictive drugs during hospitalization. Scant regard is paid to what happens after such patients are discharged. Addictive behaviors are known to follow such practices. Addiction to narcotics is a not a pleasant picture.

This trend is by no means restricted to Western societies. A Hong Kong study by Dr. Lam and colleagues showed that almost 100 percent of patients were given a drug prescription despite a sizable portion (25 percent of patients) who felt that their illness needed no drug treatment.[32] The majority of Hong Kong's doctors are trained under British and American medical school systems, but these same attitudes are prevalent among doctors worldwide. Over-prescribing is a global one phenomenon.

Looking for Quick Fixes

Positive and lasting results will occur only when we address the root causes of diseases. It is unreasonable to expect decades of indulgence to be magically reversed by an injection or a pill. Lifestyle problems require lifestyle solutions.

In December 2000, CNN's *Your Health* program hosted a panel that reveled in the exciting new treatments on the horizon for obesity. One participant declared that up to 70 percent of obesity in human beings was to be blamed on our genes. Based on their assumption, they concluded that gene-based anti-obesity drugs were the best way to tackle the modern obesity epidemic. Such futuristic drugs would be designed to switch on or switch off the genes responsible for obesity. In principle, these sounded like brilliant ideas, but they do not reflect the truth about the real causes of obesity.

Doctors yearn for successful treatments for obesity especially since it occupies such a central place in the development of type II diabetes and cardiovascular diseases. Our attempts to treat this condition have been frustrating and largely unsuccessful. Obesity cannot be treated in a doctor's office. It cannot be treated the same way you treat a headache. Long-term successful weight management demands lifestyle and dietary changes. This is the unanimous verdict of nutritionists and obesity experts. Being the creatures of habit that we are, making long-term lifestyle changes are more easily said than done. A successful outcome needs effort, discipline, and perseverance. Such commodities are in short supply in this modern age of "instant coffee and instant tea."

Aiming for quick results is not a problem in itself, but such attitudes will never work in our quest to control obesity. People do not go to bed one night and awake thirty pounds heavier the following day; obesity is not an overnight affair. Lifestyle changes, weight loss, and weight maintenance are not quick fixes. At the Royal Victoria Infirmary and the Freeman Hospital in England, morbidly obese patients were sometimes admitted for supervised low-calorie (500-calorie) diets. In such controlled environments, short-term weight loss was easy to achieve, but the greater challenges awaited patients after they exited the hospital doors. Weight regain was the rule in the majority of patients.

Why is there such an overwhelming failure rate in the treatment of this growing public health problem? For a comprehensive answer, we must examine why people gain weight in the first place. Individual details may vary, but the obesity epidemic is at its core a reflection of changing lifestyles. People do not gain weight simply because of their genetics. Genes can and do influence the tendency to gain weight, but genes do not lie at the heart of the problem. Just think about those countries where war and famine reign—you do not see hordes of obese people flooding the television screens, except for the greedy warlords and gunmen who control food and relief supplies.

The previous paragraphs highlighted obesity, but the same quick-fix attitude applies to our approach to heart disease and type II diabetes. As mentioned in the previous chapters, these diseases are heavily intertwined. Many still demand new cures for diabetes and heart attacks, with long-term lifestyle changes receiving scant attention. The television networks are obsessed with sensational therapies and "new" medical breakthroughs. In the interim, too many of us continue to whine, dine, and sit on the sidelines (waiting for that pill that will solve every ill).

Is It Really Your Genes?

Majoring on the Minors

Our genes are not the reasons behind the epidemic
of lifestyle-related diseases.
People's genes have not changed … their lifestyles have.

The successful sequencing of the human genome in early 2001 made international headlines. Researchers had successfully analyzed for the first time the human genome—all those genes that are found in human beings. The buzz in the scientific community was infectious. Hurrah! "We are on the brink of a new revolution in the way that doctors understand and treat most diseases." According to the genetic pundits, scientists would now develop futuristic treatments by going to the brain of the matter—the genes themselves. Celera Genomics and other participating companies raced to patent the human genome. In my opinion, they had their fifteen minutes of fame. The last time I heard of their flamboyant CEO was that he was no longer employed by company.

Honest researchers will say that gene treatments are promising in principle, but the reality is an entirely different matter. Sequencing and isolating human genes is one thing—understanding their full significance and developing treatments that work is an entirely different matter. At best, effective treatments based on such research lie several decades away. Ignoring risk factors and putting emphasis on gene therapies to solve the epidemic of chronic diseases is misguided. Such therapies and innovation hold medical promise, but they will fail as viable treatment options for diseases that have wayward lifestyles at their roots—not wayward genes.

Let us suppose for a moment that these scientists are right. How much would such therapies cost and who could afford them? Did you notice the mad rush to patent human genes? These companies look forward to their pay day. You can get it if you can pay for it. The current pharmaceutical wars over anti-HIV drugs is not about who needs it; it is about who can pay for it. It is not about medicine or ethics; it is about investments and dividends. A major magazine cover featured pictures of new HIV drugs accompanied by a stark admission—this (meaning the picture) is as close as most HIV-positive patients would ever get to these new therapies.

After all the talk about gene therapy and stem cell research, have no doubt that if and when successful therapies arise, these will be far more expensive than regular pharmaceuticals. Remember that "the money is in the medicine." You can get it only if you (or others) are prepared to pay for it. Your genetic endowment is a done deal. What happens after birth and during our lifetime is about the only thing we have some control over.

> We are products of our genes,
> but we become victims of our lifestyles.

Is It Nature or Nurture?

> Obese husbands tend to have obese wives.
> Obese people tend to have obese dogs.
> Nature matters, but nurture matters more.

Much money and research have been invested in finding cures for cancer, Alzheimer's disease and heart disease. In the three decades since Richard Nixon declared war on cancer, the United States has spent billions on devising better ways of fighting this scourge. Several new therapies have arisen and tremendous new knowledge acquired. However, we have failed to make a huge impact in reducing death rates from cancer since the 1970s.

In spite of great scientific efforts, breast, colo-rectal, and prostate cancers afflict Americans 5 to 30 times the rates seen in other countries around the world. In Asian countries, 2 to 5 out of every 100,000 women die from breast cancer. In America the figure is closer to 40 out of every 100,000 women.[33] Inevitably, speculations do arise over the genetic differences, and those who champion genetic differences as the cause of this observation receive lots of funding for such research. The rationale is convincing: scientists will identify the cancer genes, and then employ designer drugs to target them and prevent or cure breast cancer. The evidence, however, is far less convincing.

A report in the *New England Journal of Medicine* showed that the risk of a woman developing breast cancer, if her sister has it, is less than 9 percent. The risk of getting breast cancer if a genetically identical twin sister does is only 13 percent. This means that the role of genes in breast cancer is far less than proponents would have us think. Dr. Robert Hoover of the National Cancer Institute reported that, "The fatalism of the general public about the inevitability of genetic effects" on cancer is unfounded. Of course there is a genetic contribution, but it plays a minor role. The American Cancer Society and the Human Genome Project consider breast cancer genes to be responsible for only a small portion of breast cancers.[34]

Japanese and Asian women with different nutrition and lifestyle patterns than American women exhibit only 10 percent the breast cancer rates as their American counterparts. This is what should capture our attention, not the common fixation on racial and genetic possibilities. Japanese women and their descendants who live in America and Hawaii exhibit breast cancer rates that approach those seen in American women. Is it nature (genes) or is it nurture (environment)?[35] This trend applies not just to cancer, but equally to cardiovascular diseases. Professor Paul Whelton and colleagues at John Hopkins highlighted the primary role of environments in preventing hypertension and cardiovascular diseases:[36]

> Although BP [blood pressure] tends to rise with age in most countries, this is not a uniform finding. Populations with a low average BP and little evidence of age-related change in their BP have been described in several parts of the world. Typically, these "normotensive" [normal blood pressure] populations tend to be found in relatively isolated societies who have a high level of physical activity and consume a natural diet, which is low in sodium and high in potassium. The infrequency of hypertension in such populations is extremely interesting since it indicates that age-related increases in blood pressure are not a biologic necessity. When these populations have adopted a Western lifestyle, their blood pressures have begun to rise with age, and they have lost their immunity to hypertension. The explanation for this change in blood pressure pattern must lie in an alteration of environmental rather than genetic influences. Dietary changes, including consumption of processed foods with relatively high sodium/potassium ratios and more calories, as well as an increase in emotional stress have frequently been suggested as etiological factors of greatest importance in this change.

So here we see, coming from eminent experts, clear references to the pre-eminence of nurture over nature. This same pattern applies to many traditional populations. The Koreans, who are known for their low incidence of cardiovascular diseases at home, exhibit (along their American-born progeny), a higher incidence of hypertension and cardiovascular diseases after migrating to the United States.

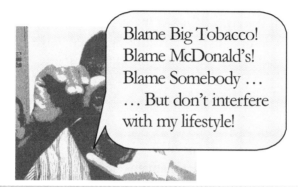

Blame Big Tobacco!
Blame McDonald's!
Blame Somebody …
… But don't interfere
with my lifestyle!

We came here by nature,
but we can become messed up by nurture.

Doomed by What Happened In the Womb?

There is another story that has come to light recently about the causes of chronic diseases. Some scientists call it fetal programming. In UK public health circles, it is known as the Barker Hypothesis, so named after the professor who first described the association between low birth weight and disease in later life. Professor Barker was puzzled when the records showed that the poorer areas of England (with higher infant mortality rates) were the same environments with more deaths from heart disease later in life.[37] His team then studied the relationship between low birth weight and heart disease by selecting 13,249 men born in Hertfordshire and Sheffield in the early 1900s. They discovered that if a man weighed less than 5.5 lbs at birth, he had a 50 percent greater chance of dying from heart disease compared to a similar man with a higher birth weight. This was true even after taking other possible causes into account. Death rates from stroke and coronary heart disease were also generally highest in men who weighed the least at birth.

These findings have been confirmed in subsequent studies, including a Harvard study by Dr. Janet Rich-Edwards and colleagues that examined the records of over 70,000 American women. Women with birth weight lower than 5.5 lbs were 23 percent more likely to develop cardiovascular disease compared to women who weighed more than 5.5 lbs at birth. This observation has been duplicated in other studies that examined the relationship between birth-weight and diabetes, and birth-weight and obesity. [38]

There are exceptions to these findings. Dr. Karin Michels and colleagues of the Harvard School of Public Health found that women who weighed 9 lbs at birth had twice the risk of developing breast cancer than women who weighed only 5.5 lbs at birth, even after all other contributing factors wore considered.[39]

Although these findings raise another possibility of an intrauterine contribution to diseases later in life, please do not ignore the huge gap that exists between date of birth and development of disease later in life. Here again, what happened in-utero is a done deal. There is nothing that you or I can do to redress our past lives in the womb. The only "cards" we can play are the choices we make about good nutrition and healthy lifestyles.

Despite all these academic observations, a person is not doomed to develop diabetes or heart disease later in life simply on what happened in the womb. Our subsequent lifestyles have a greater impact on what happens next.

The Root of the Matter

People don't just "get" diabetes or heart attacks

Having a check-up and getting normal blood sugar (glucose), cholesterol and EKG results do not mean that everything is okay.
If you are overweight, physically inactive, and smoke, you are well on your way to develop complications
even if your doctor says that "everything is ok."
It is like what happens to a car. Not because it has not broken down means that everything is okay. Behind-the-scenes damages accumulate with little warning, long before the final breakdown takes place.

Personal responsibility and lifestyle have been relegated to the back seat in our fight against lifestyle chronic diseases. Far too much demand has been placed on health care providers. As we examine the chapters that follow, it will become clear that we can do a lot, not just to prevent disease, but also to maximize health. We are not accidents waiting to happen. Once we have grasped the ABCs of chronic diseases and identified those big risk factors for the common lifestyle diseases, we will be able to intelligently embark on meaningful and effective changes.

We should not be interested in "band-aid" therapies. These have a place in the short-term, but are bound to fall short unless they are followed up by strategies that minimize risk. Results are what we aim for. It is undesirable to see patients continue in poor health year after year, from one problem to another, simply because the root causes of their problems have not been tackled. Root causes must be tackled with the same intensity that we tackle the symptoms.

Healthcare programs must emphasize education, prevention, and personal responsibility. This shift will pay great dividends that far outweigh the initial sacrifices. Doctors must challenge the person that weighs 350 lbs that the answer to their arthritis is not simply a prescription for painkillers. We need to help people see the big picture—that being overweight means that the entire body (and not just their knees)—is under serious strain. Down this road lie high blood pressure, diabetes, and related complications like heart attack, stroke and cancer (Figure 2-4).

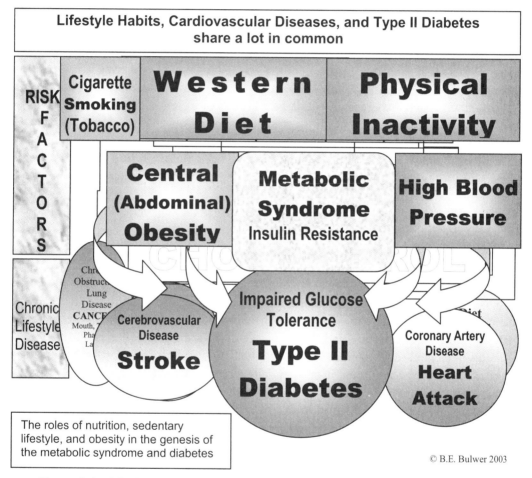

Lifestyle Habits, Cardiovascular Diseases, and Type II Diabetes share a lot in common

RISK FACTORS

Cigarette Smoking (Tobacco)

Western Diet

Physical Inactivity

Central (Abdominal) Obesity

Metabolic Syndrome Insulin Resistance

High Blood Pressure

Chronic Lifestyle Disease

Cerebrovascular Disease **Stroke**

Impaired Glucose Tolerance **Type II Diabetes**

Coronary Artery Disease **Heart Attack**

The roles of nutrition, sedentary lifestyle, and obesity in the genesis of the metabolic syndrome and diabetes

© B.E. Bulwer 2003

Figure 2-4. A look at the roles of nutrition, sedentary lifestyle, and obesity in the development of the metabolic syndrome and type II diabetes

Long before diabetes becomes manifest, there exists a pre-diabetic stage called impaired glucose tolerance (IGT). This is detected when a person has a normal fasting blood sugar and no diabetes complaints, but the sugar readings are abnormally high during an oral glucose tolerance test (OGTT). Obesity leads to resistance to the action of insulin. In response to this resistance, the pancreas (the gland below the stomach that produces insulin) has to work harder to compensate. This increased level of circulating insulin (hyperinsulinemia) is the cardinal feature of the metabolic syndrome (insulin resistance syndrome). It can trigger a family of diseases connected to obesity—cardiovascular diseases (high blood pressure, heart disease, and stroke), type II diabetes, and cancers (e.g. uterine cancer). [40-49]

The term "metabolic syndrome" is now the most popularly accepted nomenclature to refer to this condition that affects 50 million Americans. It has nicknames like the "beer-belly" syndrome or the "roti-belly" syndrome (Trinidad). [50] The term "metabolic" is important to understand because too often, many erroneously believe that diabetes is merely a problem of blood sugar. Diabetes mellitus is a metabolic disease. The word "diabetes" refers to the passage of large quantities of urine, and "mellitus" comes from the Latin word "miel," meaning honey or sugar. The marked weight loss that accompanied uncontrolled diabetes was described by medical historians as the "melting of the bones and the flesh into the urine." [51] People with severe uncontrolled diabetes can lose large amounts of weight very rapidly.

Metabolism encompasses every aspect of body chemistry—how the body handles not just sugars, but also fats, proteins, minerals and all body fluids. Indeed diabetes mellitus affects almost every bodily function. It is therefore not surprising that the number one killer of diabetes sufferers is not diabetes itself, or the blood sugar elevations. Most people with diabetes die from heart attacks. There are enough scientific grounds upon which to declare that diabetes and coronary heart disease are largely different faces of the same coin.

Many people go for their check-ups and assume that because their blood sugar is normal, everything is okay. Blood sugars (glucose) become elevated only after the pancreas can no longer cope—after the insulin-producing beta-cells of the pancreas have become exhausted. Behind-the-scenes damage accumulates long before type II diabetes is diagnosed. In a normal weight adult, the insulin-producing beta cells need to produce only 30 to 40 units of insulin daily to control blood glucose and the body's metabolism. In an overweight or obese adult, those same beta cells need to double or quadruple their insulin production to do the same job. If this strain of obesity persists, the pancreas suffers exhaustion and high blood glucose—the hallmark diabetes mellitus—becomes manifest. The problem, however, began long before this detectable elevation in blood glucose levels. Those overtly diabetic readings are just the final straw in a worsening spiral brought about by overweight, sedentary lifestyle and unbalanced nutrition (Figure 2-4, see also Introduction and Chapter 5). [52-54]

All is not bad news since the converse is also true. Individuals who embark on personal education and positive lifestyle changes will control not only their type II diabetes, but can simultaneously control their weight, lower their blood pressure, and reduce their risk of developing complications. It's the proverbial killing of many birds using one stone, with the one stone being "healthy lifestyles."

The same measures that are effective in preventing and controlling type II diabetes are the same measures that are effective in preventing and controlling obesity, hypertension, heart attack, stroke, and related diseases. These diseases are fundamentally disorders of nutrition and lifestyle, and tackling the root causes using non-pharmacologic measures (improved nutrition, weight reduction, and increased physical activity) are central to long-term success. Adrianne Bendich, Ph.D. and Richard Deckelbaum, M.D. underscored the importance of a concerted approach to prevent cardiovascular diseases, type II diabetes, and cancer:[55]

> An increasing body of evidence suggests that there are far more commonalities relating to how nutrition reduces risk factors for varied chronic diseases than differences. Different diets are not required to reduce the risk of cancer compared to cardiovascular disease (CVD)…Preventive nutrition strategies, increasing intake of fruits and vegetables has been linked to decreased prevalence of cardiovascular diseases [hypertension, coronary heart disease], stroke, and also cancer. Foods rich in other dietary components, including fiber, complex carbohydrates, and micronutrients, appear to decrease the risk of certain forms of cancer, as well as coronary heart disease and the manifestations of diabetes.

Adopting a preventive strategy does not decry the use of medicines or high technology therapies. It is a matter of setting priorities. Although prevention is not an exact science (and indeed no part of medical science is), we can never go wrong by advocating lifestyle solutions to lifestyle-related diseases. This calls for "regime change" (Chapter 8).

The prevention agenda is not an anti-pharmaceutical crusade. It is a pro nutrition and a positive lifestyle campaign.
It is neither at odds nor in conflict with the use of pharmaceuticals.
It is about patient education and empowerment; it is about enabling people to make better decisions for better outcomes.

How Pharmaceuticals Work

There is a fundamental difference between
the way foods work and the way pharmaceutical drugs work.
Food and nutrients make up every structure of the body.
Every living cell in our body gets almost everything it needs
for growth and repair from the foods we eat.
Pharmaceuticals drugs, on the other hand, are mainly alien substances
that act on body chemistry and function. Unlike foods, however, they
play no normal roles in building and repairing body tissues (Figure 2-5).

Our modern era has been characterized by tremendous strides in pharmaceutical research. Drug companies have invested vast fortunes in isolating and modifying chemicals found mainly in plants and other organisms. People in the tropical rainforests are continually bombarded by armies of Western researchers and scientists looking for insights into native and medicinal folklore. These habitats are renowned for their biodiversity and herbal concoctions have served as remedies for thousands of years. Modern scientists have tapped into this body of traditional knowledge and have since isolated and modified thousands of pharmacologically active compounds from nature's vast resources. Studying their effectiveness in hi-tech laboratories is often a lengthy and an expensive process, but the drugs so engineered are highly potent, and exert prompt and measurable effects on human body systems. Drugs have been designed to deliver intended therapeutic effects, but they also carry great potential for negative and unintended adverse drug reactions.

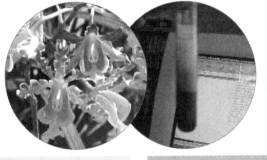

Figure 2-5. Contrasting food and nutrients vs. pharmaceuticals, drugs and medicines

Pharmaceutical drugs include a vast array of both prescription and over-the-counter (OTC) medicines. These are formulated to act on organ systems of the body such as the central nervous system, the cardiovascular system, and the endocrine/hormonal systems. Drugs vary in potency and effectiveness. Some drugs are primarily for short-term use only (e.g. antibiotics) and others are meant to be taken daily for the rest of a patient's life.

To appreciate how differently drugs work compared to food and nutrients, an illustration from a common herpes simplex virus infection can make this clear. The herpes simplex virus frequently causes a painful cold sore or blister that erupts near the margins of the lips or nostrils during times of stress. The herpes virus acts like a sleeper-agent in the central nervous system and wages guerrilla-type warfare when the body's defenses are lowered. This results in the typical disgusting cold sore.

Two different approaches can counter this viral attack—one that uses drugs and the other that uses nutrients. The common medical approach uses the antiviral drugs acyclovir (Zovirax) tablets or penciclovir cream early in the attack. The other option employs vitamin C (ascorbic acid) and citrus bioflavonoids, both nutrients that are plentiful in citrus fruits. When given in the early or prodromal phase, the vitamin C and bioflavonoid combination can abort or greatly reduce the duration of these lesions.[56,57]

Vitamin C is an essential nutrient that mammals (except guinea pigs) cannot produce. It must, therefore, be obtained from food. It plays a critical role in healing and repair of connective tissues. Vitamin C is found in all organs and tissues, but is most highly concentrated in the adrenal glands, the brain, pancreas, spleen, kidney, liver, lung, and the heart.[57] Vitamin C also circulates in the blood where its levels are best measured within the white blood cells (leukocytes). These leukocytes play indispensable roles in defending our bodies against infections. Taking megadoses of vitamin C boosts their levels in the leukocytes and greatly enhance the body's ability to fight certain viral infections. High doses of Vitamin C can be safely tolerated with no significant side effects except in very few cases.[58]

Acyclovir, the second option for treating cold sores, effectively works by preventing the herpes virus from multiplying within the body. It does not destroy the virus but reduces the viral load thereby allowing the body's own defenses to subdue the viral attack. The drug merely tips the odds in favor of complete recovery. Acyclovir is foreign to the body and has no essential function. It is potentially toxic when taken and side effects frequently occur. The entry of foreign substances into the human body handled by detoxification and elimination systems that reside within the liver and the kidneys.[59]

Drug safety in the United States is regulated by the U.S. Food and Drug Administration (FDA). Pharmaceutical drugs must first be approved by the FDA before being allowed for public consumption. The serious matter of adverse drug reactions (side effects) was highlighted in a 1998 report in the *Journal of the American Medical Association (JAMA)*. Fatal drug reactions claim the lives of an estimated 100,000 hospitalized patients each year in America and cause at least 2 million serious (but non-fatal) side effects in hospitalized patients. On the basis of these findings, fatal drug side effects rank as the fourth leading cause of death after heart disease, cancer, and stroke! This is far beyond the number of Americans who die from illegal drugs.[60]

In fairness to the pharmaceutical industry, what those statistics do not show are the countless millions who have benefited from the positive effects of drugs and pharmaceuticals. I think it is less of a nightmare living with the potential dangers posed by prescription drugs than living in a world without them. Give credit where credit is due, but do not pull the wool over your eyes. Pharmaceutical drugs can play important roles, but they are not the best first line agents in the fight against chronic lifestyle-related diseases.

Placebo Effect

> For some patients, though conscious that their
> position is perilous, recover their health
> simply through their contentment with the physician.
> Hippocrates

There is another principle at work that determines the effectiveness of a drug, herb or any other treatment. It is the placebo effect. The word "placebo" comes from the word placate, which means to appease or pacify. Placebos are drugs or neutral substances that have no logical or scientific usefulness, but they are often used in medical research to compare the effectiveness of prescription drugs. Placebos are sometimes prescribed to patients when nothing else works, or when a patient demands such treatment. Placebo medicine is not bogus medicine. Placebos have been effectively used to "treat" a long list of conditions including anxiety, headaches and pains, to the common cold, arthritis, peptic ulcer, and high blood pressure.

Indeed there is an element of placebo in virtually every thing that a doctor does for a patient. The effectiveness of the same drug can vary from patient to patient and from one physician to another. The placebo effect is most marked when patients have confidence in their doctor, or if the physician is caring and sensitive.[61] Placebos work better when both patient and physician believe the medicine will work, even if there is no logical medical reason for using the drug (e.g. giving vitamin D to treat diabetes). When good chemistry exists between physician and patient, the treatment is often considered effective. Tonics and vitamin injections are among the most widely used placebos for patients with multiple, recurrent complaints.[61]

What roles do placebos play in chronic lifestyle diseases? Over time, most patients will recover from acute illnesses whether they receive medical treatment or not. Even though chronic diseases are commonly believed to require lifelong medications, the human body has the capacity to heal itself when given the proper tools: good food, healthy lifestyles, and a good attitude.

Natural vs. Synthetic; Herbs vs. Prescription Drugs

"Natural" does not mean healthier or safer. Many poisons are, in fact, natural. Most medicinal drugs did not fall from the sky; they are derived from natural sources.

Many people fail to appreciate that everything on earth, living and non-living, is essentially a chemical substance. Most drugs occur naturally, in one form or the other. Therefore, strictly speaking, most drugs are natural. Few drugs could be considered truly man-made. Popular perception is that natural is better or safer, but even these terms need to be clarified, because many poisons are in fact natural. This argument can be taken further about discussions on food. Despite genuine concerns over drug safety, herbs are not better than pharmaceutical drugs on the basis that they are more "natural."

The plant kingdom is the primary origin of most drugs and medicines. Of the 300 or so families of plants, only two dozen families are the source of the major pharmaceutical drugs. In Central America, boiled senna leaves are the traditional purgative, but senna tablets are among the most widely used laxative in the United Kingdom. Many pharmaceutical drugs have a similar history—they were first used by the natives, and the active principles subsequently identified, extracted, and packaged.

Aspirin came from the bark of the *Salix* species of the willow tree. It was popularized by Felix Hoffman, a chemist with the Bayer Company in 1899, who used it to treat his father's arthritis. Lignocaine or lidocaine, a widely used local anesthetic, was synthesized from barley in 1943 after a researcher noticed that it anesthetized his tongue. Lidocaine was first introduced into cardiology practice by Harvard cardiologist, Bernard Lown M.D., founder of the Lown Cardiovascular Center and Research Foundation. Cocaine needs no introduction and neither does caffeine. The Andean Indians chewed coca leaves for its energizing and pleasant mental effects long before it gave rise to the billion-dollar drug cartels. Cocaine was first isolated in 1860 from the South American plant *Erythroxylon coca.*. Theophylline, a relative of caffeine that is prescribed for asthma, originally came from the tea plant.

Ergotamine, used to prevent uterine bleeding and control migraine headaches, came from the fungus *Claviceps purpurea*. Brand name drugs like Lipitor (atorvastatin) and

Zocor (simvastatin) owe their origins to fungi. Coumadin or warfarin, used for preventing blood clots, was first harvested from molds found on the sweet clover, a legume. Morphine and its stronger relative heroin (diamorphine) are widely used drugs in the intensive and coronary care units in Europe and North America. They originate from the poppy plant, *Papaver somniferum*. Their weaker narcotic relatives include meperidine/pethidine (Demerol), codeine, and oxycodone (Oxycontin).

Cinchona bark from South America produces quinidine that is used to treat irregular heart rhythms. Its identical twin, quinine, is an effective treatment for malaria and is used in England to treat nocturnal leg cramps in the elderly. Atropine, used in anesthesia, cardiology, and in counteracting the effects or certain nerve agents, originated from the leaf and berries of the deadly nightshade, *Atropa belladonna*. Digitalis medicine (digoxin) came from the foxglove plant that was used as a traditional English folk remedy for heart failure or dropsy.[62]

The composition of herbal medications fluctuates widely, depending on the type of soil and the growth environment. Barley from Iraq is well known for its high chromium content. This mineral is essential for optimal insulin activity. Barley grown elsewhere, however, does not exhibit a similar high chromium content. Herbal medicines also vary according to source and are thus far more difficult to standardize. This is a major drawback in comparing their usefulness in scientific trials. Better standards are needed to protect consumers.

On the other hand, pharmaceutical drugs, because of their purity and potency, can deliver quick results, but they also have a greater potential for adverse drug reactions. Herbal products, though generally considered safer than pharmaceutical drugs, are not exempt from side effects. Ephedra, a herbal preparation, had to be withdrawn from the market because of fatalities related to its use.

Turf War

Consumers need to be aware that they are in the midst of a turf war. In this war between the herbal industry and the pharmaceutical drug companies, billions of consumer dollars are at stake.

Most drugs come from herbs … legal and illegal. They have something in common. They both make good business. Heroin, morphine, and cocaine were mentioned earlier. Medicinal marijuana or cannabis is being hotly debated in many quarters of America. Some European countries have decriminalized marijuana use. Some states like California and Colorado have medical marijuana laws permitting its use where conventional drugs have failed or where nausea, vomiting, and pain may be troublesome symptoms. Dronabinol (nabilone, UK), a drug with superior anti-nausea and anti-vomiting effects compared to other drugs in this category, is derived from cannabis. It is a cannabinoid. A twenty-capsule pack of nabilone costs more than one hundred and fifty dollars! Illegal cannabis costs far less.[59] It is evident that both the legal and the illegal marijuana trade are quite profitable. Cocaine itself has a history of both medicinal and recreational use. In the case of marijuana and cocaine, both the herb and the refined drug have been mass-produced and marketed by drug companies, both legally and illegally. These examples deal with the extremes, but a similar scenario exists with today's dietary supplement and pharmaceutical industries.

Consumers are in the midst of a turf war. In this war between the herbal industry and the pharmaceutical companies, billions of consumer dollars are at stake. Annual revenues of the pharmaceutical industry topped 100 billion dollars in the United States and some 300 billion dollars worldwide. In 1996 alone, U.S. consumers spent more than 6.5 billion dollars on dietary supplements. The herbal industry has steadily increased its market share with a near 400 percent increase in sales between 1991 and 1997, a reflection of the new interest in complementary and alternative medical therapies.[7]

Pharmaceutical companies complain that the herbal industry can sell their products as dietary supplements while, at the same time, making health claims for their products. Dietary supplements are exempt from FDA regulation. This spares them multiple millions and years of conducting research to ensure the efficacy and safety of their products.[63-70] In this feeding frenzy over the consumer dollars, it becomes less of an issue whether herbs are better than pharmaceuticals. "If you can't beat them, join them." Just examine who now own and manufacture much of the dietary supplements and herbal products. Do not be surprised to find the big pharmaceutical names and their subsidiaries listed on the fine print.

Blurred Distinctions: Condiments, Spices, Beverages, Herbals and Pharmaceutical Drugs

Herbs and pharmaceutical drugs share some commonalities, but there are important distinctions.

Herbs, spices, condiments, and beverages have played important roles in the diet of many cultures for millennia. The spice trade between Europe, the Middle East, India and the Far East is a testament to the historical importance of herbal commodities. These herbs were used primarily for their organoleptic and gastronomic qualities, and not as medicines. Traditional societies did not always make distinctions between foods and medicines, but scientific analyses reveal that condiments, beverages, and spices are packed with pharmacologically active compounds that exert beneficial effects on health (Figure 2-6). Many such herbs enjoy global popularity.

Pharmaceutical Drugs

Herbs, Homeopathy

Foods, Dietary Supplements

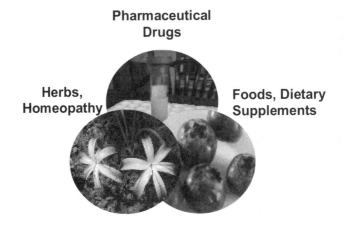

Figure 2-6. Overlap between foods, herbs and drugs

The herbal tea industry is one such example. Traditional teas are grown in over 30 countries and are the most widely consumed beverage other than water.[71] Commercial teas are sold in three broad categories: green or un-oxidized tea, oolong or partially oxidized tea, and black or oxidized tea. Fresh tea leaves are rich sources of polyphenols, especially catechins, which are especially plentiful in green teas. They are potent anti-cancer agents (see Chapter 8). Black teas also protect against cancer, but are less effective than green teas.[72-78]

Garlic, chives, onions, and leeks, members of the *Allium* family, are rich in organo-sulphur compounds. These have been shown, in several studies, to suppress the development of many cancers (see Chapter 8). These include cancers of the breast, colon, lung, skin, esophagus, and uterus.[79] They are particularly effective at neutralizing cancer-causing nitrosamines that are generated from the nitrites in foods like bacon, ham, and sausages.[80-81]

Citrus peels, mint, cardamom, coriander, thyme, mint, and caraway contain a powerful groups of chemicals called the terpenes.[82] D-limonene, one of these terpenes, has generated a lot of interest because of its ability to halt the growth of skin, breast, and lung tumors. It possesses an impressive ability to cause regression of existing tumors (see Chapter 8).[83]

If this broad definition of herbs is compared to pharmaceutical drugs, herbs undoubtedly possess superior benefits over pharmaceuticals agents. Such herbal foods have the potential to prevent and even reverse disease, something that is not an intrinsic property of pharmaceutical drugs. Incorporating such herbal foods and beverages as a part of everyday nutrition choices is therefore recommended (Chapter

8). But note that many herbs exert their benefits through pharmacologically active ingredients.

Although food, herbs, and drugs may share some things in common (Figure 2-6), the main message must not get lost. It is not an argument about herbs or drugs; it is instead the message about disease prevention and optimal health. This is best achieved by good nutrition and healthy lifestyles, not from popping either herbal capsules or pharmaceutical pills.

"The Future Is Food"

There is a love affair between the medical establishment and cutting-edge therapies. Novel medical treatments stimulate great academic interest and respectability. Nutrition on the other hand, does not...until recently. The winds of change have now started to blow and medical orthodoxy is becoming excited about those things that they once despised, as the record below indicates:[84]

> Dr. Mitchell Gaynor knew a lot about cancer when he finished his oncology training at Cornell Medical Center, but he didn't know much about food. So he was flabbergasted when he showed up at Rockefeller University in 1986, for a postdoctoral fellowship in molecular biology, and found everyone buzzing about Brussel sprouts. Laboratory researchers had started discovering dozens of new chemicals in common fruits and vegetables. And in test-tube and animal studies, these obscure compounds were showing a remarkable ability to disrupt the formation of tumors. Today our knowledge of these compounds is exploding. And as scientists learn more about the chemistry of plants and other edibles, they grow more hopeful about sparing people from malignancy. "We've seen the future," says Gaynor, now the head of medical oncology at New York's Strang Cancer Prevention Center. "And the future is food."

The pursuit of this most basic of endeavors—healthy nutrition—will prove to be challenging and exciting in its own right. Futuristic medicine will involve making simple, yet intelligent choices, to prevent disease and optimize health. We are on the verge of a revolution in how we look at health, and a big part of this lies in what we choose as food.

Nutrition: Prompt Result, Not Quick Fixes

Nutrition and healthy lifestyle are not about quick fixes. Decades of self-indulgence cannot be reversed by a few healthy meals or a day in the gym.

Lifestyle changes mean a change in style. This is a style for life—not a passing fad. Our bodies respond quickly to positive changes, not the same magical changes you see on television, but measurable changes nonetheless. Those who have exchanged idling on the couch for active exercises can attest to the difference. A stronger body and an improved sense of wellbeing are just the start of its benefits. Blood sugars and triglycerides (a type of fat in the blood) can change within hours following a good diet and exercise. The arteries and the rest of the cardiovascular system respond almost immediately to cessation of smoking. This reduces the risk of heart attack and sudden cardiac death within 24 hours (see Chapter 6).[85]

Blood cholesterol levels and blood pressure can be lowered within days or weeks after commencing a healthy lifestyle program. It is important not to be overly excited about a single improved blood pressure or cholesterol reading. These readings must be understood within the context that it took years for arteries to become narrowed, and these changes will not be arrested or reversed overnight. They will take time. However, studies have convincingly showed that even people who have suffered heart attacks can benefit dramatically within months after commencing positive lifestyle changes (see Chapter 8).

A landmark report in the *British Medical Journal* investigated 27 medical studies that involved more than 30,000 healthy adults. It revealed that low-fat diets cut heart disease deaths by 9 percent, and heart attacks and strokes by 16 percent.[86] The benefits, however, took two years to kick in. A diabetes prevention program involving over 3,000 volunteers concluded that nutrition-and-exercise was twice as effective as the diabetes drug (metformin) in preventing full-blown diabetes. [86]

The Dietary Approaches to Stop Hypertension (DASH) study, the Lyon Diet Heart Study and the Lifestyle Heart Trial (see Chapter 8) have convincingly shown that good nutrition and lifestyle deliver benefits that can be prompt as well as progressive. These measures can both prevent and reverse established diseases. Data from the Harvard-based Nurses' Health Study and the Physicians Health Study provide a wealth of information on the benefits of changes in nutrition and lifestyles. Perhaps 75 percent of diabetes and cardiovascular diseases are preventable by healthy lifestyles.[88]

The Problem with Doctors

Doctors often dismiss nutrition's effectiveness in treating obesity, diabetes, and cardiovascular disease simply because they fail to see dramatic results. This "quick-results mentality" is entrenched in a medical education program that teaches doctors to treat, rather than prevent disease.

The mind-set of the average Western-trained physician could be described as one of impatience. It works only if it works quickly enough. While that is not a bad standard in itself, it certainly clouds the assessment of the effectiveness of nutrition-based therapies. Aiming for quick results can sometimes be a bad thing, as is seen when blood pressure is lowered too rapidly by sublingual nifedipine—a drug that can be placed under the tongue. Clinical authorities condemn such practices because of documented life-threatening heart attacks, strokes, and irregular heart rhythms that have resulted from rapid lowering of blood pressure.[89]

A drug often needs to demonstrate its effectiveness while the patient is still in hospital. This gives only a few days for a drug to show its effectiveness. This is quite understandable, as patients in severe pain do not want any preaching; they want pain relief. A patient in a diabetic hyperglycemic coma with very high blood sugars needs immediate insulin therapy to control a potentially fatal condition.

Doctors extend this same attitude extends to the treatment of chronic diseases. Many dismiss nutrition interventions precisely because they fail to see measurable results after a few days of nutrition-based therapies. Such mindsets reflect a fundamental failure to appreciate how healthy lifestyles restore health as compared to pharmaceuticals. Pharmaceutical drugs generally act quickly with easily measurable results. Nutrition-based therapies tend to take effect more slowly with measurable results seen only after weeks, months, or years of therapy—long after a patient leaves a hospital or a doctor's surgery. Pharmaceutical drugs (used to treat chronic diseases) generally "work" without removing the root causes. Therefore, such drugs must be taken for life. Healthy lifestyles generally act more slowly, but provide a future prospect of living without dependence on prescription drugs. This is because such changes addressed the root of the matter. Again, lifestyle problems demand lifestyle solutions.

Taking the time to teach nutrition to a patient can be like writing a message in a bottle and throwing it into the ocean. It may take a long time for the message to reach its target and you may never be aware of the response. This is one reason why angioplasty (using a high-tech balloon to widen arteries) is sexy and teaching people how to eat is not. But time and experience have taught me how gratifying it is to see people take charge of their health. It is rewarding to equip patients, who in times past were like accidents waiting to happen, but who now enjoy a new lease on life. This was achieved by patients making simple, but life-changing choices. These are they who fret less about prescription benefits and the future of healthcare, and focus instead on the only thing over which they have control—their lifestyles.

> ## Doctors need to stop looking at nutrition the same way they look at drugs.

CNN Health ran a headline segment declaring that a high fiber diet does nothing to lower a person's risk of developing cancer. This was the media's verdict on the results of a study appearing in the *New England Journal of Medicine* (2000). The ability of high fiber diets to prevent the recurrence of pre-cancerous colon polyps (growths in the large intestine believed to precede colon cancer) was unceremoniously dismissed. Their conclusion, based on a four-year of study of some 1900 patients, was that "adopting a diet that is low in fat and high in fiber, fruits, and vegetables does not influence the risk of recurrence of colorectal adenomas." [90,]

Such sweeping declarations are prime examples of what the media frequently feeds their audience—half-baked reports that fail to present the big picture. Drawing sweeping conclusions based on limited studies is a common mistake in the nutrition debate. If doctors keep looking at nutrition-based therapies as they look at drug therapies, then they have failed to understand how nutrition prevents diseases. Unfortunately, this has been the fundamental flaw in medical education as the following chapter will indicate.

Summary

Drugs and potions are as old as man. This has been the legacy of mankind's struggle to survive. The modern pharmaceutical industry has made unprecedented strides in treating diseases. The evidence of this is everywhere. The triumphs have been remarkable, but so have been the victims.

A prime casualty has been the prevalent mentality, pushed by pharmaceutical companies and nurtured by doctors and the media, that there will be a "pill for every ill." Therefore, in the fight to tackle the modern epidemic of chronic diseases that result from unhealthy lifestyles, a system that promotes profit over principle has given rise to a "drug culture" that has failed to address the root causes. Lifestyle problems demand lifestyle solutions.

Herein is the need for balance. Drugs for chronic diseases should complement, not substitute for changes in nutrition and lifestyle. Let us therefore place at least as much emphasis on nutrition education and prevention. This is a "regime change" that is long overdue.

******

Chapter 3

How Much Does Your Doctor Know About Nutrition?

Chapter Outline

Introduction 107
On Automobile Mechanics and Doctors 108
What gets taught in Medical Schools 110
Postgraduate, Specialist or Residency Training 112
Important Historical Backdrop..113
The Early 1900s: Nutrition Awakened 113
The Mid 1900s: Nutrition Forsakened 114
The Years Since: Nutrition Disregarded 116
Prestige, Influence and Credibility...117
Who Dictates Research? 118
Increased Professional Awareness...120
Growing Public Awareness 121
Nutrition Education in U.S. Medical Schools 122
Nutrition Education Elsewhere...125
Conclusions and Recommendations...126
The End-game..127
Summary...127

As healthcare As healthcare begins to focus on early identification of risk, preventive health, and early management of disease, it is crucial that healthcare professionals recognize the essentiality of nutrition in total patient care.[1]

Nutrition Education for Health Care Professionals
American Diabetes Association (1998)

Most Americans say that they regard their physician as their primary source for reliable nutrition advice, yet many physicians are poorly trained in this area.[2]

Nutrition in Medicine Project—University of North Carolina (2000)

U.S. physicians are "widely believed to be poorly trained in human nutrition with only few medical schools offering formal nutrition training as part of the required curriculum."[3]

Journal of the American Medical Association(1990)

§§§§§§§§

Introduction

> There is an assumption that doctors are nutrition experts, but nutrition is a veritable outsider to medical practice. Doctors regard it the same way many people relate to distant relatives—they are aware of its existence, but they keep their distance.[4]

Most patients trust their doctors. The opinions given by doctors have historically been held in high regard, but these long-held views are changing. Although there is still the assumption that doctors are the most knowledgeable people about nutrition and health, it has become evident that the U.S. public's interest and knowledge of nutrition has surpassed that of their doctors.[5,6]

Despite this shift in interest and knowledge, few dare to challenge doctors' knowledge of nutrition. Consumer programs on nutrition often advise listeners to let the doctor have the final say. This mainly reflects medico-legal concerns. This chapter aims to provide the reader with a view that doctors, despite their noble intentions, are not enthusiastic about instructing the public on this vital area of health. Nutrition is medicine's stepchild.

Western medical education enjoys an colorful history. What began, in essence, as an apprenticeship, has now evolved into a highly competitive profession that is based on a structured education curriculum. My own observation is that people often make erroneous assumptions about doctors' expertise and training. Many fail to understand the complexities of medical education. Although physicians possess a large database of knowledge, there are important areas where significant gaps persist. Practical nutrition education, and understanding its crucial role in preventing and managing chronic lifestyle disease, is one of them.

A closer look at medical school education reveals why most doctors adopt the attitudes they do towards healthcare. Medical education has focused on treating rather than preventing medical problems. The overcrowded medical school program leaves little room for the introduction of any new subject material.[7] Therefore it should come as no surprise that changes to the medical school program will be no easy matter. A testament to this uphill struggle for change is that more than 30 years have passed before U.S. medical schools began revising their curricula.[8] Since doctors play leading roles in deciding health policies and priorities, it is important to have insight into why they have not championed nutrition and primary prevention programs. This is the basis for the title of this book.

> The medical profession does not consider nutrition as an effective weapon in the war against obesity, type II diabetes, cardiovascular diseases, and cancer. Doctors are trained to treat these health problems, not to prevent them.

This lack of nutrition awareness has, in times past, resulted in malnutrition in hospitals. Neglect of the nutritional status of hospitalized patients led to malnutrition and poor patient outcomes. This was especially true of patients undergoing surgical procedures who required extended periods of starvation.[9]

Thanks to the advent of enteral (via the gut) and parenteral (via the veins) nutrition, doctors can now provide patients with adequate nutrition support during times of prolonged starvation. This has led to improved outcomes in patients who are unable to eat for prolonged periods following surgery. These forms of nutrition are hospital-based and therefore expensive, but they highlight the important role of nutrition in healing and recovery.

On Automobile Mechanics and Doctors

> Automotive engineers know that the quality of fuels used can affect engine performance, engine wear, and maintenance schedules. It is time that we humans, who possess far more

> delicate structures, pay closer attention to the quality of the foods (fuels) that enter our bodies.

Nutrition is a pivotal subject on which swings the balance of health. All living things must feed, and in humans, we call it food. The foods we eat are the building blocks of every cell in the human body. The daily remodeling and repair of our body tissues come from the foods we eat. Just as the integrity of a building is contingent on the quality of its construction materials, so is the integrity of our bodies contingent on the quality of those building blocks we call food. If we want to pay attention to health and performance, we must pay attention to food.

Auto mechanics and operators of heavy-duty equipment pay careful attention to the fuels and mixtures they use in those engines. They know that the composition of these fuels affect performance and wear. In like manner, the composition and mixtures that enter our bodies affect performance and wear. Unlike engines and mechanical objects, our bodies possess far more delicate structures that are not supplied with spare parts. Even "spare parts" that come in the form of organ transplants can never make perfect matches, and all the talk about cloning is more hype than reality. Those fortunate enough to get near such transplants will discover that they are not as glamorous as the picture that is often painted. Transplant recipients are condemned to a lifetime of anti-rejection drugs. In these scenarios, the cure can sometimes be as bad as the disease.

We should applaud medical advances and technologies, but people need to know that the closest most of us will ever get to the AbioCor artificial heart, if we needed one, are the clips that appear on television or in magazines. Such procedures make headlines, but are unlikely to become routine if you consider the six-digit price tag that is attached. Even if money is not a problem, the artificial heart can never match the complexity and the efficiency of the healthy one that beats inside your body. Therefore, nourish and look after the only one that you have.

Despite its complexity, our physical bodies obey physical laws. Can you imagine how an engineer would react if a foundation and structure designed to carry three floors, carried an additional floor or two? What would be your thoughts if your car was loaded with bricks that it was never designed to carry? You would be confronted with a reality check—a check that will hurt your wallet. These scenarios describe obesity. It should come as no surprise that peoples' knees creak and bodies malfunction when we overload them with excess weight. Through the years, I have developed a healthy respect for the design and purpose of things. Forgetting such basics can lead to much damage and very costly repairs.

There is need for caution. Although we have made great strides in our understanding of lifestyle diseases, the complexity and the dynamics of the human body still makes it impossible to adopt a one size-fits all approach to their management. We are all unique. Risk factors for these diseases may vary somewhat from individual to individual. Two individuals with the same age, weight, cholesterol, and blood pressure levels, and lifestyle habits, may result in one person affected with a disease, and the other without. Despite individual variations, the totality of evidence supports the observation that what we eat heavily influences the balance between good health and disease.

What Gets Taught In Medical Schools

Most medical students quickly absorb the mythology that it is more emotionally rewarding to "do" things to patients than to teach them what they can do to help themselves. Behind the white jacket and the reserved clinical facade, many of us physicians want to be the knight on the white horse who "saves" his patients from death and disease. Patients expect the doctor to "do" something. So there is a subtle but real bias against approaches that lessen the patient's dependence upon the doctor and his procedures.

Alexander Leaf, M.D. Jackson Professor of Clinical Medicine Emeritus, Department of Preventive Medicine & Clinical Epidemiology, Emeritus, Harvard Medical School, USA.

The medical school program in the United States and other industrialized countries has not undergone any significant changes until recently.[10] There are currently 125 accredited medical schools in the United States. At the start of the 1900s, very few of these schools had any ties to existing universities. Some had affiliations, but many were free-standing schools run by private doctors who devoted spare time to teaching medical students. Clinical education for medical students during this era was "put together out of scraps," with teaching scattered among affiliated doctors offices. Medical education has since evolved into a highly structured program that is an integral part of teaching hospitals and universities. The evolution from an ad-hoc apprenticeship program to today's extremely competitive program, was summarized in the *Journal of the American Medical Association*.[11]

> In the early 20th century, a conceptual model of medical education was proposed in which the medical school would control all the resources needed to ensure quality medical education. In this model, articulated by Abraham Flexner, the medical school should employ full-time faculty members in the basic and clinical sciences whose attention should be devoted to teaching and not distracted by the necessity of providing clinical care unrelated to their education and research responsibilities. The medical school also would own or control one or more hospitals to serve as training sites for its students and laboratories for its clinical faculty. Funding for the medical education enterprise would come from the university with which the medical school was affiliated. In this model, the medical school would be a self-contained system, with all the components aligned toward congruent goals of educating the next generation of physicians and contributing to new knowledge…The extent to which this model was realized during the 20th century is a matter for debate.

The basic U.S. medical school program averages four years. Medical students gain acceptance following completion of college or higher degrees. The subjects taught in the early pre-clinical years covers the basic medical sciences on the structure (anatomy), function (physiology), and chemistry (biochemistry) of the human body. Other foundation courses, such as pharmacology (study of drugs and medicines), microbiology (study of microscopic agents and infections), pathology (study of disease processes), and various courses in epidemiology (study of the distribution and determinants of diseases), and community or social medicine, are introduced during this period and continued into the clinical years.[12]

The clinical years involve hospital-based training that gives medical students the practical opportunity to learn about diseases and their treatments. A problem-based approach, the core of the medical program, teaches students to diagnose and treat diseases. This clinical period includes medical clerkships or rotations in the major branches of medicine, ambulatory care, family practice, internal medicine, neurology, obstetrics/gynecology, pediatrics, psychiatry, general surgery, and surgical subspecialties. Students learn good clinical skills (on how to take a good medical history and conduct a proper physical examination) and methods of diagnosis and treatment during these rotations (Figure 3-1).

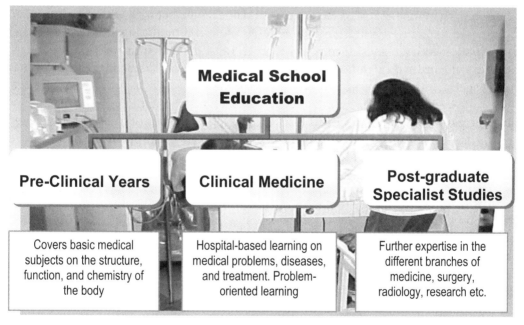

Figure 3-1. A Glimpse at Medical School Education

Doctors are then granted their medical degrees following successful completion of the required courses and examinations. These include the former National Board of Medical Examiners (NBME) exams, assessment of students' clinical skills using standardized patients (SPs), objective structured clinical examinations (OSCEs), and the United States Medical Licensing Examinations (USMLEs).[11] Foreign medical graduates working in the United States have undergone training programs in their home countries based on a similar Western model of training. Foreign doctors must pass the USMLEs and the Clinical Skills Assesment (CSA) before being granted certification to practice clinical medicine in the United States.

Postgraduate, Specialist or Residency Training

A specialist is one who gets to know more and more about less and less until he finally comes to know everything about nothing.
Anonymous

Residency training follows basic training. This is the time when a doctor defines him/herself. This period involves in-depth training in different medical specialties. It now comprises an ever-increasing number of disciplines and sub-specialties. As unprecedented spheres of knowledge and technology developed, so have the fields of medical specialties.

The lines separating many of these new specialties have become increasingly blurred as new subspecialties venture into areas that were the traditional domains of other specialties. Kidney stones, formerly the preserve of general surgeons and urologists, are now also treated by radiologists who may use lithotripsy to shatter kidney stones using special ultrasound equipment.

In the treatment of coronary heart disease, occluded coronary arteries may be dilated by cardiologists using invasive balloon angioplasty procedures, or by insertion of metallic stents to maintain arterial patency. Heart surgeons employ even more aggressive surgical procedures to bypass clogged arteries, although these are being supplanted by minimally invasive procedures. Newer techniques that involve energy therapies to evaporate cholesterol plaques are on the horizon. Large tertiary hospitals and institutions employ highly skilled personnel who combine their best talents to perform cutting-edge therapies for their patients.

Postgraduate training is rigorous, with demanding schedules, and varying degrees of involvement in medical research. For some doctors, this signals the start of a never-ending treadmill as doctors move from one level to another in the quest for respect, recognition, and greater contributions to medical understanding. For many, it is a prelude to a long overdue vacation to relax and enjoy the fruits of their labor.

Important Historical Backdrop

A careful and balanced analysis of history will indicate that the neglect of nutrition was in part the result of evolving health priorities.

Many believe there has been a deliberate plot by the medical profession to kick nutrition out of the practice of medicine. But a careful and balanced analysis of history indicates that this neglect of nutrition was largely the result of evolving health priorities.

The late 1800s and the early 1900s ushered in new health realities that compelled the medical profession to re-define its role. The early decades of the twentieth century served the profession with a platter full of malnutrition and infectious diseases. Scarlet fever, rheumatic fever, diphtheria, polio, measles, whooping cough, smallpox, and tuberculosis claimed the lives of millions. These were all infectious diseases. The bulk of their victims were malnourished children and adults living in impoverished environments in Europe and North America.[13]

With greater understanding of infectious diseases, the advent of antibiotics, immunization, and improved living standards, massive strides were made in the fight against malnutrition and these communicable diseases. Towards the middle of the twentieth century, industrialized countries moved through their "epidemiological transition." Malnutrition and infection became increasingly replaced by problems due to longer life expectancy, material prosperity, and profound changes in lifestyles. As life expectancy increased, industrialized societies became more pre-occupied with the diseases of aging, nutritional excesses, and physical inactivity. These then became the medical profession's new priorities.

The Early 1900s: Nutrition Awakened

Despite new discoveries in medical science, it was improved living standards—better nutrition, better housing, clean water supply, and improved sanitation—that were the real driving forces behind improved health of industrialized populations.

The diseases of malnutrition that gripped much of the Western world had its roots in urban poverty, inadequate sanitation and hygiene, lack of clean water supply, and a paucity of fresh fruit, and vegetables. Working class people in several European cities survived in crowded city slums, often infested with pests and vermin. This sad state of affairs came up for discussion in the boardrooms of Great Britain following the near defeat of the British in the 1899 South African Boer War.

Undernourished British military recruits performed poorly in the battlefield and forced Britain to declare this matter a public health crisis. A fact-finding committee convened to investigate this crisis concluded that "the main causes of ill-health and poor physique were to be found in the homes of the poor. The poor quality of food was to blame. Life expectancy of the average British worker was 46 years during those days![14,15]

Vitamin and nutrition research became frenzied and food science was pursued with the same vigor and attention as computers that the internet receive today. Nutrition and food science was the new frontier. This led to important breakthroughs in our understanding of the composition of foods. It is from this era that scientists learned about carbohydrates, fats, proteins, vitamins, and other food nutrients. American scientists like Wilbur Olin Atwater (1844-1907) at Yale and Francis Gano Benedict (1870-1957) at Wesleyan University made great strides in our understanding of the energy content of different foods. They gave us the unit of heat or energy we call the calorie (from the Latin word *calor* meaning heat).

It was during this same era that the concept of "protective foods" was developed.[15] Such foods protected people from infections and vitamin-deficiency diseases. Milk, cheese, meat, eggs, fruit, and vegetables were classified as protective foods. They enriched peoples' diets and protected against infection. These foodstuffs were a luxury, but became the prescription for good health. People of privilege who had access to such foods were physically more robust and largely untouched by the ravages of infections and deficiency diseases.

It must be underscored, however, that it was not the scientific nutrition renaissance that was most responsible for improved health status of these populations. Improved living standards—better nutrition, better housing, clean water supply, and improved sanitation—were the real catalysts for their improved health status.[16]

The Mid 1900s: Nutrition Forsakened
A New Love Affair with Technology and Therapeutics

Increased prosperity, lots of money for research, and hi-tech medicine, relegated nutrition studies to "Third World" status. Nutrition education tumbled from its pedestal and was given low priority, receiving only passing mention in medical circles.

The post-World War II era heralded unparalleled economic expansion and technological progress in the United States. Poverty and nutritional-deficiency diseases were no longer on the list of national health priorities. Fortification of staples like flour and cereals with vitamins and minerals became established policies. Technological improvements in food and agriculture led to tremendous strides in the production of milk, meat, and butter. Intensive farming and animal husbandry for meat and poultry amplified production. Food security in Europe and North America were now ensured.

The farming revolution gave rise to massive agro-industry, industry multinationals, and a proliferation of supermarkets and convenience foods.[17] Agricultural advances led to high-yield seeds, new farming methods, and massive specialized single-crop farms. States were given nicknames like "the corn and hog state" or the "land of famous potatoes" according to their major agricultural output. In short, food in America became plentiful and cheap. Excesses became the order of the day and Americans became famous for doing everything in a big way. Government policies in Europe, which included generous government subsidies, led to excesses on the other side of the Atlantic. Massive surpluses of wine, cereals, milk, and butter in Europe led to those scandalous food dumps infamously known as "butter mountains" and "milk ponds." The United States itself became the world's greatest agricultural nation ever, not just in consumption, but also in terms of food exports.[18]

Concurrent with the prosperity in the industrialized West were the famines that blighted the lives of millions in Africa, China, and India. Malnutrition had become a distant memory in the industrialized world. The name "Third World" underscored how great the economic divide had become between the West and the rest. Far removed from the problems of malnutrition, Western medical institutions needed to resort to overseas collaboration to keep in touch with such diseases. The British, for example, established medical research units to study malnutrition (marasmus and kwashiorkor) in the former colonies of Jamaica, India, and Uganda.

The economic boom of the post-war era provided a huge boost to medical research, and here began in a new love affair with new technologies and fancy therapeutics. Generous government grants and private funds fueled research at unprecedented levels. The new research focused on finding cures for the prevalent diseases in the industrialized world. Billions were spent on cancer research and heart disease. "Real medicine" was no longer about malnutrition and vitamin deficiencies; these were Third World problems. Nutrition education became a scientific discourse taught within biochemistry and physiology courses. Medical educators no longer saw the need to entertain nutrition as a separate discipline in Western medical education. Therefore nutrition tumbled from its pedestal and received only passing mention in medical circles. Richard Nixon declared war on cancer and pledged billions for research and development of new cancer-fighting tools. No serious attention was paid to nutrition and primary prevention. Despite the tremendous new knowledge gained, and despite almost unlimited funding, deaths from cancer in America failed to fall significantly since the 1970s.[19]

The Years Since: Nutrition Disregarded

As life expectancy increased, industrialized societies became preoccupied with the diseases of aging and lifestyle excesses. Doctors' energies were directed accordingly.

The virtual abandonment of nutrition education by the medical establishment was addressed by the American Medical Association's (AMA) Council on Foods and Nutrition as far back as 1961. This investigative panel documented that nutrition education in U.S. medical schools received "inadequate recognition, support and attention." This was true at both undergraduate and postgraduate levels of medical education.[20] They urged medical schools to designate nutrition committees to develop teaching programs at every level of medical training, including internship and residency.

Despite these proddings, the call to focus on nutrition education was ignored. The frequent excuse given by medical administrators was that the medical school program was already overcrowded, with little room for any additional subject. Schools also blamed insufficient funds as another important reason for their failure to implement the recommended nutrition programs. Therefore, the verdict was issued—American medical schools no longer equipped their students with a sound background in nutrition. This situation persists to this day, but there are signs of meaningful changes. The University of North Carolina's (UNC) Nutrition in Medicine (NIM) Project noted that nutrition is still taught in a haphazard fashion, without a comprehensive plan to teach nutrition-related skills to physicians, researchers, and teachers.[21] The majority of medical graduates are aware they received insufficient training in nutrition.[12]

> Of medical students graduating in 1990, almost two-thirds perceived that their nutrition training was inadequate. This perception by medical students still persists. In 1991, the Association of American Medical Colleges reported that, of 138 U.S. Medical Schools, only 29 (23 percent) had a required nutrition course, and that was, on average, less that 6 hours; 25 percent failed to offer nutrition education.

The numbers of schools offering formal nutrition programs have since increased, but this does not automatically translate into changed attitudes towards nutrition. The result is that the majority of physicians are inadequately equipped to offer people the nutrition advice they need.[22]

Prestige, Influence, and Credibility

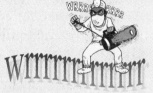

The more high-tech... the more respect!

In medical circles, prestige is given to those specialties that involve more rigorous training programs, advanced technology, and expensive therapies. Heart and transplant surgeons receive far more recognition than their colleagues in public health and preventive medicine.

Doctors would jump to deny this, but the more expensive your research and the more fancy your technology (especially those that your other colleagues can't afford), the more distinguished you become. This attitude extends to the general public. People may not be shocked, but most are certainly in awe when they realize the truly fantastic work that is being done in several medical specialties. I have been to several medical conferences around the globe where such attitudes reign. In addition to the distinguished academic exchange and excellent research presented, it is evident that the boys (and increasingly the girls) enjoy showing off their new toys.

In postgraduate medical circles there is an adage that says "publish or perish." This means that unless a doctor participates in respectable program or does meaningful research, he or she risks losing respect in the eyes of their fellow colleagues. Medical research and publications are the steps to climb the academic ladder. Publications improve the odds of landing that dream job and the perks that follow.

I shared a flat with a brilliant Scottish academic who performed with distinction at both the medical school and postgraduate levels. Dave Motwani became one of the youngest senior residents in cardiology in the UK. His résumé was first-class. Dave did intervention cardiology that involved balloon angioplasty and insertion of flexible metallic stents to keep coronary arteries open. He frequently organized academic presentations and meetings sponsored by pharmaceutical companies. I engaged him frequently in discussions on prevention of heart disease using nutrition and lifestyle changes. In cardiology circles, this hardly went beyond using the latest prescription drugs.

Cardiologists are held in high esteem by their fellow medical colleagues, because their specialty involves highly sophisticated medical techniques. Nutrition-oriented physicians, on the other hand, find their views ignored or simply dismissed by the politically dominant medical establishment. An in-house estimate of published material in the *New England Journal of Medicine* over the past ten years—by pioneer Harvard cardiologist and founder of the Lown Cardiovascular Research Foundation, Bernard Lown, M.D.—revealed that a pitiful one percent of all publications was about prevention, or about problems relevant to the developing world. This Boston-based journal is easily the most highly respected medical journal in the world. Most doctors would dare not admit it (at least publicly), but most do not have a clue about the overwhelming bulk of the research material that appears in this journal. It is full of lofty research, far beyond the reach of the vast majority of the world's doctors. Herein can be aptly declared—"The more high-tech … the more respect!"

Medical students quickly develop the attitude that "real medicine" is about lofty therapies and techniques, and not about banal matters like nutrition and prevention. A certain attitude prevails—nutritional approaches for treating diseases are dismissed as "unsubstantiated," or "ineffective." Attempts to break ranks with such current medical thinking, and any challenge to medical orthodoxy, can result in a loss of credibility—a price that many would-be dissenters find too high to pay.

Who Dictates Research?

He who has the gold makes the rules

There is a dilemma in medical training. Despite attempts by scientists to use the best research methods to achieve trustworthy results, serious bias is introduced by very nature of the funding process. Scientists investigate what they receive funding to study. As the saying goes, he who pays the piper always calls the tune.

To conduct medical research you need money. Where does the money come from? It comes from those who have it. The United States leads the world in medical research with almost 40 percent of all published medical research originating here. America spends more billions more on medical research than several of the leading industrialized nations combined. The federal government and private organizations invest huge sums to investigate better ways of understanding, diagnosing, and treating diseases. Apart form government-sponsored agencies like the National Institutes of Health (NIH) and the Center for Disease Control and Prevention (CDC) in the U.S., and the Medical Research Council (MRC) of the UK, and private philanthropic foundations, funding for medical research is largely underwritten by the private companies that sponsor research on their products.

Consider this scenario. ... the case of antioxidants for the treatment of cold sores that was discussed in Chapter 2. Vitamin C and citrus-derived compounds called flavonoids have been recommended as very effective treatments. In the popular medical book called the Merck Manual (1992 edition), they compared therapies for the treatment of cold sores or fever blisters caused by the herpes simplex type 1 (HSV1) virus.[23] A combination of citrus bioflavonoids (200 mg) and ascorbic acid tablets (200 mg), given early, can abort or greatly reduce the appearance or the duration of these blisters.

Interestingly, the newer 1999 edition of the same book completely dropped all references to vitamin C. The new editors mentioned only oral acyclovir (Zovirax) and topical penciclovir—both expensive patented anti-viral drugs for the treatment of this viral infection.[24] This omission was not for lack of effectiveness of vitamin C and flavonoids. Rather, medicines and substances without patents have few friends in the medical profession to extol their virtues. No drug company owns the patent to exclusively manufacture vitamin C, and funding is not readily forthcoming to study non-patented drugs. Reserpine is an exceedingly cheap, effective, safe, once-daily, antihypertensive drug—the ideal requirements for any drug. The new generation of U.S. doctors or cardiologist have never heard of it, or heard only of the negatives— its potential to cause depression. Institutions won't even bother to conduct new research on reserpine, despite hypertension being a major public health problem. The truth about reserpine and the reason why it is no longer used in America is because of one thing, and one thing only: Reserpine has no commercial sponsor.[25] The list of effective therapies that have been sidelined for similar reasons can be extended.

Dean Ornish M.D. and colleagues demonstrated the effectiveness of aggressive nutrition and lifestyle changes in reversing heart disease in the Lifestyle Heart Trial and follow-up studies (1990, 1998). The Dietary Approaches to stop Hypertension trial (DASH, 1997) showed that simple dietary changes were as effective as medications, in lowering blood pressure, after just 2 months. The Lyon Diet Heart study showed a striking 70 percent reduction heart-related deaths in people who consumed a Mediterranean-style diet (see Chapter 8 for further details on these studies). Such studies, however, receive scant mention in cardiology circles, but you are bound to hear a lot about statins (Zocor, Lipitor etc.), stents, and stylish procedures. The saying, "he who has the gold, make the rules," reigns. The politically dominant medical establishment still disregards excellent research that lies outside of their scope and interest.

In the previous section, I referred to my cardiology flat-mate Dr. Motwani. Without exception, every cardiology presentation and conferences was sponsored by a pharmaceutical company. Drug company sponsorships of medical meetings are the norm, not the exception. This has lead to major conflict-of-interest concerns mentioned in the previous chapter. Doctors with scientific integrity are aware that such influences have insidiously hijacked the course of medical education and research. Doctors have been warned against such influences. A article in the *New England Journal of Medicine* (2000) spelt out this concern:[26]

> Medical schools should adopt formal rules that prohibit all gifts from drug companies to students, whether books, stethoscopes, or meals. Medical training should not include acquiring a sense of entitlement to the largesse of drug companies. Finally, teaching hospitals should enforce these same restrictions, proscribing drug-company sponsorship of lunches, conferences, and travel for house staff, and should also make it clear that accepting birthday presents, Christmas gifts, or food and drink off the premises from drug-company representatives violates the ethical norms of the profession.

Pharmaceutical companies can play helpful roles in medical education and research, but clear policies must define the nature of this relationship. There is a lot of debate over the future of these relationships, but conflicts of interest are bound to arise as the relationship between doctors and drug companies is a very cozy one indeed.[27-30]

Increased Professional Awareness

Nutrition-related diseases demand nutrition-related solutions. These diseases kill more that 50 percent of Americans.

In 1974 Dr. Charles Butterworth Jr.'s article "The Skeleton in the Hospital Closet" highlighted the previously unrecognized problem of malnutrition in hospitalized patients.[31] Most attention was centered on providing the best surgical procedures and powerful drugs inside the hospitals, but the fundamental role of nutrition in healing and recovery were largely ignored. Patients had successful surgeries, but they were dying from malnutrition and related consequences. Doctors have since paid closer attention to nutrition in hospitalized patients. However, diet's role in promoting healing is still glossed over by many in the medical profession.

Proper nutrition leads to better health and better outcomes for patients. Malnutrition increases complications and length of hospital stay. Patients that are starved prior to surgery have additional nutritional needs, not just to maintain body tissues, but also to repair damaged tissues following surgery.[32] Doctors caring for cancer patients know that both cancer and anti-cancer treatments frequently insult the digestive system. Chemotherapy can severely diminish appetite and digestion. Failure to notify patients about this is often perceived as the cure being even worse than the disease. The whole patient must be treated, and not just their disease.

Many doctors are now more aware, and have taken the steps to promote nutrition solutions for nutrition-related problems. Type II diabetes was treated primarily by endocrinologists—doctors specializing in hormones. Insulin is indeed a hormone, but type II diabetes relates far closer to obesity, nutrition, and cardiovascular diseases than it relates to thyroid, pituitary, and other hormonal problems. Enlightened medical institutions have forged a compatible marriage between diabetes and nutrition departments to replace the traditional union of diabetes and endocrinology departments, a relationship that still lingers because of entrenched medical traditions.

The metabolic syndrome (Chapters 1, 2, 5, and 8) and the picture on this book's cover highlight this new relationship. This is the way these diseases relate. Together, these nutrition-related conditions are responsible for more than 50 percent the deaths in the industrialized world. The time has come for public health authorities and prevention-oriented physicians to rise to this new challenge.

Growing Public Awareness

Consumer groups are the vital catalysts in the nutrition debate. They have forced government, industry, and the medical profession to pay attention to their health concerns.

Since the 1960s, the American public has become increasingly aware of the connection between diet, lifestyle, and disease. Generated by increased public awareness of the connection between diet and heart disease, the food industry made the switch from animal-based fats to vegetable-based varieties in response to consumer demand. In 1990 McDonald's stopped cooking its french fries in a beef-fat mixture, and switched to pure vegetable oil following increased public outcry. Businesses listen to people who spend their money. This is how they grow and survive, thanks to competition.[33] The billions of dollars spent by consumers on health foods and alternative therapies has forced everyone—government, industry, and the medical establishment—to pay attention.

Healthier choices began springing up in supermarkets, cafeterias, and public places in response to increasing consumer demand. In 1990, Congress passed the Nutrition Labeling and Education Act (NLEA) to provide the public with greater insight into the composition of processed foods (see Chapter 7). Since 90 percent of the money Americans spend on food goes into buying processed varieties, the addition of a food label was a welcome addition for health-conscious consumers.

And it has not stopped here. Television, magazines, and now the Internet, regularly keep the public abreast of the latest developments about health and disease. The post-war baby-boomer generation became as interested in better health, as they we in better healthcare. As the generation that reaped the material benefits of the American dream, it seemed that the logical next step was to cultivate new ideals. Optimal health and quality of life became the new frontier.

The dietary supplement industry, the organic food industry, holistic medicine, and healthy lifestyle programs have become increasingly popular. But in the midst of this increased popularity, important challenges arise to separate fact from fiction, and hype from reality. This is a matter of public health concern, but it is made more acute by the shortage of doctors seasoned in comprehensive nutrition knowledge. Claudia Plaisted, clinical assistant professor and Steven Ziesel, professor and chair of the department of nutrition, University of North Carolina(UNC) at Chapel Hill, summed up some of these challenges:[34]

> It is difficult as a topic for credible preventive nutrition to compete with headlines touting the latest dramatic medical miracles or the whirlwind of activity around the changing healthcare system itself. Physicians, like any other individuals, are exposed not only to nutrition facts, but also a plethora of fraud and quackery, which often capitalizes on pseudo biochemical language to promote its legitimacy. Without adequate nutrition training, it can be difficult for any healthcare provider to discern fact from fiction when it comes to new alternative nutrition and botanical supplements and practices.[34]

Therefore, despite this new era the personal computer, the Internet, and the unprecedented democratization of health information, there is great need for guidance in separating hype from reality on the www—the world wide web. Despite cynics calling it a "web of deceit," the Internet continues to provide mind-boggling access to health information. It will continue to revolutionize the way people inform, educate, and empower themselves.[35,36]

Nutrition Education in U.S. Medical Schools

Despite an increasing number of medical schools starting separate nutrition programs, the success of such programs depend on more than window dressing. It requires a fundamental shift it attitudes from a disease-care program towards a prevention-oriented model.[37]

Medical education currently operates within an overcrowded curriculum.[38] The high cost of training doctors prevents any attempt to lengthen the current medical education program. Therefore, the call to increase the nutrition content of medical education goes largely unheeded. Even if time and resources allowed its inclusion, relevant nutrition would still face major dilemmas. Among them is the major challenge of recruiting qualified teachers. The prolonged deficiency in nutrition education has left a legacy of generations of doctors that are ill-equipped to train the doctors of tomorrow.[39] Doctors are aware of nutrition's relevance. Surveys have indicated that 60 percent of them willing to learn more.[40] Most who so desire teach themselves nutrition through conferences, scientific literature, and the popular media.[41]

> Scientific discoveries have solidified the role for nutrition in medical practice. Medical students want more nutrition education, and have suggested core content. The great increase in the health consumer's interest in nutrition and nutrition supplements has made it mandatory that physicians be able to give their patients sound nutrition advice. Changes in national priorities, including revision of the healthcare system so that it emphasizes prevention of diseases, are giving nutrition a more important role in medical schools.

In 1991, the Association of American Medical Colleges (AAMC) looked at the current situation among 128 U.S. medical schools. There is a small but increasing trend in nutrition education, but a quarter of all medical schools offered absolutely no nutrition instruction. Of the remainder, 25 percent of schools offer separate nutrition courses, and 45 percent provide electives or optional courses as part of medical students' training (Figure 3-2).[42]

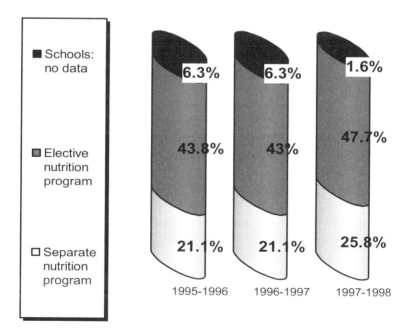

Figure 3-2. U.S. medical schools offering a separate nutrition program (1995 – 1998)
Source: Association of American Medical Colleges (AAMC, 1997). [42]

Although this trend appears encouraging, it is misleading to assume that increased in nutrition hours translates into improved nutritional education. Successful integration of nutrition education goes beyond the hours allotted to nutrition subjects. Professor Maurice Shils of Cornell University, a pioneer advocate of nutrition education, declared that the AAMC yardstick for assessing nutrition education is useless as it gives no information on "how well clinical nutrition has entered into the knowledge base of the graduating student."[43,44] Merely combining nutrition within the basic science courses of anatomy, physiology, and biochemistry obscures medical students' appreciation of nutrition concepts.

Even schools that increased nutrition content in their programs fail to graduate doctors who appreciate the crucial role of nutrition in preventing and managing chronic diseases. The success of nutrition programs, therefore, depend on far more than the mere hours allotted to nutrition; it must be measured by the changes in attitudes and practices of graduates towards the central role of nutrition in preventing and managing nutrition-related diseases.

It is mandatory that schools go beyond a cosmetic inclusion of nutrition topics. In their essay, "Incorporating Preventive Nutrition into Medical School," appearing in *Primary and Secondary Prevention of Nutrition* (Humana Press, 2001), Claudia Plaisted and Steven Zeisel summarized the uphill battle faced by those who strive to refocus the pivotal role of nutrition. Such a role demands a major shift in emphasis, a shift that some critics view as wishful thinking:[45]

> Traditionally, westernized medicine has focused on a systems approach, as opposed to a whole-person approach to health. Medical students have been taught to fix a health problem rather than to prevent one. The scope of time for the practice of medicine lasted from minutes to hours, perhaps weeks to months in worst cases, but certainly not over a lifetime. To alter this scope from a crisis management mode to a public health approach requires a shift in the actual conceptual framework of medicine. Such large paradigm shifts often take time and are slow to progress.

Therefore it should come as no surprise why the repeated calls (since the 1961 Congressional recommendations to focus on nutrition) have fallen on deaf years.[39] Prevention is not a priority in the medical profession.

The University of North Carolina at Chapel Hill must be commended for their pioneer efforts to change all this. They have embarked on an ambitious Nutrition in Medicine (NIM) Project (http://www.med.unc.edu/nutr/nim). Their aim is to offer a more systematic approach to the teaching of nutrition in U.S. medical schools.

The American Medical Student Association (AMSA, http://www.amsa.org) should also be commended for their efforts. They established the Nutrition Curriculum Project that created a framework for integrating nutrition in medical education (1996).[46] Several problem-based learning (PBL) methods are in vogue in medical schools in the United States and around the world. These can empower both students and patients to grasp real-life scenarios and tailor solutions to suit.[47-64]

Nutrition Education Elsewhere

British Nutrition Foundation (BNF) Report

A key player in setting global trends for medical education has been the United Kingdom. Indeed, it was in the United Kingdom where the doctors in colonial North America were trained. For historical reasons, British medical education serves as the model for in Canada, Australia, New Zealand, South Africa, and former British colonies in Asia, Africa, the Middle East, and the Caribbean. Most foreign medical graduates coming to America were educated under this system of education. The lack of nutrition education in the British medical system has had a multiplied effect on nutrition education elsewhere.

The status of nutrition education in UK medical schools was published in a landmark report by the British Nutrition Foundation (BNF) titled, "Nutrition in Medical Education: Report of the British Nutrition Task Force on Clinical Nutrition." It summarized the status of nutrition programs in undergraduate and postgraduate medical training. Their sentiments mirrored the verdict delivered on nutrition education in the United States:[65]

> It is apparent that nutrition is not at present accepted as a clinical research discipline within the teaching or district hospitals and does not generally play a major part in training in most hospitals and medical schools. Nevertheless, it is recognized that there are both organizational and financial constraints influencing the universities and health services and that, in fact, it would probably be undesirable to introduce another separate discipline into the medical curriculum.

Undergraduate and Postgraduate Nutrition Education (UK)

> Medical schools worldwide are based on North American and European models. Both are disease-oriented systems where doctors have very little interest in prevention.

During my tenure at the Nutrition Department at King's College, University of London, nutrition was headed by non-medical researchers. On the nutrition faculty was a single medical doctor, and he was not actively involved in day to day patient care. A few British medical students pursued elective programs in nutrition as part of an intercalated program; virtually no practicing British doctor did postgraduate degrees in nutrition. Such a degree was not even considered as a part of your "real" medical education. I know this from experience; my postgraduate degree in nutrition does not appear (it was not considered relevant) on my full registration certificate issued by the General Medical Council (GMC) of the United Kingdom. Very little collaboration exists between hospital-based doctors and researchers in the nutrition departments. This is a marriage that is long overdue.

Nutrition education in postgraduate medical training in the United Kingdom remains largely frozen in time. The London and Cambridge nutrition schools have outposts overseas in the Caribbean and Africa, but most of the research is about malnutrition. The BNF acknowledged this slant, even in the way nutrition was assessed in postgraduate medical examinations. In a sense, this is a reflection of prevailing medical attitudes towards nutrition in Britain—it is a problem that exists, but far, far away:[65]

> With the exception of the faculty of Community [Public Health] Medicine, it was apparent that questions on nutrition appeared rather infrequently in the examinations of all the Royal Colleges [UK postgraduate bodies] and in general, where questions on nutrition did appear, they did not seem to reflect current thinking in nutrition and often related only to problems arising from vitamin and mineral deficiencies.

The United Kingdom has excellent nutrition foundations and societies. The reputed *British Medical Journal* (BMJ; http://bmj.com) published the *ABC of Nutrition*, but this is a relatively short dossier by Professor Stewart Truswell of Australia and Professor Christopher Pennington of Scotland. I had the great privilege of working in the diabetes unit headed by Professor Sir KGMM Alberti, president of the Royal College of Physicians and the former dean of the medical school, University of Newcastle-upon-Tyne. To my knowledge, this was the first British university to pioneer a two-week undergraduate program in nutrition, thanks to Professor Alberti's efforts.

Conclusion and Recommendations

Many attempts have been made to yoke doctors to the nutrition bandwagon, but the wheels of change in medicine grind ever so slowly. There remains entrenched institutional resistance to changes that emphasize nutrition and prevention.

The *Nutrition Education in U.S. Medical Schools (1985)* report and the British Nutriton Foundation Report provide a good assessment of the past.[12,65] The American Dietetic Association (ADA) and other interest groups point to the future.[66,67] I recommend the essay "Nutrition Education in Medical Schools: trends and implications for health educators," by Jessica Schulman, MPH, RD of the University of Florida at Gainesville. She gave good advice that could pave the way for nutrition literacy among doctors. Good organization, a committed faculty, and better collaboration between medical disciplines, were prominent among her recommendations.[68] Any change in the status quo will depend on the willingness to commit money and resources to develop nutrition programs.[69-71]

I salute the great efforts by Professor Walter C. Willett and colleagues from the Department of Nutrition at the Harvard School of Public Health. They have done so much to bridge the considerable gap in nutrition education among doctors, and have propelled the nutrition to the center of the health debate.

The End Game

> If doctors continue to ignore the primacy of nutrition in the fight against the global epidemic of nutrition-related diseases, it could spell a dismal future for healthcare.

Major health and economic issues are at stake.[56-57] Many will continue to entrust the future of their health to the medical and political establishments, but changes take a long time in medicine, especially changes like nutrition education that will reduce patients' dependency on their doctors. My parting words to my patients who complain about the sorry state of healthcare is this: Doctors were trained to treat your illness, politicians promise to look after your healthcare, but *only you* can look after your health. Good nutrition is a crucial link to good health.

Summary

Nutrition plays a central role in the global epidemic of obesity and chronic diseases. Yet doctors around the globe receive poor training in nutrition at all levels of medical education. The medical profession, despite recent moves to include more nutrition subjects, remains largely stuck in a disease-treatment mode. The voices that champion a paradigm shift towards prevention are still being drowned out. External influences and entrenched attitudes will prevent any such shift any time soon.

Consumer groups have spearheaded a growing demand for prevention. Many have taken the initiative, and have taken more responsibility for their health. They now spend billions in this pursuit. This consumer-led demand has forced governments, industry, and the medical profession to pay attention their nutritional concerns. It behooves the serious student of nutrition to follow this lead towards nutrition education and empowerment.

******

Chapter 4

Complementary and Alternative Medicine (CAM)

Chapter Outline

The Gripe and the Hype about CAM 131
Of Egos and Attitudes 133
Why so many are turning to CAM 135
How popular is CAM? 138
Disquiet in the Mainstream Ranks 139
All those Names! 142
Definitions: CAM and Integrative Medicine...143
NIH Classification of CAM 146
    6.   Alternative Medical Systems: Chinese, Ayurveda, etc............. 146
    7.   Mind-Body Interventions: Hypnosis, Religious healing, etc.................. 148
    8.   Biological-Based Therapies: Herbal, Special Dietary, etc. 149
    9.   Manipulative and Body-Based Methods: Chiropractic etc............... 149
    10. Energy Therapies... 150
Doctors: Mixed Reviews about CAM...150
Doctors: Concerns about CAM...152
Responsibility and Regulation of CAM 154
Conclusion and Summary..155
Addendum: Personal Perspectives 157

Complementary and Alternative Medicine is the fastest growing area in healthcare today. A Harvard study estimated that twice as many consultations were with complementary medicine practitioners as with mainstream family doctors. Out-of-pocket expenditures for alternative medicine were 27 billion dollars compared to 29 billion dollars for all U.S. physician services. This figure increased to 38 billion for alternative care services in the year 2000.[1]

For profit healthcare is essentially an oxymoron. The moment care is rendered for-profit it is emptied of genuine caring…Healing is replaced by treating, caring is supplanted by managing, and the art of listening is taken over by technological procedures.[2]

Bernard Lown, M.D.,
Professor Cardiology Emeritus (Harvard), Lown Cardiovascular Center
Author: The *Lost Art of Healing—practicing compassion in medicine*

We know from research that people are drawn to complementary and alternative therapy mostly out of a desire for a more humanistic, "holistic" approach. Medical education should re-examine the emphasis it places on the importance of the integration of mind, body, and spirit and acknowledge the role of social, cultural, and environmental influences and the power of self-care and healing. Healthcare professionals, patients, and our healthcare system can only benefit if medical education bridges the gap with complementary and alternative therapy.[4]

Brian Berman, M.D. Professor of Family Medicine and Director
Complementary Medicine Program, University of Maryland School of Medicine

§§§§§§§

The Gripe and the Hype about CAM— Complementary and Alternative Medicine

An awakening is taking place in the healthcare arena. It is fueled by millions of consumers who are unhappy with the current system of healthcare. Many dissatisfied, disaffected, and desperate individuals have turned their backs on modern medical practice and now participate actively in alternative healthcare.

The longer I live, the more I realize that life is essentially about relationships. As human beings, there exists an inborn desire to be loved and respected—to be cared for and appreciated. Whether the relationship is horizontal or vertical, casual or professional, the same desire essentially applies.

Under the present system of managed care in the United States, there is growing resentment because consumers have very little control over many aspects of their healthcare, while "corporate medicine" dictates how care is delivered.[5] Many of the dissatisfied, and sometimes desperate patients, are turning their backs on the style of modern medical practice that increasingly regards patients as cases or numbers. This has led millions to seek alternatives.

The medical profession itself, has been at odds with the current approach to healthcare. Doctors resent being categorized as "providers" by health maintenance organizations (HMOs).[6] Many see the use of this word as deliberate ploy by the insurance industry to undermine the doctor-patient relationship. This minimizes the physician's role in healthcare and lessens their control over medical decision-making. Indeed, managed care organizations could be more aptly referred to as "managed cost" organizations.

Despite the distaste for HMOs by doctors, this bitter pill is a direct result of the unbridled escalation in healthcare costs. These arose primarily due to over reliance on curative medicine at the expense of prevention. Doctors in America now find themselves caught in the middle and express their increasing dissatisfaction with the current regime which, incidentally, is a by-product of their own making.[5] Insurance companies and their policies of reimbursement now largely dictate the way medicine is practiced in America.[7]

As people weigh their options for healthcare, many have resorted to alternatives that have become increasingly popular. How much of this is hype or a passing fad is yet to be seen, but what is clear is that many are dissatisfied. Fundamental questions need to be asked about what constitutes good medical practice. Is the modern healthcare system in America, considered by some to be the best in the world, the standard by which others be judged? Is good medicine merely a matter of making use of the best technology and the best therapies that money can buy? Is it just about healing bodies? Are our maladies merely biochemical and physical disorders for which drugs or surgery alone are sufficient? Does one size fits all?

The answers to these questions may delve into the fundamental concepts about human life and existence. It goes to the core of our definitions of human health and well-being. Human health and healing involves more than pharmaceutical and technological fixes. People are influenced by variables that go far beyond what is measured in a doctor's office or a science laboratory. Human dynamics involve people, it involves culture … it involves belief systems. Even the World Health Organization (WHO) acknowledges that health as "a state of physical, mental, and emotional well-being and not simply the absence of disease or infirmity."[8]

Of Egos and Attitudes

If it isn't happening in medical circles, it isn't happening!

Many doctors are content to propagate disparaging second-hand opinions about alternative therapies without paying serious attention to why many patients opt for, and subscribe to complementary and alternative therapies.

Historically, the medical profession has enjoyed almost demigod status in most societies. Doctors have, for a long time, been spared interference in the way they practice their profession. They do not like non-medics intruding in the way they practice their art. Therefore it came as no surprise when the medical profession deeply resented being relegated to the category of "providers." The American Medical Association (AMA) requested that the word "physician" rather than "vendor" or "provider" be used and vowed zero tolerance towards any further attempts to debase the medical profession.

I empathize with my colleagues in this matter. Most doctors have made great personal sacrifices in their academic and professional pursuits, and it is understandable that AMA would do what it takes to guide how medicine is practiced. Traditionally, the medical profession has been held in high regard, and with good reason. People confronted with the fear and vulnerability that accompanies illness express great appreciation to all who participate in their healing, especially towards their doctors. Wonderful strides have been made in medical care and all caregivers are deserving of accolades.

There is another side to healing that is known to all experienced physicians. Doctors sometimes joke that patients recover despite their doctors. Books can be written on this subject, but it is clear that healing is more than a matter of drugs and surgery. We should be humble enough to acknowledge that we may be agents of healing, but not really the healers. There is a big difference. Our bodies were designed with an innate ability to heal itself, especially if exposed to a conducive environment—good facilities, a concerned and caring staff, and proper attention to medical protocols.

Elderly people are good at providing a much needed perspective on this. Many grew up in times when they had to fend for themselves. They were far less spoiled than the generations of today. A *Newsweek* article titled "How to live to 100" quoted a centenarian, Angeline Strandal, who did not place much confidence in doctors. "If they start poking around you," she was reported as saying, "they'll only make you sick."[9] There is not much anyone could say to dispute a centenarian, but she certainly had a clear understanding that health takes more than a medical prescription.

The respect and trust traditionally given to the medical profession is being challenged. A Harvard study has shown that Americans have been moving away from mainstream medicine in droves and now actively pursue alternate approaches to healthcare.[1] When television personality Suzanne Somers went public with her decision to forego conventional medical treatment for breast cancer, and opted instead for alternative treatments, this drew a lot fire from the medical establishment. Respected medical organizations accused her of being irresponsible and sending the wrong message to the public.[10]

The medical profession has, up until recently, largely dismissed alternative health practices. Doctors were never taught these practices during medical training. With our overcrowded medical schedules, we had a hard enough time keeping up with our own information overload, much less learning about unorthodox practices. Doctors have largely condemned, or at best evoked skepticism at all strange and unfamiliar therapies. This reflects an entrenched bias against everything not taught in medical schools.

Disparaging opinions against CAM also reflects a lack of exposure. Doctors can be so caught up in their own little worlds that they ignore the realities of what is happening on the outside. I spent the last eighteen years of my academic life studying, working, and interacting with various peoples and cultures in several countries. This has been an extremely educational and enriching experience—a true eye opener. Traveling broadens your scope and can give you a better appreciation for other people and their worldviews. It has been a teacher without parallel. Mature individuals know the value of the saying, "Never criticize a man until you have walked in his shoes." I have often speculated on the reasons why almost half the world's population are Chinese and Indians, and how they thrived and survived quite well without Western medicine. They have for millennia pioneered their own forms of traditional Chinese and Indian Ayurvedic practices. We should be more humble, rather than dismissive, about practices we do not fully comprehend. Dr. Mike McClure summed up the attitudes of the mainstream medical community towards such CAM practices:[11]

> Part of it is a gut reaction that it's not scientific, that there's not enough hard data to prove its effectiveness... Here again, we are venturing outside the paradigm of the traditional medical community, and so there's a tendency to downplay any method of medical treatment that doesn't fit the accepted model.

Such misunderstandings also extend into other areas of CAM practice. Take the example of cultural and belief systems. Faith and prayer are impossible to accurately quantify, but they play important roles in the lives of most people. This extends into what people believe about health and healing; they provide comfort and hope for many in times of sickness. Doctors need to avoid ignoring or dismissing the important roles that complementary adjuncts play in the healing process. Everything important for people's health cannot be written on a prescription or treated in a hospital.

Why So Many Are Turning to CAM

…According to some doctors, technology has become a sufficient substitute for talking with a patient. The decline in respect for doctors is accelerated by the extraordinary hubris instilled in medical students. They are taught a reductionist model in which human beings are presented as complex biochemical factories. … current medical practice focuses on the acute and the emergent and is largely indifferent to preventing disease and promoting health.

Bernard Lown, M.D.
Professor Cardiology Emeritus (Harvard),
Lown Cardiovascular Center / Brigham and Women's Hospital
Author: *The Lost Art of Healing—practicing compassion in medicine* [2]

Most CAM users in the United States are the baby boomer generation between the ages of 30 to 50. They represent a well-educated section of American society that has tremendous purchasing power. About half the population of most industrialized countries regularly uses complementary medicine. Although higher education, higher income, and poor health are predictors of CAM use, many who engage in CAM are not just interested in treating disease. Many are keen to preserve their health and optimize their quality of life.[13]

The majority of CAM users pay out-of-pocket for services without any expectation of re-imbursement.[13] Despite this constraint, the number of CAM users continues to increase. Many doctors remain unaware of this trend, particularly those who express hostility towards CAM and believe that only the gullible and the ignorant are adherents of such practices. Surveys have indicated that doctors who harbor such attitudes are less likely to be told by patients about their CAM exploits.[14]

CAM users are not doltish. There is no question about where people should go following a motor vehicle accident, severe burns, a gun-shot wound, a bleeding ulcer, or a heart attack. The great skill of emergency room doctors and surgeons are not on trial. What disenchants many are primarily those chronic medical conditions that just will not go away—chronic pain, headaches, and those lifestyle related diseases that are the primary focus of this book.

There are many converts to CAM for those medical conditions that modern medicine fails to resolve, especially if these leave people dependent on pills for life.

> Most people, if given the option, would prefer therapies that empower them and prevent them from remaining trapped in the disease-mode, or being heavily dependent on hospital-based therapies.

Doctors have been taught in medical and postgraduate school that "once diabetic, always a diabetic." This same view is generally held about high blood pressure and coronary heart disease. Abundant evidence exists that these diseases can be controlled, and sometimes reversed, by changes in lifestyle. Most people, if given the option, would prefer therapies that empower them and prevent them from remaining trapped in the "disease-mode" or in physician-dependent, hospital-based therapies.

Most people resent being labeled, especially with a diagnosis of an incurable condition. This is a natural defense mechanism and is a primary reason why many patients remain in denial following diagnosis with a chronic disease. This is no small matter. This in no way suggest that doctors should deny the truth; a person diagnosed with diabetes needs to be told so. However, it is also important that people understand that the old dogmas of being "diabetic for life" do not necessarily hold true. The evidence is to the contrary—that diabetes and the metabolic syndrome are preventable and reversible conditions, providing patients are provided with the right tools.

> Resorting to diabetes medications and excellent diabetes care, as good as that may seem, does very little to get to the root causes of type II diabetes.
> A patient with diabetes must be taught to manage their diabetes using the best standards of practice.
> However, patients would be severely short-changed if doctors neglect to tell them *how to look after their health.*
> This is not a trivial matter. ... There is a powerful distinction between the two.

The diagnosis of type II diabetes should primarily be a wake-up call for lifestyle change rather than a rush to treat with diabetes drugs. A recently concluded diabetes prevention study confirms the superiority of lifestyle changes over pharmaceutical drug therapy for the pre-diabetic condition.[15]

> The short time available for medical consultations robs patients of a crucial ingredient necessary for better outcomes—their doctor's time. When the doctor-patient relationship suffers, health and healing becomes short-changed.

In an article "CAM: Complex Reasons for Popularity" appearing in the *British Medical Journal*, Dr. Edzart Ernst, chair of the Department of Complementary Medicine, University of Exeter, UK, tabled several reasons for the increasing popularity of CAM in the United Kingdom (Figure 4-1).[16] He stated that the reasons people seek CAM therapies "... are complex; they change with time and space, they may vary from therapy to therapy, and they are different from one individual to another. For example, a patient with AIDS will have different motives from someone who is 'worried well'." Regardless of the individual reasons, it is evident that they amount to a serious deficiency within our modern healthcare system.

Motivations for resorting to CAM

Positive motivations

Apparent effectiveness and safety
Holistic approach
More natural
More patient centered
More control over treatment
"High touch, low tech"
Good patient/therapist relationship
Sufficient time
Non-invasive nature—less emphasis on drugs and surgery
Pleasant therapeutic experience

Negative motivations

Dissatisfaction with mainstream healthcare:
Ineffective for certain conditions
Fear of serious adverse effects
Poor doctor-patient relationship
Insufficient time with doctor
Anti-science and technology
Anti-establishment
Desperation

(modified from E. Ernst, University of Exeter, UK. http://bmj.com/cgi/content/full/321/7269/1133)

Figure 4-1. Reasons for choosing CAM practices.[16]

Conventional medical practitioners should take such motivations to heart. According to Rees and Weil, UK-based researchers, most patients turn to complementary medicine out of frustration. Therapies like dietary supplements are not taken because of illness, but primarily as a kind of insurance for health. Other patients' concerns, such as too little time spent with the doctor during consultations, are causes for dissatisfaction with the current system of care. Patients are more satisfied when they can spend more time with their doctor.

How popular is CAM?

By 1998, about 42 percent of people in the United States reported using CAM therapies. This translates into an excess of 20 billion dollars in annual expenditures.[1]

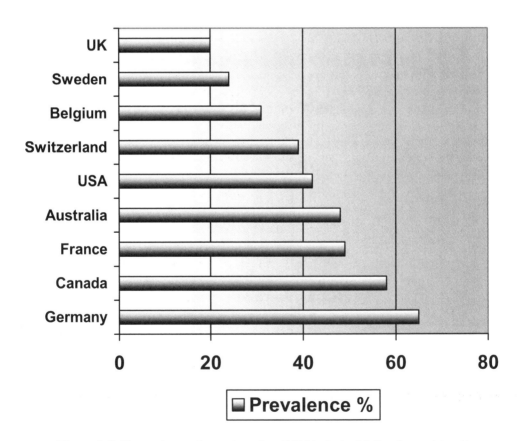

Figure 4-2. Percentage of people using CAM in industrialized countries.[16]

(Data from E. Ernst, University of Exeter, UK. http://bmj.com/cgi/content/full/321/7269/1133)

CAM is now the fastest growing area of the U.S. healthcare industry. David Eisenberg's article, "Trends in Alternative Medicine Use in the United States 1990-1997,"[1] documented CAM's growing popularity. He and his Harvard colleagues conducted random household telephone surveys of 1,539 adults in 1991 and 2,055 adults in 1997, and assessed the prevalence, costs, and patients' disclosure of CAM use to their doctors. These CAM practices included herbal medicine, massage therapies, megavitamins, self-help groups, folk remedies, energy healing, homeopathy, chiropractic, and acupuncture. Here is a summary of their findings:

- 46% of survey respondents (1997) said they had visited an alternative medicine practitioner, compared to 36% in 1991.
- 42% reported at least one alternative therapy, compared to 34% in 1990.
- Over 600 million visits to CAM practitioners were made in 1997, compared to less than 400 million visits to primary care doctors.
- CAM use was most popular with persons between the ages of 30 to 50.

CAM users paid out-of-pocket for these services totaling 27 billion dollars in 1997 compared to 29 billion dollars for all U.S. physician services over the same time period. Herbal medicines experienced an astronomical increase in popularity between 1991 and 1997 in the United States. It grew by almost 400 percent. Vitamin supplements purchases grew by 130 percent.[1]

Within the industrialized world, Germany heads the pack. Almost 70 percent of German adults surveyed engaged in some form of CAM therapy. CAM also enjoys great popularity in Canada, France, and Australia (Figure 4-2). In the British Isles, there is less enthusiasm for CAM therapies. Nevertheless, its popularity throughout the industrialized world has been astounding. People who have more disposable income are the chief consumers of CAM services in the West.[17-19]

Data for much of the developing world is not readily available, but alternative medicine in the industrialized West actually reflects traditional forms of medicine in many countries. The resurgence in interest by Westerners to many traditional forms of medicines has led to a new appreciation (by the natives) for their heritage. For many, this is the only medicine they have known, and it may be the only type of medicine they may ever know.

Disquiet in the Mainstream Ranks: What Some Doctors Are Saying

Organized medicine has surrendered to an overbuilt and overused political-industrial complex that underfunds

> prevention, undermines scientific research, and overlooks patients' needs—with disastrous results for doctors and patients alike.
>
> George Lundberg
> Former editor (JAMA) and author: *Severed Trust: Why American Medicine Hasn't Been Fixed*

The criticisms levelled against mainstream medical practice are not just coming from fringe groups. There are prominent voices that are unhappy with the current trend in medical practice. Prominent among them is the former editor of the *Journal of the American Medical Association*, for seventeen years, Dr. George Lundberg. His book titled: *Severed Trust: Why American Medicine Hasn't Been Fixed* (2001), blasted aspects of the modern medical practice. One reviewer summed it up this way:[20]

> … organized medicine has surrendered to an overbuilt and overused political-industrial complex that underfunds prevention, undermines scientific research, and overlooks patients' needs—with disastrous results for doctors and patients alike. High costs and managed care are the least of our problems, … the greatest threat is the pervasive erosion of professional standards.

Bernard Lown, M.D., professor of cardiology (Harvard) and pioneer in the use of DC (direct current) for cardiac arrest and cardioversion, Nobel Peace Prize laureate (1985), and a host of other accomplishments, has delivered a timely message for today's cadre of doctors. In his book, *The Lost Art of Healing—practicing compassion in medicine*,[2] he counseled that "the art of healing does not mean abandoning the spectacular advances of modern science, but rather incorporating them into a sensitive, humane, and enlightened approach to medical care." This book is a must read. Many in the mainstream have increasingly incorporated CAM therapies into their practice. Dean Ornish M.D., and Andrew Weil M.D., both Harvard-trained physicians, are advocates of a new vision of healthcare. Dr. Ornish advocates changes in diet and lifestyle as a scientifically proven alternative for arresting and reversing heart disease. Aspects of his program appear in his book, *How to Reverse Heart Disease without Drugs or Surgery*.

Andrew Weil M.D., professor of Integrative Medicine at the University of Arizona in Tucson, has authored a number of national bestsellers. In the chapter, "Prescriptions for Society" of his book *Spontaneous Healing*, he offered this vision of healthcare:[7]

> Imagine a future world in which medicine was oriented toward healing rather than disease, where doctors believed in the natural healing capacity of human beings and emphasized prevention above treatment. Except for urgent care facilities, hospitals in such a world might more resemble spas, where patients could learn the practice and principles of healthy living, where they would learn to eat and prepare healthy food, learn to take care

of the physical needs of their bodies, learn to use their minds in the service of healing, and become less rather than more dependent on health professionals ... In such a world doctors and patients would be partners working toward the same ends, with malpractice litigation a rare event rather than a commonplace.

In a *British Medical Journal* editorial on "Integrated Medicine," Andrew Weil, M.D., director or the Program in Integrative Medicine, University of Arizona and Lesley Rees, director of education at the Royal College of Physicians, London, issued a joint statement on the case for CAM: [21]

> Conventional medicine has become dependent on expensive technological solutions to health problems, even when they are not particularly effective. In its enthusiasm for technology, it has turned its back on holism and simple methods of intervention, such as dietary adjustment and relaxation training, which are prominent in many alternative systems of medicine and are often effective.

Professor Nick Read and Dr. Jack Czauderna of the United Kingdom addressed their desire to offer patients more than what is provided by the current healthcare system. They challenged the current trend where patients are increasingly objectified as "ill stomachs, sick lungs, or damaged kidneys." [22] Many patients often complain that doctors do not listen to them, but this is not surprising. The current system of medical care is increasingly caught up in its own pursuits, to the detriment of arguably the most important relationship in healthcare—the doctor-patient relationship. If you don't spend sufficient time, it is hard to build meaningful relationships. It is quite easy for a patient to know the difference between a doctor who cares, compared to a doctor who is simply doing a job. It does make a difference.

Many doctors who are cognizant of these deficiencies in modern healthcare, have resolved that they will not compromise their standards and simply to follow the dictates of those institutions that now govern the practice of medicine:[22]

> Therapists using complementary and alternative treatments do what doctors have so little time to do. They try to understand the sick person, and they use techniques that relax the emotional tension that often keeps the illness going. We all know from experience in childhood that getting better is not just a matter of taking the medicine: it requires time, rest, compassion, understanding, and care.

Professor Stephen Wright of Lancaster, England lamented what he referred to as the descent into "soulless medicine." Citing the Hippocratic maxim that "some people recover simply because of their satisfaction with the goodness of their doctor," he pointed to evidence that the quality of the doctor-patient relationship plays an important role in reducing patients' "stress of disease." [23]

Fortunately, such voices are no longer crying in the wilderness, CAM practices are now being taken seriously by the National Institutes of Health (NIH). The NIH is now firmly entrenched in partnerships with prominent mainstream academic medical institutions. Participating institutions include Columbia University, Duke University, John Hopkins University, Harvard University, the University of Maryland, Stanford University, and Memorial Sloan-Kettering Cancer Centre, and the University of North Carolina at Chapel Hill. In response to consumer interest, the U.S. Congress created the National Center for Complementary and Alternative Medicine (NCCAM) at the NIH, with the mission to explore, educate and train CAM researchers. Their additional plan was to identify and disseminate information on CAM that are safe and effective.[24]

All Those Names!

CAM practices range from beneficial and scientifically-sound therapies (e.g. behavior therapy, nutrition, and patient education), to those that are ridiculous, outlandish, and downright dangerous.

One of the challenges faced by a pluralistic democratic society is the freedom of expression. This generates many voices that peddle their ideas, regardless of how strange these may seem. The practices that are identified as alternative medical practices are legion! Those therapies with promise and reason have stood the test of time. Fly-by-night therapies often vanish as quickly as they appear. Nutrition and acupuncture are CAM therapies that have been, to varying degrees, incorporated into mainstream medical practice. Others, like chelation therapy, are now being investigated by the NCCAM.[25]

This chapter introduces CAM practices, but they will not be discussed here in any individual detail. The names are legion. Included among them are acupuncture, aromatherapy, Ayurvedic and Chinese medicine, biofeedback training, bodywork and somatic therapies, chelation therapy, chiropractic, colonic cleansing, detoxification therapies, energy medicine, expressive art therapies, fasting, flower therapies, guided imagery, herbal medicine, homeopathy, integrative dentistry, meditation, mind/body medicine, naturopathic medicine, nutritional medicine, osteopathy, Qi gong and taiji, sound healing and music therapy, yoga, and believe it or not … this list is far from complete!

There may be some confusion as modern medical practice is referred to variously as Western mainstream medicine, conventional, allopathic, orthodox, scientific, or the politically dominant medical establishment. You may see the term "traditional" used for either alternative or conventional medicine, depending on the point of view. Asians refer to their own practices as "traditional," which Westerners refer to as "alternative."

In the United States, conventional medical practice includes allopaths and osteopaths. This is medicine as practiced by holders of either M.D. (doctor of allopathic medicine) or D.O. (doctor of osteopathy) degrees, some of whom also practice complementary and alternative medicine. Osteopaths in America are, for all intents and purpose, indistinguishable from M.D.'s in their practice of medicine. Osteopaths enjoy the same rights and privileges as allopathic physicians and are fully licensed to perform surgery and prescribe medicine in all fifty states. Historically, osteopaths were trained with an additional skill to treat patients with osteopathic manipulative medicine (OMM) , but today this is true of only a small minority of practicing osteopaths.

Definitions: CAM and Integrative Medicine

Complementary and Alternative Medicine

...includes all "those treatments and healthcare practices not taught widely in medical schools, not generally used in hospitals, and not usually reimbursed by medical insurance companies."

National Center for Complementary and Alternative Medicine (NCCAM)[21]
National Institutes if Health (NIH)

Integrative Medicine

...integrated medicine is not just about teaching doctors to use herbs instead of drugs. It is about restoring core values which have been eroded by social and economic forces. Integrated medicine is good medicine, and its success will be signaled by dropping the adjective. The integrated medicine of today should be the medicine of the new millennium.

Andrew Weil, M.D.; Lesley Rees[21]

Complementary and Alternative Medicine

The Cochrane Collaboration group based at Cambridge University, England defines CAM as follows: [26]

A broad domain of healing resources that encompasses all health systems, modalities and practices and their accompanying theories and beliefs, other than those intrinsic to the [politically dominant health] system of a particular society or culture of a [given historical period.] CAM includes all such practices and ideas self-defined by their users as preventing or treating illness or promoting health and well being. Boundaries within CAM and between CAM and that of the dominant system are not always sharp or fixed.

Reference to the politically dominant health system is an important addition to this definition because, in many foreign countries, alternative medicine is not "alternative" at all. Here, these therapies are the norm. They constitute the traditional medical practice in these healthcare systems. In the Western world, alternative medicine is medicine that is not taught in medical schools. Therefore Western doctors remain largely unfamiliar with such practices. Even respected forms of CAM such as nutritional therapies are considered alternative by the average U.S.-trained doctor. This is because, in most doctors' frames of reference, these therapies are not a part of their training.

Yesterday's cures may be tomorrow's quackery. Therefore, placing the definition of CAM within its historical context is important. This definition must take into account what is the acceptable medical practice of the day. You may be aghast at what doctors of yesteryear gave patients for peptic ulcer disease and gastritis. Cannabis (weed), mercury, carbolic acid, arsenic, massage, and electricity were the established medicines for these stomach maladies just 100 years ago (Merck 1899 Manual)![27] And this was not in some far away place; this was the established treatment in 19th century America! Today's doctors would be absolutely horrified at just the thought of such therapies for stomach ailments, but this was standard medical practice in those days.

The NCCAM defines CAM as those disciplines that include a broad range of healing philosophies, approaches, and therapies that are not a part of mainstream medical practice: [24]

> ... healthcare and medical practices that are not currently an integral part of conventional medicine. The list of practices that are considered CAM changes continually as CAM practices and therapies that are proven safe and effective become accepted as "mainstream" healthcare practices.

Many CAM therapies are referred to as holistic. These therapies endeavor to address the totally individual's mental, emotional, and spiritual concerns in addition to their physical or medical condition. Preventive CAM therapies focus on education and health optimization. CAM therapies may be used alone (alternative), in combination with other alternative therapies, or in addition to conventional therapies (complementary).

Zollmann and Vickers in their book, *ABC of Complementary Medicine* indicated that even though CAM practices are grouped together as healthcare outside of the mainstream, much uncertainty over its definition remains: [26]

> Complementary medicine is an increasing feature of healthcare practice, but considerable confusion remains about what exactly it is and what position the disciplines included under this term should hold in relation to conventional medicine.

Integrative Medicine

There is another proposition that is gaining wider acceptance in the medical community on both sides of the Atlantic. It has been called Integrative (U.S.) or Integrated (U.K.) medicine. This approach to medicine makes sense. Indeed it is not a new phenomenon. It aims to combine the best of what medical science has to offer with the best of what care should be all about—the health of the whole person. In his book the *Lost Art of Healing*, Bernard Lown, Professor Emeritus at Harvard made this confession:[28]

> In my own practice as a highly specialized cardiologist, the problems of more than half my patients do not relate to their heart conditions but to the stresses of living. I have learned that few patients search for alternative therapies when physicians focus on healing as well as using the powerful scientific tools at their disposal … Sometimes a doctor may have to resort to unconventional techniques in order to improve a patient's well-being. These are not taught in medical school but are discovered through clinical experience and sanctioned by common sense.

A related agenda has been gaining adherents in the practice of medicine in the United States and Europe. At a recent conference held in London under the auspices of the Royal College of Physicians of the UK and the U.S. National Center for Complementary and Alternative Medicine, a concerted attempt was made to raise the profile of integrated or integrative medicine. Advocates of integrative medicine define it as follows: [21]

> … practicing medicine in a way that selectively incorporates elements of complementary and alternative medicine into comprehensive treatment plans alongside solidly orthodox methods of diagnosis and treatment. Integrated medicine is not simply a synonym for complementary medicine. Complementary medicine refers to treatments that may be used as adjuncts to conventional treatment and are not usually taught in medical schools.
> … Integrated medicine has a larger meaning and mission, its focus being on health and healing rather than disease and treatment. It views patients as whole people with minds and spirits as well as bodies and includes these dimensions into diagnosis and treatment. It also involves patients and doctors working to maintain health by paying attention to lifestyle factors

such as diet, exercise, quality of rest and sleep, and the nature of relationships.

It is helpful to realize that integrative medicine does not aim to replace conventional medical practice, nor is its intention one of simply adding or combining CAM to conventional practice: [21]

> … integrated medicine is not just about teaching doctors to use herbs instead of drugs. It is about restoring core values which have been eroded by social and economic forces. Integrated medicine is good medicine, and its success will be signaled by dropping the adjective. The integrated medicine of today should be the medicine of the new millennium.

Proponents of integrative medicine stress that their aim is not simply a matter of adding a few CAM courses to current medical education program. This will not change the focus of medical education from a fix-it mode to a prevention mode. A sincere quest to care for patients goes far beyond the customary physical examination and treatment of disease. The best medicine and the best care is what good medicine should be all about. This demands a major shift in focus that expands the horizon of medical practice beyond the mere treatment of disease.[29]

NIH Classification of CAM

The National Institute of Health has attempted to group the multitude of CAM practices under five major groups or domains (Table 4-1).[30] The practices listed as CAM are frequently updated and therapies that are proven safe and effective become accepted into mainstream healthcare. Currently included in the list of CAM practices are: (1) alternative medical systems, (2) mind-body interventions, (3) biologically-based treatments, (4) manipulative and body-based methods, and (5) energy therapies. This categorization is simply an attempt to classify the myriad of alternative medical practices, and should not be taken as an exhaustive list.

I. Alternative Medical Systems

Alternative medical systems include many traditional medical practices: Chinese, Indian, and those of other indigenous cultures. Migration, travel, and globalization have made such practices increasingly popular in North America and Europe.[31-35]

Table 4-1. Complementary and Alternative Medicine (NIH classification)

CAM Therapies (NIH classification)	Subcategories of CAM Therapies
Alternative Medical Systems	Traditional Oriental medicine, Qi gong, Acupuncture, Herbal medicine, Massage Ayurvedic medicine; Native American, Aboriginal, Middle-Eastern, Tibetan, Curanderismo (Latin America), Homeopathic medicine, Naturopathic medicine
Mind-Body Interventions	Patient education, Cognitive-behavior therapies, Meditation, Hypnosis, Prayer, Faith and mental healing
Biologically-Based Treatments	Herbal therapies, Special diet therapies: (Atkins, Ornish, Jenny Craig, Weight-Watchers, The Zone, Schwarzbein, Low-Carb, Sugar busters, Suzanne Somers, Pritikin) Orthomolecular therapies: (multivitamins, mega-dosing, shark cartilage, melatonin), EDTA chelation therapy
Manipulative and Body-Based Methods	Chiropractic therapy Osteopathic manipulation, and Massage Therapies (Oriental, Shiatsu)
Energy Therapies	Qi gong (Chinese) Reiki (Japanese), therapeutic touch Bio-electromagnetics

Traditional Oriental medicine emphasizes the proper balance or disturbance of Qi (vital energy) in health and disease. Chinese medicinal practices include acupuncture, herbal medicine, oriental massage, and Qi gong (a form of energy therapy). Acupuncture involves stimulating specific anatomic points in the body by puncturing the skin with a needle. It has won many converts in Western medical institutions. Ayurveda is India's traditional system of medicine. Ayurvedic medicine (meaning "science of life") places equal emphasis on the body, the mind, and the spirit, and strives to restore what it calls the inborn harmony of the individual. Ayurvedic treatments include diet, exercise, meditation, herbs, massage, and yoga. Chinese and Indian practices dominate this group, but other traditional medical systems have developed by Native American, Aboriginal, African, Middle-Eastern, Tibetan, and Central and South American (Curanderismo) cultures. They have their own devotees, especially among immigrant communities.

Homeopathic and naturopathic medicines are additional examples of complete alternative medical systems. Homeopathic medicine is an unconventional Western system that is based on the principle that "like cures like". The same substance that in large doses produces the symptoms of an illness can, in very minute doses, effect its cure. In one sense it is comparable to the principles underlying vaccinations or immunization. Giving a small dose of a disease-causing agent can prevent the subsequent development of the real disease. Homeopaths use small doses of specially prepared plant extracts and minerals to stimulate the body's defense mechanisms and healing processes in order to treat many illnesses.

Naturopathic medicine views diseases as the failure of the body's natural healing processes. Restoring health, rather than treating disease is the primary emphasis. Naturopathic physicians use a wide assortment of healing practices that include diet, clinical nutrition, homeopathy, acupuncture, herbal medicine, hydrotherapy (the use of water in a range of temperatures and methods of applications), physical therapies involving electric currents, ultrasound, light therapy, counseling, spinal, and soft-tissue manipulation.

II. Mind-Body Interventions

Mind-body interventions like patient education, cognitive, and behavior therapies have become well-established in mainstream medical practice. Others like meditation, hypnosis, prayer, and faith healing remain categorized as alternative practices.[36-40]

Mind-body interventions employ a variety of techniques. They underscore the mind's ability to influence bodily function and symptoms. They tap into the understanding that the mind is the battleground between health and illness, between victory and defeat. There have been a number of investigations that indicate the benefit from such therapies. But because of the very nature of the mind, the effectiveness of these therapies is often a highly subjective matter and therefore, very difficult to precisely quantify.

III. Biological-based Therapies

This is the most popular category of CAM practice in the Western world. It includes dietary supplements, herbal therapies, popular diets, and orthomolecular therapies.[41-48]

Herbal therapies champion the use of herbs in place of pharmaceutical drugs. Special diet therapies include diets made popular by Dean Ornish, M.D., the late Dr. Robert Atkins, and the Hawaii Diet. They focus on nutrition to prevent and manage diseases as well as to optimize health. The word "orthomolecular" was made popular by the late Professor Linus Pauling, two-time Nobel laureate, who championed the use of vitamin C. Orthomolecular therapies primarily advocate the use of chemicals normally found in the body, like magnesium, melatonin, and mega-doses of vitamins.

Also included is the employ of conventional drugs for non-conventional uses. EDTA (ethylenediaminetetraacetic acid) chelation is a standard medical treatment to remove excess lead and heavy metals from the blood. EDTA chelation therapy as a CAM adjunct for treating coronary artery disease is currently being evaluated by the NCCAM. Recent surveys indicate that more than seventy million Americans use herbal medicines, the fastest-growing segment of CAM services. Sales of herbal medicines increased by almost seventy percent in 1997, including a ten-fold increase in sales of St. John's wort, a popular herb used for mild depression.[49]

IV. Manipulative and Body-based Methods

These methods employ manual techniques that use pressure and movement of the musculo-skeletal system, as well as various schools of massage therapy. They have proven particularly useful in the management of a variety of chronic pain syndromes.[50-55]

Chiropractors have traditionally focused on the relationship between structure (primarily the spine) and function, and how this relationship affects the preservation and restoration of health. Such practitioners use manipulative therapy as an integral treatment tool. Many of today's chiropractors have adopted a combination of mainstream and alternative medical practices. This form of medicine has become useful for chronic pain and chronic headaches.

Many osteopaths place emphasis on the musculoskeletal system. Osteopathy teaches that all of the body's systems work together and that disturbances in one system may have an impact upon function elsewhere in the body. They are not to be confused with Osteopathic physicians (D.O.'s) who are indistinguishable in training and practice from M.D.'s. Today's osteopathic physicians have all but abandoned the practice of osteopathic manipulation.

Massage therapy and soft tissue manipulation have become increasingly popular. Practitioners are represented by a variety of schools in America ranging from Asian, Indian, European, and Near East techniques.

V. Energy Therapies

> These forms of CAM use energy fields that originate within the body (biofields), as well as those from external sources (electromagnetic fields).[55-60]

Qi gong is a Chinese therapy that combines movement, meditation, and regulation of breathing to enhance the flow of vital energy (Qi) in the body. This is said to improve blood circulation, and enhance immune function. Reiki, the Japanese word representing universal life energy, is based on the belief that by channeling spiritual energy through the practitioner, the spirit is healed and this in turn heals the physical body.

Therapeutic touch is derived from the practice of "laying on of hands". It is based on the premise that the healing force of the therapist can impart healing to the recipient. This should be distinguished from the belief in many parts of Christendom that subscribes to divine healing through the medium of the laying on of hands.

Bioelectromagnetic-based therapies use magnetic fields and electrical currents to treat asthma, cancers, chronic pain, and headaches. They sometimes use gadgets and techniques that some may find quite scary, but I guess the same could be said about placing a patient under a gamma-knife to zap brain tumors or into the belly of an MRI (magnetic resonance imaging) machine—both highly sophisticated technologies employed in modern medical practice.

Doctors: Mixed Reviews about CAM

> Despite vigorous debates by both supporters and opponents, there is an overall shift towards integration and accommodation of CAM by mainstream medical practice.

Consumer interest and expenditure in this fastest-growing area in healthcare has forced the medical profession, which has nurtured great historical prejudices against CAM, to adopt such a stand.

There is a growing list of advocates who seek rapprochement between the contrasting views of CAM. Medical purists condemn any move to cater to CAM as nothing but a sell-out of true scientific pursuits by adopting unproven therapies. Brilliant minds, as exemplified by Bernard Lown, M.D., put CAM use in perspective. He describes "another dimension in medicine beyond the uncertain, one that derives from its scientific infrastructure." In his book, the *Lost Art of Healing,* he expounded an honest personal perspective on the subject:[61]

> At present, about 25 percent of patients who visit an American doctor are successfully treated. The other 75 percent have problems that scientific medicine finds difficult to resolve. After being shuffled among a bevy of specialists and subjected to costly and invasive technologies, many patients, frustrated, turn away from conventional medicine … n my own practice as a highly specialized cardiologist, the problems of more than half of my patients do not relate to their heart conditions but to the stresses of living. I have learned that few patients search for alternative therapies when physicians focus on healing as well as using the powerful scientific tools at their disposal. Healing and improving a patient's well-being frequently require imagination in devising approaches that assuage discomfort or relieve a complaint. Sometimes a doctor may have to resort to unconventional techniques in order to improve a patient's well-being. These are not taught in medical school but are discovered through clinical experience and sanctioned by commonsense.

Nevertheless, CAM continues to be vilified by many doctors as superstition practiced by quacks and charlatans. The recent moves to merge, complement or integrate CAM with conventional medical practice have been regarded by the purists as downright betrayal. Dr. Roger Fisken, consultant physician in England, expressed such view:[62]

> If we join forces with alternative medicine we are not only betraying our scientific heritage but we are also a short step away from betraying our patients. It has taken hundreds of years to pull medicine away from the quagmire of superstition, witchcraft, mumbo-jumbo, and sheer quackery and turn it into something resembling a scientific pursuit...There is no necessary opposition between scientific medicine and humane, holistic, clinical practice, and the best clinicians throughout history have been skilled at combining both elements. To suggest that one cannot be a good scientist and a caring, compassionate doctor is nonsense.

CAM practitioners, on the other hand, are equally wary and suspicious of the new attempts to accommodate or integrate CAM with conventional medical practice. David St. George, director of the Center for Integrative Sciences in Complementary and

Alternative Therapies (CISCAT) in London, sees this new interest by the medical profession as nothing more than an "attempt to shore up its monopoly by bringing the professions working in complementary therapy under its wing."[63] There are grounds to support the view that the medical establishment feels threatened by CAM's growing popularity, and is seeking ways and means to exert control. CAM purists view this new embrace from the mainstream as a veiled conspiracy by the medical establishment to invade and dominate the lucrative CAM practice.

Despite such opposing views, there are growing trends towards accommodation, cooperation, and integration. Consumer interest in CAM has undoubtedly sparked this new interest on the part of physicians. Dr. Terrence Steyer, professor of Family Medicine at the Medical University of South Carolina in Charleston, has been pressing his fellow doctors to have at least a basic knowledge of CAM. He referred to surveys that showed that as many as 50 percent of patients visiting doctors were using at least one form of alternative therapy.

This is the reality that doctors must face, and they would be better off getting on board or risk alienating the very people for whom the profession exists. Many patients, largely because of mainstream skepticism towards CAM, have deliberately concealed their CAM exploits for fear of being chided by the attending physician.[14] But in the final analysis, people adhere to what they perceive as effective, CAM or not. Michael Katz of the University of Arizona gave this advice:[64]

> Clinicians need to be open-minded and understanding about patients' use of these products. One should review with the patient what evidence exists for a particular product. Ultimately, we will no longer be discussing alternative versus conventional treatment. We will discuss treatments that work and those that do not. The "beef" is in the evidence.

Doctors: Concerns about CAM

Doctors have been taught to tackle diseases in a systematic and rational way. We were taught that we should always be in control. This is not necessarily a bad thing in itself if we were always right. The trouble with this view is that we are not. Despite the shortcomings of the medical profession, it is undeniable that a lot of dishonest practitioners are on-the-loose whose sole intentions are to deceive the gullible and to make a fast buck. The public needs to be protected from this. There has to be standards and checks and balances, and it is best to start with the consumer. It is obligatory that individuals make informed decisions, but for them to do this, they must first be informed.

In *ABC of Complementary Medicine*, Zollmann and Vickers summarized the major concerns of doctors regarding the practice of complementary and alternative medicine.[26] They include:

1. Patients should seek only qualified CAM practitioners. A list of qualified practitioners should be sought in each area before trying unfamiliar therapies.
2. Patients risk missing or delaying medical diagnoses because they may chose to visit non-medical practitioners before consulting their doctor.
3. Patients may stop or refuse effective medical treatment and substitute instead unproven therapies.
4. Patients may waste money on treatments that are ineffective. Ingredients of herbal medicines vary widely and unpredictably, from brand to brand and from bottle to bottle, even within the same brand. This has led to charges of false labeling and deception against the manufacturers of many such products. Herbal products do not require FDA approval as they are marketed as dietary supplements.
5. Patients may experience dangerous side effects of CAM. Ephedrine-containing beverages can worsen blood pressure control and trigger strokes. The immensely popular St. John' wort was shown to reduce the effectiveness of anti-HIV drugs. Ephedra, used for allergies, asthma, colds, and other respiratory ailments, has been connected to a number of deaths. Some, but not all brands of Ephedra have since been banned by the FDA.[65]

Physicians and pharmaceutical companies remain unhappy with the Dietary Supplements and Health Education Act of 1994. This act still allows herbal medicines to be marketed as dietary supplements. This exempts the herbal industry from investing in extensive research to ensure proper standards and the safety of their products.[66] This is essentially a turf war (see Chapter 2). It is therefore not surprising, that a number of companies which initially cried foul ended up producing their own brands of herbal products and dietary supplements. In the drug arena, it seems to ring true that "if you can't beat them, join them."

Despite the ingrained biases and prejudices against CAM by the medical profession, they do have cause to be concerned. Historically, the medical profession has had to tackle witches, superstition, and their many victims. Therefore, doctors could be excused for harboring a high degree of skepticism regarding a number of CAM practices.

Responsibility and Regulation of CAM Practice

Given the confusion, claims, and counter-claims in this growing trend in healthcare, there is much need for transparency and accountability to inform and protect the consumer. Just as the regular practice of medicine is regulated, so must the practice of CAM therapies. Although CAM may involve practices that are not easily evaluated, this should not prevent concerted action to ensure that these practices are safe.

In the Western world, most osteopaths and chiropractors have their own accreditation institutions. Other disciplines are yet to follow. However this form of regulation may be inappropriate for practices such as prayer and meditation which carry deep religious and cultural underpinnings. Even in this area, organizations like the National Federation of Spiritual Healers (NFSH) have been set up to provide standards of practice and accountability.[67]

Public safety must be the overriding concern, and in response to this a number of consumer watchdog groups now do their own policing. Among them is the National Council Against Health Fraud, Inc., a non-profit group of health and nutrition professionals, researchers, lawyers, and concerned citizens who actively seek out misinformation and health fraud in the marketplace.[68] In the United States, three federal agencies have responsibility for addressing consumer concerns related to frauds and quackery. The U.S. Postal Service has jurisdiction over products (and their misleading claims) sold through the mail. The Federal Trade Commission (FTC) has authority over the advertising of non-prescription products and services, and the FDA has jurisdiction over the labeling of food products and drugs.

The Internet is a wild and yet untamed frontier. Spam or junk e-mails and pop-up ads are a major nuisance. They are a law unto themselves. While laws and regulation will take years to catch up, consumer sites like Quackwatch (www.quackwatch.com), seek to combat health-related frauds, myths, fads, and fallacies.[69] It must be stated that the internet is as much a source of empowerment and democratization of information, as it is a conduit to undesirable material.[70]

> The key message for CAM enthusiasts is to make informed choices. Individuals must choose certified practitioners in their areas of interest and carefully weigh their options.

Conclusion and Summary

CAM's new popularity is actually a wake-up-call for something more. It should not really about adding acupuncture to aspirin, or replacing pills with prayer. It should herald a new challenge to shift focus from sickness to wellness, and from healthcare to health.

CAM has arrived, and millions now spend billions annually for such therapies. This new trend is not fueled by the desperate and the gullible, but by intelligent people with money to spend, who are dissatisfied with the deficiencies of mainstream medical practice.

Modern medical practice has been strong on technology but weak on touch, gaining the world while slowly losing its soul. As exists in any relationship, people gravitate to where they feel their needs are being met, regardless of the establishment norms. It has left some doctors feeling like jilted husbands, who work doubly hard to provide the best that money could buy, only later to realize the estranged wife needed his time, more than his things.

This is not an isolated event. The majority of people in the industrialized world now demand more from their doctors. The medical establishment can either continue to steer this present course and scoff at the need for change, or left sulking over why patients opt for CAM therapies. As long as the overwhelming emphasis continues on the path of a profit-driven, "low-touch, high-tech, disease-care" system, the search for alternatives is bound to continue.

Many doctors within in the medical profession itself are unhappy with current trends in modern healthcare, and have sought to restore those core values that promote a more meaningful doctor-patient relationship. Even at the institutional level, the National Institutes of Health in conjunction with respected academic institutions, have now moved beyond historical attitudes, and now openly consider therapies that can complement current medical practice.

In the midst of this new embrace, there remain skeptics on both sides. The unsuspecting public needs protection through improved access to information and better regulation of CAM practice. This should not be seen as an attempt by the establishment to dominate or hijack the practice of CAM.

The real challenge is really not about names or labels. The real challenge is about care. In the quest to halt the current global epidemic of obesity, cardiovascular diseases, type II diabetes, and several forms of cancer, the real challenge is to complement the best of mainstream medical practice, with an alternative approach to prevention. What we have done thus far has clearly not helped.

But even in this drive to complement the best of what we have, with the best of what we should have, it should be a fitting reminder that what we need is more than the addition of acupuncture to aspirin, or prayer to pills. We need to shift from a doctors-centered model, towards one where prevention-conscious individuals take the primary responsibility for their own health.

We need to address the reasons why we now face a mountain of diseases that has still not peaked. The alternative that we need is to seek ways that work, and abandon those ways that have not worked. Knowledge and action go hand in hand. That is what this book is about. That is why it takes you, and not your doctor, to make you healthy.

§§§§§§

Addendum:

Personal Perspectives

> The health of the patient is his or her primary responsibility, but patients must first be empowered before being given the responsibility to handle this task.

The previous decades have given me a deep appreciation for diversity, especially for peoples, cultures, and belief systems. I grew up in Belize, a country with a population of some 250,000 until life's journeys, academic and otherwise, took me to the countries of the Caribbean, Central and North America, Europe, the Middle East, Africa, and Asia.

There was so much to learn about people, customs and cultures. I am now a self-confessed junkie with a taste for things exotic. My kitchen is very Chinese; my cupboard has its share of Afro-Caribbean, Indian, Middle Eastern and Oriental flavors. Some of my favorite dishes are from Ethiopia and the Sudan. This appreciation for diversity was not just from a distance, but also as a participant. Curiosity, coupled with sincerity and a willingness to learn, proved to be great teachers.

My return to practice medicine in Belize after postgraduate training in the United Kingdom was a great challenge. It proved to be a watershed in the focus of my practice of medicine. The epidemic of lifestyle-related diseases in a country with a third-rate healthcare budget, meant that there was urgent need for a "regime change." Rather than being militaristic, or challenging the government or the medical profession, I launched a unilateral assault on unhealthy lifestyles. The captive audience was my patients. My first priority was to educate, as ignorance appeared to be the biggest public health problem. In this setting, prevention was the only option as the cost of curative medicine for the average citizen could easily lead to financial ruin. The insurance schemes were until recently, exclusively the domain of the private sector. Technically, primary health care was free, but as the saying goes—you get what you pay for. There was no doubt in my mind that primary and secondary prevention strategies were the way to go.

Yet there was one great benefit. It was the freedom to chart an intellectually-independent and relevant course in the provision of healthcare. This was free from the academic shackles and entrenched protocols that guide medical practice in industrialized societies. The aim was simple—to arrange a harmonious marriage between the best medical care guidelines I learned, along with aggressive preventive strategies in a primary care setting.

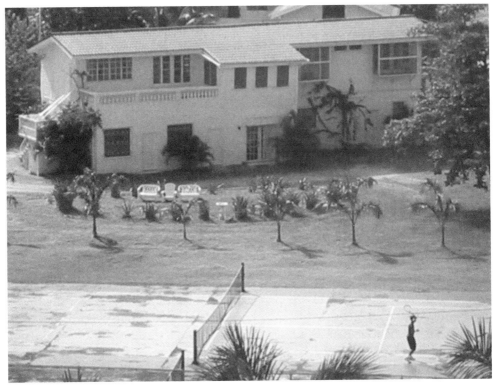

The clinic on the breezy Caribbean Shores in Belize, Central America.

Education of the individual and populace was the first task. This took on a variety of forms including weekly newspaper articles in the Amandala ("power to the people"), educational videotapes, and a mini-library. Medical advice is often shrouded in jargon that people find difficult to translate into practice. Nutrition is not a theoretical subject; it must be consumed. It must nourish and people must be able to experience the difference. This is where my kitchen came in. It is a clinic that was unorthodox, but I took countless patients upstairs to experience a different way of cooking quick and tasty meals and my favorite carrot juice (later to be replaced by West African palm oil—the richest natural source of beta-carotene—in Boston). It came as no surprise that I won the local cooking contests for my cosmopolitan entrées★, albeit second place prizes (To soothe my bruised ego, I reasoned that they were not first prizes for fear of completely discouraging the other contestants).

On a more serious note, my passion was to promote practical nutrition and lifestyle prevention programs that people could both follow and afford. We were militant in pursuing a patient-centered or shared decision-making approach, with emphasis on tackling root causes of many of the chronic lifestyle diseases. This was something that was well received both at home and abroad.

Many doctors express skepticism about patients' ability to make major nutrition and lifestyle changes. This takes time and effort, but in our experience, it was time and effort well spent. Our average consultation for new patients with lifestyle related problems may take an hour or maybe two, at the initial visit—this is impossibility in any HMO setting. We were determined to go far beyond the customary medical consultation. Our services were organized to look after a patient's health, as much as to look after their disease. Most people can embark on lifestyle changes if sincere effort and continued support are provided.

I will single out my former patient, a morbidly obese (285 pounds) expatriate who first consulted with me in the late 1990s. He had an acute infection with lots of pus literally exuding from his abdomen. This complication resulted from self-inflicted, uncontrolled type II diabetes. He smoked and drank in excess. Our custom was traditionally one of gently prodding our patients to see diabetes as a wake-up call to start paying attention, not just to diabetes, but to their overall health. In my patient's condition, time was a luxury he simply could not afford. He seemed like an accident waiting to happen.

In rather uncustomary language, I told him exactly that. He took my advice to heart, we worked closely together, and he did what was needed to achieve the desired results. He lost more than one hundred pounds in a little over a year, and the last saw him in 2003, he remained highly motivated. For him, he did not lose out on the good life, and if he lost anything, he would quickly admit that it was his weight, or the need to constantly check his blood sugars. He was diagnosed as type II diabetes, but all his checks (blood glucose, glycated hemoglobin levels, blood pressure, and lipid levels have returned to normal, and they have remained so). He no needs medications for diabetes, and leads a normal life, albeit a healthy life without resorting to his former indulgences.

Such cases are said to be the exception and not the rule, but it underscores the reality that lifestyle-diseases demand lifestyle solutions. Lifestyle changes are effective and can lead to lasting benefits—not just in controlling diabetes, but in promoting better overall health. Adopting such a perspective towards healthcare is bound to deliver great benefits to the practice of medicine and the people we serve.

★ See Chapter 8 for recipe

******

PART III

The Burden of
Lifestyle Diseases

There are two major reasons for
the rising burden of chronic diseases:
The first is unhealthy lifestyles
(smoking, unbalanced diets, and physical inactivity).
The second is the impact of our aging populations.

Chapter 5

Common Risk Factors in Chronic Diseases:

The Western Diet and Negative Lifestyles

Chapter Outline

Observations...165
The Concept of Risk 167
Framingham Heart Study...168
Risk Factors Defined..169
The Primary Risk Factors in Lifestyle Diseases 171
    Common Risk Factors…Multiple Outcomes............................171
    Tobacco Use 172
    Overweight and Obesity 173
    Sedentary Lifestyle (Physical Inactivity).................................173
The Western Diet: A Closer Look 173
    Excess Food, Excess Calories 175
    Should Women Eat More During Pregnancy? 179
    Too Much Highly Processed Foods...181
    Excess Total Fats, Saturated Fat and Trans-Fats 183
    Tropical Oils: Are they as bad as some believe?.........................187
    Meaty Matters 190
    Poultry...192
    Seafood 193
    Misunderstandings about Dietary Cholesterol............................194
    Milk and Dairy Products 195
    Milk, Dairy Products, and Prostate Cancer 197
    Cured, Smoked, and Charcoal-Grilled Meats.............................198
    Excess Sodium; Reduced Potassium and Magnesium 199
    Too Much Alcohol: Weighing Risks and Benefits 200
    Reduced Fruits, Vegetables, Greens, Grains, and Fiber.............202

Risk Charts and Tables.. 203
The Metabolic Syndrome—the Insulin Resistance Syndrome......... 204
Beyond Risk—Towards Maximized Health 206
Towards Aggressive Prevention 207
Summary.. 208

"At least one-third of all cancers are attributable to poor diet, physical activity, and overweight. Thus, if our goal of reducing cancer incidence by 25% in the United States by 2015 is to be reached, cancer prevention efforts must include strong programs for healthy eating and physical activity. Such programs will also help to reduce the incidence of many other chronic diseases."

Dileep G. Bal, President, American Cancer Society, 2001

"Fighting Heart Disease and Stroke"

The American Heart Association (AHA)

Recent studies have found a connection between a high-cholesterol diet and an increased risk of Alzheimer's, a disease caused by the destruction of nerve cells in the brain "We're seeing more and more that what is bad for your heart is bad for your brain…Any risk factor linked to heart disease, you need to pay attention to it for Alzheimer's as well."[1]

Rudolph Tanzi, Professor of Neurology, Harvard Medical School

§§§§§§§

Observations

Doctors traditionally treat obesity, cardiovascular diseases, and diabetes as separate medical problems. These diseases are, in essence, simply different faces of the same problem. Failure to tackle the root causes has focused too much attention on disease and too little on lifestyles.

The chronic diseases that affect 90 million Americans and hundreds of millions worldwide share much in common.[2] Changes in dietary habits and lifestyles have led to a global epidemic of obesity, heart disease, type II diabetes, and several forms of cancer. Almost 60 percent of Americans are overweight, and the figure is higher in minority communities and many emerging countries.[3] Smoking, high-calorie convenience foods, and sedentary lifestyles have fueled a global epidemic of obesity, the metabolic syndrome, and related diseases (Figure 5-1 and 5-6).[3-5]

I became heavily involved in the care of people with diabetes following my medical internship, and it was plain to see that the majority of them were obese. A large percentage of these obese, diabetic patients were also hypertensive and hyperlipidemic (elevated blood lipids—cholesterol and triglycerides) compared to their normal-weight counterparts. These obese, diabetic individuals are four times more likely to suffer heart attacks and strokes. This scenario is repeated globally and is heavily influenced by modern urban living.

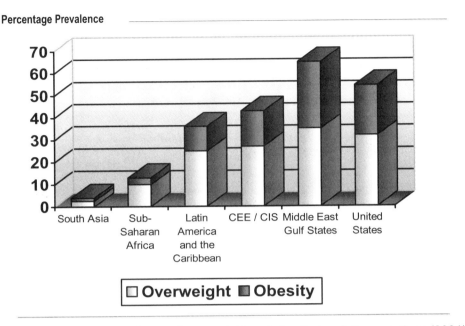

Percentage Prevalence

Figure 5-1. Global prevalence of overweight and obesity in adult populations (2001)

Source: B.E, Bulwer M.D. http://www.procor.org/nutrition and obesity [4]

We are witnessing the globalization of lifestyle patterns as the world's becomes linked by travel, telecommunication, and trade. Rapid urbanization and market forces have resulted in major changes in traditional dietary and occupational patterns. A detailed discussion of urbanization is outside the scope of this book, but it has had a major impact on the way people eat and live. One inescapable consequence is the increasing dependence on highly-processed and convenience foods.[6,7]

Decades of lifestyle indulgences incrementally build up and destroy body tissues and organ systems, and then make their presence known in the form of lifestyle diseases. Unfortunately, by the time most people are medically diagnosed with these diseases, much damage has already taken place. Treating a disease without treating the root cause is like inserting band-aid over a sore that refuses to heal. The challenge is to halt those factors that lead to these difficult-to-manage and expensive-to-treat conditions. We will fail in our efforts if we fail to address the root causes.

The major chronic non-communicable diseases were globally responsible for 52 million deaths in 1996.[7] They today cause 40 percent of all deaths in developing countries. Historically, these were considered diseases of older adults and the elderly, but today they increasingly afflict much younger individuals as early as in their teens and 20s. The blame for much of this rests with the massive drop in physical activity levels that accompanied modernization and urbanization, together with the increasing indulgence in high-calorie, high-fat convenience foods.[5]

Today about two-thirds (64 percent) of deaths in some developing countries are due to chronic diseases. Diabetes rates are expected to double to 300 million by the year 2025, with the bulk of all new cases occurring in the developing world. In the United States, chronic diseases are responsible for almost 70 percent of deaths and disability.[8,9]

The Concept of Risk

Why Study Risk?
Risk factors help us identify and measure the likelihood or odds of developing a disease. Some risk factors are well known, some are not yet known; some we have control over (e.g. behavior), and some we have no control over (e.g. age or sex).

Why do certain people have a greater likelihood of developing a particular disease compared to others? This is what the discussion of risk is about. The study of risk is not an exact science like mathematics, physics, or chemistry. Risks have to do with the odds or probabilities of developing certain diseases. The reason for its imprecise nature is that there are so many things that vary from one individual to another. This picture is further fuzzed by the length of time it takes for chronic diseases to manifest. These diseases often take several years or decades before they are diagnosed.[10]

Many dismiss attempts to link behavior and disease, and preoccupy themselves instead with genetic or esoteric influences. They point to people who engage in unhealthy behavior yet remain "well" throughout most of their life. For them the word "well" means that there has not been the need for hospital admissions, surgery, or prescription drugs. I beg to differ. Wellness is more than the absence of sickness. It is presence of health, vitality, and wholeness of body, mind, and spirit.

Skeptics may doubt the clear evidence that supports the indisputable relationship between lifestyle and disease. Many still debate on whether cigarette smoking causes lung cancer. They ignore health warnings and point to the fact that most smokers never develop lung cancer, chronic bronchitis, and heart disease, but "a man convinced against his will is of the same opinion still." However, for those who are genuinely interested in optimizing their health, we will address those factors that dramatically increase your risks of developing disease.

Risks indicate the likelihood, not the certainty, of developing diseases. For example, most people who drink (alcohol) and drive do not have motor vehicle accidents, but drinking while driving leads to such increased risks of accidents, that it forced the law to prohibit such behavior. The reason is in the statistics. Drinkers have more accidents than non-drinkers. Therefore, drinkers are statistically at increased risk of having motor vehicle accidents. The greater the odds, the more likely it is for a problem to occur. This assists in detecting those at risk, thereby enabling early measures to prevent a catastrophe.

Medical researchers have long observed that people with risk factors for chronic diseases go on to develop these diseases later in life. Obesity, smoking, and physical inactivity all increase the risk of developing diabetes and heart disease. The risks for diabetes and heart disease can be minimized, and a significant percentage of catastrophes avoided, if we take appropriate measures to eliminate or minimize the prevalence of these factors.

We will examine the factors that increase the risks for chronic diseases.[5] There are clear answers rooted in scientific research that has studied populations and disease trends over extended periods of time. We will also delve into the details of several aspects of behavior and diet that led to this modern epidemic (that has still not peaked) of chronic diseases. Always bear in mind the need to focus on the totality of good evidence rather than on isolated or anecdotal studies. Too often, we get caught up in headlines propagated by the media and self-styled mavericks, who may sound sensational, but promise far more than they can deliver.

The Framingham Heart Study

The Framingham study helped us to define the major risk factors for cardiovascular diseases. High blood cholesterol, high blood pressure, and diabetes were found to be major risk factors for heart attack and stroke.

Any discussion of risk factors would be incomplete without an acknowledgement of the Framingham Heart Study.[12,13] The town of Framingham, Massachusetts, was chosen in 1948 by the U.S. Public Health Service as the cohort for "the study that changed America's heart." The organizers recruited 5,209 healthy male and female adult volunteers between ages 30 and 60.

Before the findings of this landmark study, doctors had believed that the hardening of the arteries (atherosclerosis) was an inevitable consequence of aging. The same view was held of hypertension in industrialized populations. It was widely thought that these were normal features of the aging process, and as a result, there was little medical insight into modifying risk factors for cardiovascular diseases. Arresting or reversing coronary heart disease through aggressive prevention or management of risk factors was an unknown concept. Therefore, prevention was given little or no attention.

The Framingham Study sought to understand "which biologic and environmental factors were contributing to such a rapid rise in cardiovascular death and disability. They settled on an epidemiological approach—a novel idea at the time—that was designed to learn how and why those who developed heart disease differed from those who escaped it." It is from this study that doctors first understood that high cholesterol, high blood pressure, and diabetes were risk factors for heart attack and stroke. The Framingham study established a clear relationship between high blood cholesterol levels and the risk for heart disease. It further established the strong artery-clogging effect of LDL (low density lipoprotein cholesterol) with coronary heart disease, as well as an equally strong protective effect of artery cleaning HDL (high density lipoprotein cholesterol). Framingham made it possible to refer to LDL cholesterol as "bad cholesterol" and HDL as "good cholesterol" (see further discussion on LDL and HDL cholesterol in Chapter 5, "Excess total fats, saturated fats, trans-fats").

The Framingham Heart Study provided clear evidence that the changes in American lifestyles were heavily responsible for the high rates of cardiovascular diseases. The American lifestyle, epitomized by nutritional excesses and increasing sedentary lifestyles, had given rise to the epidemic of obesity. Negative habits, led by cigarette smoking, were shown to be major risk factors for heart attack and sudden death. There was a clear relationship between the number of cigarettes smoked and the duration of smoking with the incidence of heart disease. The greater the "smoking years," the greater was the risk of cardiovascular disease.

On a positive note, Framingham also provided evidence that smoking cessation promptly halved the risk of heart attacks. Positive lifestyle changes such as exercise were noted to be effective in reducing the risk of heart attack and stroke.

Risk Factors Defined

Unbalanced nutrition and physical inactivity have given rise to obesity, the metabolic syndrome, dyslipidemia, and hypertension. These risk factors increase the likelihood of dying from a heart attack, stroke, type II diabetes, and cancer.

Risk factors estimate your future risk of developing diseases. A risk factor may be a behavior (e.g. smoking, an unhealthy diet, or a physically inactive life), or an inherited trait (e.g. a strong family history of premature heart disease before age 50), or a laboratory measurement (e.g. abnormal cholesterol levels). Risk factors vary in strength and degree and are classified as major or minor depending on the strength of association between the factor and the disease.

For type II diabetes, obesity and physical inactivity are the major risk factors. However, every obese person will not develop diabetes, and every diabetic person is not obese. Nevertheless, obesity places an individual at much greater risk of developing type II diabetes compared to people who are of normal weight. Obesity is, therefore, a major risk factor for type II diabetes. The major risk factors that contribute to the six leading causes of death are cigarette smoking, obesity, unbalanced diets, physical inactivity, hypertension, and high blood cholesterol (Table 5-1 and Figure 5-2).[16-20]

Table 5-1. The Six Leading Lifestyle Diseases and their Major Risk Factors (U.S.)

The Leading Six	Deaths (1998)	Major Risk Factors
Heart Disease	460,000	C,H,S,O,P,D
Stroke	158,000	C,H,S,O,P,D
Lung Cancer	155,000	S
COPD (chronic lung disease)	113,000	S
Diabetes	65,000	O,P,D
Colon Cancer	57,000	S,O,D,P
All Causes	2,337,000	-

RISK FACTOR ABBREVIATIONS: **C** = high serum cholesterol; **H** = hypertension; **S** = smoking; **O** = obesity; **P** = physically inactive; **D** = diet (unbalanced Western diet)

The greater the number of risk factors present, the greater is the tendency to develop disease. An obese, inactive person has a greater risk of becoming diabetic than an obese, but physically active person. At the other extreme, an obese, inactive hypertensive smoker with high cholesterol and a family history of heart attacks and stroke is at extremely high risk for a heart and stroke. This latter example is like "an accident waiting to happen."

Some risk factors are controllable. These pertain to behavior. But there are also risk factors over which we have no control. They are not controllable—such as our age, gender, and family history. The controllable risk factors are amenable to lifestyle changes—doctors refer to them as the "modifiable risk factors." These are the focus of this book. Risk factors amenable to lifestyle changes are listed in Figure 5-2. The chief purpose of identifying them is to adopt strategies to prevent and manage diseases in people at risk. In heart disease, doctors are now paying attention to more recently recognized risk factors like C-reactive protein (CRP), fibrinogen, homocysteine, and lipoprotein (a).

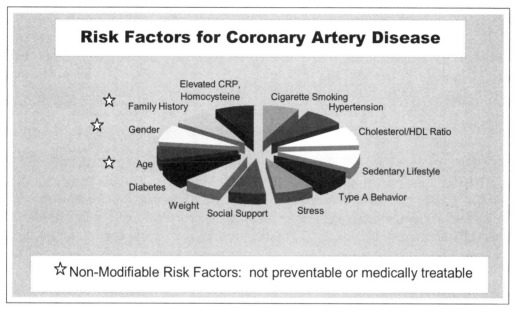

Figure 5-2. Chart Showing Risk Factors for Coronary Heart Disease

The Primary Risk Factors in Lifestyle Diseases

Common Risk Factors—Multiple Outcomes

Behavioral Risk Factors for Cardiovascular Disease Among U.S. Adults

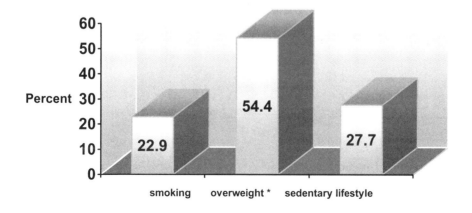

Figure 5-3. The Major Behavioral Risk Factors for Cardiovascular Diseases (U.S. Adults)
Source: Center for Disease Control and Prevention (CDC)[21-22]

Tobacco Use

Cigarette smoking is the single most important preventable cause of death and disease in the United States. The statistics are staggering: Smoking kills more than 400,000 Americans annually, almost 50 million Americans smoke; 500 million people alive today will die from tobacco-related diseases (Figure 5-4). Smoking carries a 50 billion dollar price tag in direct medical expenses and another 50 billion dollars in indirect healthcare costs.[22-24]

On the global scene, Europeans smoke more cigarettes per capita than Americans, and China's smoking population exceeds 300 million![25] Analysts fear that the problem will grow worse in developing countries as tobacco multinationals seek overseas markets where the anti-smoking lobby is decidedly absent, or less hostile. A Turkish patient once told me, "All Turkish men smoke!" I will confess that it took me several days while traveling through Turkey, before I came across a non-smoking Turkish male. The recent adoption of the World Anti-Smoking Treaty in May 2003, however, heralds a new global conscience, but what actually happens on the ground will be an entirely different matter.

The medical implications of cigarette smoking are indisputable. Smoking greatly increases the risk of several cancers, lung diseases, heart attack, stroke, high blood pressure, type II diabetes, and impotence. Tobacco smoke contains more than 3,800 compounds, more than 40 of which are known carcinogens. Smokeless tobacco (chewed or snuffed tobacco) and cigars are not safer tobacco alternatives to cigarette smoking. These can cause cancers of the mouth, larynx, esophagus, and lungs. Passive or environmental tobacco smoke (ETS), also known as second-hand smoke, was originally thought to be relatively innocent but ETS increases the risk of coronary heart disease. In the United States exposure to ETS causes 5,000 non-smokers to die from lung cancer each year.[26]

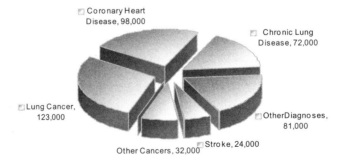

Deaths (430,000) from cigarette smoking (U.S., 1997)

Figure 5-4. Annual Deaths from Smoking (United States)

Overweight and Obesity

Obesity is the fastest growing health threat in America, and is set to overtake tobacco as the number one cause of death. Sixty percent of Americans are now considered overweight or obese. In 1991, only seven states showed obesity rates of over 15 percent of the population. Seven years later, only seven states did not! Obesity now affects up to 15 percent of American youth under age 18.[27-28]

Overweight and obese individuals are at increased risk for heart disease, type II diabetes, high blood pressure, osteoarthritis, cancer, and a host diseases and quality of life issues (Table 8-12 and 8-13).[29] The classification of overweight and obesity, and strategies for control are discussed in Chapter 8.

Sedentary Lifestyles (Physical Inactivity)

Industrialization, urbanization, motorized transportation, and the computer age have caused a revolution in the way people live and work. We are now the least physically active generation in history. In the United States, more than 200,000 deaths annually can be attributed to physical inactivity, making it a risk factor second only to tobacco use as a preventable cause of death. Regular physical activity can reduce the rates of heart attack, diabetes, high blood pressure and cancers.[30]

More than 60 percent of Americans do not get the exercise they need. This extends into the age groups that are traditionally known for their inability to keep still. More than a third of school-age children don't get the regular physical activity they need. Student participation in high school physical education classes fell from 42 percent in 1991 to 29 percent in 1999. The television, video games, computers and the internet are winning the battle for the hearts and minds of 21st century youth. These now have a virtual stranglehold on the activities of youth in industrialized nations, and increasingly so, on youth in emerging societies. Physical activity and the challenges of staying active are discussed in Chapter 9.[31-34]

The Western Diet: A Closer Look

The Western diet is a pattern of food consumption characterized by excess intake of high-fat, high-protein, and carbohydrate-rich foods (predominantly of the highly-processed variety), along with insufficient intake of fresh fruit, vegetables, and whole grains. Its popularity has been fueled by the demands of modernity and the convenience food industry.

(Figures 5-5 and 5-6)

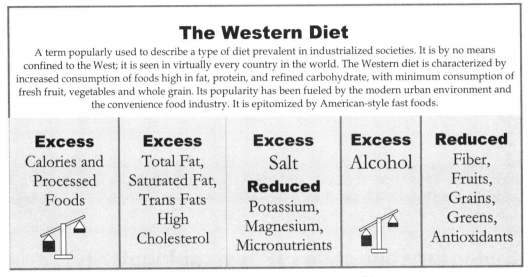

Figure 5-5. The Unbalanced Western Diet

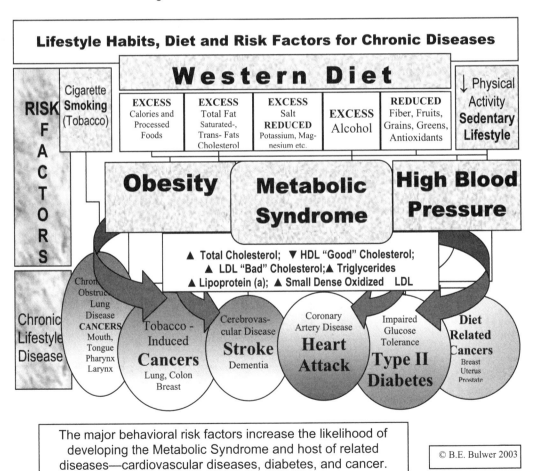

Figure 5-6. Schematic Representation of the Link between Lifestyle Risk Factors and the Major Chronic Non-communicable Diseases

Our food supply has changed drastically over the past fifty years, but most people are ignorant to this change and the impact it has had on our health. Most people in the industrialized world purchase their food from supermarkets, and 90 percent of all foods consumed in America are of the processed variety.[35-37] Market forces orchestrated all this. People are now busier, the traditional household is becoming a fixture of the past, and convenience foods are everywhere. People who have spent all their lives in a Western environment may be oblivious to the major faults of this dietary pattern. But when you compare it to the food choices of a century ago, it becomes strikingly clear that radical changes have occurred within our food supply.

Today, there are many people who live industrial as well as traditional societies, who eat strikingly different, and enjoy markedly lower rates of obesity and chronic diseases. The Western diet is the major contributor to the modern global epidemic of obesity and chronic diseases (see Introduction and Chapter 1). It is impossible to address today's epidemic of obesity and chronic diseases without paying attention to this prevalent dietary pattern.[38-39] This is the major task of this chapter.

Excess intake of fats, carbohydrates, and protein are consumed at the expense of the fruits, vegetables, and whole grains. Less than 25 percent of American adults eat the UDSA recommended servings daily of fruits and vegetables. This figure rose to almost 70 percent in Minnesota to more than 90 percent in Arizona.[40]

This pattern of food consumption reflects changes that are happening all over the world, especially among urban populations. This is what has come to be popularly known as the Western Diet (Figure 5-5 and 5-6). The discussions that follow will analyze in more detail the components of this diet and their roles in the diseases that now kill 70 percent of Americans, and an increasing percentage of people around the globe

Excess Food, Excess Calories

Overconsumption of high-energy (sugary, starchy, or fatty) foods is the major cause of overweight, obesity, and the metabolic syndrome.

The United States is the epitome of consumption excesses; it is reputed for doing everything in a big way. Portion sizes are no exception. First-time visitors to America are often left aghast by what "large" means in America. The servings of popcorn and the size of the drinks served at the movies has left many visitors literally in "shock and awe." In most countries I have traveled, a large drink equates to a small or a regular-sized drink in America (12 fluid ounces). This is what the British call standard or medium. A "large" drink in America measures 32 fluid ounces!

The Western diet with its excessive intake of highly-processed foods and huge portion sizes is the modern sin of America. It reflects a coalition of capital, technology, and marketing, never before seen in the history of the world.

All-you-can-eat and all-you-can-drink restaurants further epitomize this indulgence. Fast food chains constantly try to outdo each other to generate bigger sales. "Bigger is better." You don't have to settle for a regular burger or french fries anymore; you can "super size" for just a few pennies more. Double Whoppers, Monsters, and Triple Decker hamburgers (with cheese) are just a glimpse of the indulgent labels. Unlimited servings of ketchup and mustard that are still the norm in America are not duplicated by these same multinationals overseas.[38,39] I remember paying five British pence for my ketchup at KFC several years ago!

People eat too much of the wrong foods, and this charge is borne out by the escalating rates of obesity in America and around the world. It has been said, "we need guts to get ahead in this world," but too many people appear to take this thing too literally. It will keep us back in multiple ways rather than propelling us forwards. Central or abdominal obesity ("beer-belly") is the major trigger for the metabolic syndrome that affects 50 million Americans.[5] The recently revised figures presented by the International Obesity Task Force (IOTF, 2003) puts the global figure for overweight at 1.7 billion persons (see Chapter 8). The metabolic syndrome can be likened to a Trojan horse that hides in its bowels, a sinister gang: dyslipidemia (abnormal cholesterol ratio and triglycerides), and the ingredients for type II diabetes, high blood pressure, strokes, and heart attacks (see Chapter 2, "The Root Of The Matter" and Chapter 5, "The Metabolic Syndrome—the Insulin Resistance Syndrome).

We tend to consume far more food than our bodies can ever use. We need to eat to live, but many seem to prefer just the opposite. Judging by the present food consumption patterns, eating for health is not a real concern for most people. Gustatory gratification reigns supreme (a politically correct way of saying that we are too greedy). The average American consumes 50 gallons of soft drinks annually (12-fluid oz soft drink delivers about 160 calories)[41,42] When you do the math, this translates easily into 15 extra pounds per year (from a single extra soft drink or sweetened drink per day). We can easily substitute water for such habits, but although water is now making a comeback, untold millions will confess that flavored drinks and sodas are the only drinks that accompany their meals. The idea of drinking water with meals is, in the eyes of many, a strange proposal.

There is a never-ending barrage of temptations to eat more food, and few seem able to resist. The modern, urban lifestyle is the perfect setting where busy people are held virtual hostages to the fast-food and the convenience-food industries—that is, if they so choose.

This is what is happening in so many of our societies—we consume too many calories. Compare the daily calorie intake of the average American to the Japanese. Take a closer look at the composition of a prototype diet (Table 5-2 and 5-3).[39,43,44] Closer scrutiny will reveal why Japanese who follow their traditional diets are slimmer than Americans. Please do not attribute this to genetics. Japanese sumo wrestlers know exactly how to get fat. Slim young Japanese males become 400-pound sumo heavyweights by eating fattening foods over several years.

Compare the foods that people eat and the difference it makes to calorie intake. A first glimpse at Table 5-3 may lead you to believe that the longer column with more foods (Oriental Style Diet) would give a greater total calorie intake. This diet actually totaled 200 calories less than the American styled diet (fried eggs and bacon not included). An extra 200 calories of food daily can translate into a weight gain of 20 pounds over a year. Therefore, it should come as no surprise why Americans are fatter than their Asian counterparts. This highlights a very important principle in nutrition; you can eat more and still weigh less, but the key lies in what you eat.

The picture today is changing as the Oriental diet and most traditional diets in the world became more Westernized. Many blame this trend on the food multinationals, but it is not that simple. The pressures of modernity and globalization are powerful forces that have caused major shifts in eating patterns, even among populations where no McDonald's etcetera exists. However, this is not to deny that American influence is undoubtedly the most powerful trendsetter around the globe.

Table 5-2. Comparison of the average American vs. the Japanese diets (past and present) with respect to calorie and macronutrient intake

Nutrients	The Japanese Diet		The American Diet	
	(1950)	(1997)	(1965)	(1995)
Total Energy (Calories)	2098	2,007	2750	2800
% ENERGY from				
Carbohydrate %	79.3	57.4	38.0	41.0
Fat %	7.7	45.0	45.0	34.0
Protein %	13.0	20.0	15.0	22.0

Sources: Kaicha Kida et al. Effects of Western Diet on Risk Factors of Chronic Diseases in Asia in Preventive Nutrition 2001, p.441; and U.S. Department of Agriculture, 1965 and 1977-1978 Nationwide Food Consumption Surveys, and 1989-1991 and 1994-1995 Continuing Survey of Food Intakes by Individuals.[39]

Oriental Style Diet

Menu Sample	Calories
Breakfast	
1 cup white rice	264
1 cup chicken broth	39
½ cup broccoli	22
½ cup grape juice	64
1 orange	62
3 oz tofu	123
Lunch	
3 oz pork loin	259
1 cup white rice	264
(no added fat/oil)	34
½ cup pea pods	60
½ tbsp sesame oil	112
1 cup apple juice	112
Snack	
1 cup tea (no added sugar or milk)	2
1 pear	118
Dinner	
3 oz fish(bass)	82
½ cup bean sprouts	13
2 ½ cup cooked cellophane noodles	416
¼ cup onions, cooked	23
¼ cup mushrooms	4
¼ cup green snap beans	11
½ cup mustard greens	11
½ tbsp sesame oil	60
Dessert	
¼ cup melon, fresh	14
¼ cup strawberries, fresh	11
¼ cup grapes, fresh	15
Total	2,083

American Style Diet

Menu Sample	Calories
Breakfast	
2 doughnuts	208
12 oz coffee	7
2 tbsp cream	40
1 tbsp sugar	45
Lunch	
4 slices deli ham	208
2 oz Swiss cheese	214
4 slices white bread	264
1 small bag potato chips	140
1 apple	81
16 fluid oz cola	202
½ cup tomatoes	24
3 pieces lettuce	8
Dinner	
4 oz dinner roast	594
1 ½ baked potato	180
½ cup carrots, boiled	35
½ cup green beans, canned	13
1 cup 2% milk	121
1 tbsp margarine	101
Dessert	
1 cup frozen low-fat vanilla yogurt with 2 tbsp chocolate syrup	280
Total	2,765

Table 5-3
Comparison of Daily Calorie Intake of
Oriental Style Diet vs. **American Style Diet**

Note an extra 700 more calories daily in the American style diet (even without any mention of fried eggs and sausages etc.). An extra 200 calories of food daily can translate into a weight gain of 20 pounds in a year.

Modified from source. Prevention of Myocardial Infarction. New York, N.Y. Oxford University Press, 1996[44]

Table 5-3. Comparison of Daily Caloric Intake of Oriental vs. American Style Diets

Should Women Eat More during Pregnancy?

There is a widespread belief that women must increase their food intake during pregnancy. Caribbean women are told by nurses that they must eat-for-two during pregnancy. It is based on a common sense appreciation that women need more food to build new bones and flesh.

There is no dispute that nine months of pregnancy carries an extra energy cost. Additional energy and nutrition is needed to build extra tissues, both maternal and fetal. The major question is, however, the way these additional needs are met. Calcium is a key nutrient in pregnancy; it is needed to build new bones as well as extra milk during lactation. Does this automatically mean that women must take extra calcium or lots of milk during pregnancy?

Women do not need to take extra calcium during pregnancy. This is the view of Ann Prentice, Ph.D. and colleagues at the MRC Human Nutrition Research at Cambridge University in England: [45]

> The evidence indicates that pregnancy and lactation are characterized by physiological adaptive processes that are independent of maternal calcium intake and that provide the calcium necessary for fetal growth and breast-milk production without requiring an increase in maternal calcium intake.

Pregnancy and breastfeeding, although accompanied by a heavy requirement for extra calcium, is offset by changes in a woman's body that compensates for this. There is increased absorption of calcium from food, increased mobilization of calcium from the bones, and reduced losses of calcium in the urine.[46,47] The net effect of this is to supply the additional demands of pregnancy and breastfeeding.

Pregnancy requires additional energy and nutrients, but a similar principle applies. A woman's body has been programmed to compensate for this extra demand by making better use of the food she normally eats. This increased demand can be met even in women who eat relatively little. Studies have shown that women can meet the extra demands of pregnancy on as little as 1,000-calorie diets (the normal diet averages 2,000 calories). This is *not* a call to diet during pregnancy. This figure was derived from studies of pregnancy outcomes in women living in starving environments, such as existed during the siege of Leningrad (World War II), or women in rural Guatemala (living in malnourished environments). For want of a better description, the unborn is quite "selfish." It will extract whatever it needs to survive, even at the mother's expense. Pregnancy skews the equation in favor of the unborn. This is programmed prerequisite for its survival.[48, 49]

The World Health Organization recommends that women consume an additional 300 calories daily. The British tell their women to consume an additional 200 calories daily. But telling women to eat-for-two during pregnancy has given rise to obesity among women, especially among minority communities and within the developing world. When a woman loads up with extra food during pregnancy, the increased metabolic efficiency that accompanies pregnancy makes her gain even more weight (than she would have gained, if she were not pregnant). [50,51]

Therefore, what confronts us is a scenario where women, especially multiparous minority women, exhibit an unhealthy trend of progressive weight gain with each subsequent pregnancy. In the Middle East, Latin America, and the Caribbean, it is "normal" for women who have had their quota of children to become obese. Cultural perceptions further complicate matters because "skinny" in such communities are often associated with a lack of contentment, lower socioeconomic status, or having neglectful husbands. To make matters worse, the early return of women to the workplace following pregnancy has resulted in a decline in breastfeeding rates. This robs women of the opportunity to burn an extra 600 calories daily, thereby shedding some of the extra weight gained during the pregnancy. [52]

Regardless of the reasons, the growing rates of obesity among women is a major public health concern. The medical burden arising from increasing obesity rates places women at higher risk (than men) for type II diabetes. Minority women exhibit the highest rates of obesity in the United States, and they generally have the least access to good healthcare.

Excess food can shorten lifespan and promote disease. This was the finding of researchers who conducted animal studies. Animals fed with 60 percent of their normal food intake increase their lifespan two to four-fold. [53] According to George Roth, Ph.D., of the National Institute on Aging in Maryland, caloric restriction is the only measure that has been shown to increase life expectancy in animals. In addition to longer lifespan, such animals exhibited less diseases compared to their counterparts that were fed ad libitum. [53] Obesity and caloric excess also contributes to higher rates of death and ill-health in humans. Inhabitants of the Japanese island of Okinawa are the longest-lived persons in the world. They practice healthy nutritional habits including the self-disciplinary hara hachi bu, or eating 8 parts full out of 10. [54]

We do not need to clean the plate. We do not need to eat until we are about to burst. We live in the refrigerator age. There is always the "doggie bag" or the refrigerator that can accommodate the excess food when eating out or when dining at home. Eating large portion sizes not only leads to reduced productivity (more *siestas* and naps after meals) but also places additional stresses on the cardiovascular system. Heavy meals, especially those laden with saturated fat, are well-documented precipitants factors for angina and heart attacks.

Too Many Highly Processed Foods

Highly processed foods have provoked major changes in the nutrition landscape. These foods are the major sources of hidden salt, hidden sugars, hidden fats, and unhealthy trans-fats (partially hydrogenated fats) in the modern diet. Their increased consumption occurs at the expense of healthier alternatives: fresh fruits, vegetables, and whole grains.

Food Processing is comprehensively addressed in Chapter 7, but it is introduced here as an important component of the unbalanced Western Diet. One of the marvels of this era has been the advent of the modern food-processing industry. This has given us the ability to preserve and to transport food over long distances with little fear of spoilage or contamination. There is little need for processing or preserving food where there are plentiful supplies of fresh food year-round and where people live close to communities where fresh produce is plentiful. Indeed, benefits provided by food processing became crucial when consumers moved far away from the site of food production.

As societies became more urbanized, the need for processing, storing, and transporting food became an integral part of this change. As more women moved from the home to the workplace, less time was available for domestic food preparation. This fueled the demand for the convenience-food industry and fast-foods. For the most part, convenience foods are highly processed.

Food processing can be as basic as curing, smoking, sun-drying, and salting, but the twentieth century revolutionized this process to an entirely different level. The Napoleonic armies needed to ensure that food supply was available on the battlefront. Frenchman Nicholas Appert showed that food could be preserved if sufficiently heated in a sealed container, and the canning industry was born (1809). On the battlefront, the armies that could ensure their food supply were often the armies that won the war. Food processing drastically reduces losses from spoilage and contamination. In times of natural disasters, preserved and processed foods are lifesaving. This is great in the short term, but several methods used in the food processing industry result in changes to food that can exert long-term negative impact on the health of human populations.[55-63]

Highly processed food products contain lots of hidden fat, hidden salt, hidden sugar, additives, and preservatives. They are generally deficient in fiber. "Hidden" refers to the fact that most people are unaware of these considerable distortions and additions to the original food sources. The bulk of our daily salt intake comes not from salt-shaker, but rather from salt added at the processing plant or during food preparation. Despite the advent of food labels, most people remain generally confused about labels (see Chapter 7). For example, most people have no clue what happens to corn during processing to make corn flakes. The sodium content of the processed flakes is almost ten times that of the original corn. A cup of Kellogg's Frosted Flakes contains about 17 grams of sugar—a quantity far beyond that found the original corn food. [64,65]

Added to these concerns are the subject of food additives and preservatives. Strictly speaking almost any substance can be toxic if consumed in sufficient amounts. Even too much food or oxygen can kill. Some substances, widely used as antibacterial preservatives, colorants, and flavoring agents, have justifiably been cause for great concern. The most prominent among these sodium nitrite, still used to cure and preserve meats, BHA (butylated hydroxyansole), and BHT (butyulated hydroxytoluene). [66,67]

Sodium nitrite, responsible for the pink color of ham, bacon, sausages, and other cured meats, is used to prevent botulism food poisoning by inhibiting the growth of the deadly bacteria that causes botulism, *Clostridium botulinum*. Nitrites are converted during processing and digestion to compounds called nitrosamines. Nitrosamines are powerful carcinogens (cancer-causing). There have been efforts to reduce or eliminate the use of nitrites in food, but the risks of deaths by botulism food poisoning outweigh the potential cancer risks posed by the long-term use of these agents. BHA and BHT are synthetic antioxidants that prevent oils from going rancid. Higher doses of these have been shown to cause cancer in rats and hamsters. [68-72]

Highly processed foods are nutritionally inferior to their fresh or minimally-processed counterparts. Many processed foods are fortified with certain minerals and vitamins to protect against deficiency states, but I am not aware of any study that shows their protective effect against cardiovascular disease and cancer. On the contrary, there is evidence to show the reverse.

The strongest case against highly processed foods is not just the presence of potentially harmful ingredients,
but that excess consumption of these foods substitute for healthier alternatives that protect against cardiovascular diseases and cancer.

Excess Total Fats, Saturated Fats and Trans-(Partially Hydrogenated) Fats

There is still much confusion about fats.
Fats are not all bad, all saturated fats are not the same,
and the most dangerous of fats (trans-fats)
do not even appear on food labels.

We know about the link between dietary fat intake and heart disease. The American Heart Association (AHA) recommends a diet of less than 30 percent of daily calories from fats.[73-76] Studies consistently show that a total fat intake of less than 30 percent of the total daily calories lowers an individual's risk for cardiovascular disease. Fats contribute about 40 percent of daily total energy intake in the average American diet. An estimated 50 million Americans have high blood cholesterol, and this number continues to rise. The unbalanced Western diet is notoriously high in unhealthy fats.

There is a simplistic view of fats by the general public. Americans know that animal fats are bad, but this message has been severely corrupted by a populace obsessed with the fattening effects of fat. There has been a progressive attempt to replace saturated or animal fats (SFAs) such as lard and butter, with polyunsaturated fats (PUFAs). Polyunsaturated varieties are found in vegetable oils such as soybean and corn, and monounsaturated fats (MUFAs) as found mainly in olives, avocados, almond, cashew, and rapeseed (canola) and products derived from these (Figure 5-7).[77,78]

Volumes have been published on fats, but a brief summary is fitting before continuing this discussion. Fats or lipids could be lumped into four main groups:[77,79]

1. **Structural fats**. These dominate in the cell wall envelope of every single cell in the human body). Cholesterol is found in this group.
2. **Storage fats**. These are the reserves that gather in the wrong places around the waist and in cellulite. They are popularly known as triglycerides or triacylglycerols.
3. **Metabolic fats**. These are lipids that play important roles in nutrition and body physiology. These include steroid hormones and vitamins A, D, E, and K and the fats that are found in bile.
4. **Transport fats**. These are what is measured when you go for a check up. These lipids float around in the blood and perform functions that can be both beneficial and harmful. They circulate in blood attached to special proteins called lipoproteins. This makes it possible for these fatty/oily substances to mix easily with blood. Simply speaking, they include: LDL or

more properly LDL-cholesterol, HDL or HDL-cholesterol, triglycerides, and lipoprotein (a). The last two letters of the abbreviation (DL) stands for "Density Lipoprotein." The first letters "L" or "H" means "high" or "low." Therefore LDL has a low density and HDL has a high density. Normally about 70 percent of the cholesterol that floats in the blood is of the LDL variety and 25 percent should be in the form of HDL. There are complex interactions but the blood concentrations of these lipids are heavily influenced by diet (Figure 5-7) and aerobic exercise. Doctors request total blood cholesterol levels (the sum of at least four different types of cholesterol), but the proportion of the different types of cholesterol are more important (especially the total cholesterol/LDL ratio) than any single type. HDL is called the good form of cholesterol because it removes the waxy cholesterol from the blood. LDL forms of cholesterol are bad because these forms clog arteries by forming cholesterol plaques. Lipoprotein(a) is not routinely measured but is now known to be the worst form of cholesterol. Partially hydrogenated fats also known as trans-fats (trans-fatty acids) as found in shortenings, margarines, and many foods are the major culprits that elevate blood levels of lipoprotein (a)[Tables 5-4 and 5-5].

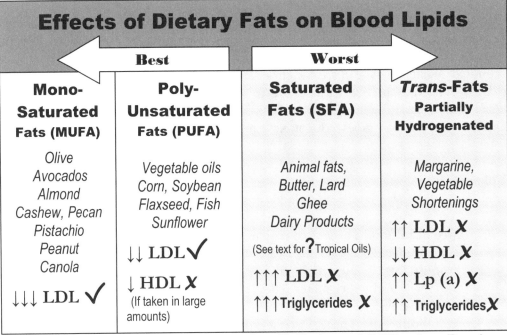

HDL—High Density Lipoprotein or "Good" Cholesterol; LDL—Low Density Lipoprotein or "Bad" Cholesterol; Lp(a)—Lipoprotein(a)or "Very Bad Cholesterol.

Figure 5-7. A Summary of the Effects of Dietary Fats on Blood Lipids: (HDL, LDL, and Triglycerides).

All fats can fatten, but all fats are not bad. Vegetable oils are healthier than animal fats, but vegetable shortenings and margarine (both made from vegetable oils and contrary to previous beliefs), are the worst (Figure 5-7). The method of extracting oils from plants and the subsequent methods of processing can exert have important health implications. Harsher extraction methods can result in the production of unhealthy chemical changes in fats.

After decades of indulging in high PUFA fats foods, researchers discovered that these PUFA alternatives are not as good as previously thought. PUFAs lower the protective HDL cholesterol if taken in excess amounts. To make matters worse, the harsh industrial processes used to extract more oil at high temperatures cause oils to chemically change from the natural cis-form to an unnatural, unhealthy trans- or partially hydrogenated form (Figure 5-7).[80] These are the now-infamous trans-fats or trans-fatty acids.

Table 5-4. Major Food Sources of Trans-Fatty Acids (TFAs)

Food Sources	TFAs (g/dl)	Relative Concentration
Fried foods	0.8	++++++++
Margarine (stick)	0.5	+++++
Breads (commercial)	0.3	+++
Cakes and related baked goods	0.3	+++
Savory snacks	0.3	+++
Margarine, soft and spreads	0.2	++
Cookies	0.2	++
Milk	0.2	++
Butter	0.1	+
Crackers	0.1	+
Household shortenings	0.1	+
Ground beef	0.1	+

Modified from sources below. Note: Partially Hydrogenated Fats on food labels refer to Trans-fatty acids. Values were based on the results of the 1989-1991 CSFII of the USDA, and the TFA composition data was adapted from Nutrient Data Bank Bulletin Board (USDA). Position Paper on trans-fatty acids. ASCN/AIN Task force on trans-fatty acids. American Society for Clinical Nutrition and American Institute of Nutrition. American Journal of Clinical Nutrition,1996. [82-83]

During industrial manufacturing of oils, they are subjected to a process called deodorization, the last step in the refining of vegetable oils. This process, in addition to converting oils into margarine and shortening, also transformed the natural cis-forms of the fat into unnatural of trans-forms of MUFAs and PUFAs. This is the process of hydrogenation or the hardening of vegetable oils. Hardened vegetable oils provide improved texture and storage of food products. Initially, these were believed to be better alternatives to butter and lard, and therefore became popular in the food processing industry:[81]

> The amount of *trans*-fatty acids in the American diet has progressively risen as the food industry has responded to consumer demands for products with

less saturated fat. The amount of *trans*-fatty acids in margarines ranges from 10% to 30% of total fat and often exceeds 25% in cookies, crackers, pastries, and deep-fried foods such as French fries and doughnuts.

They are not found in natural foods or oils made using "cold pressed" methods. Trans-fats are found in partially hydrogenated or hydrogenated oils—the most commonly used fats in the food processing industry. It is difficult to escape consuming these trans-fats in today's supermarkets. Trans- or partially hydrogenated fats are almost everywhere. Common sources of trans- or partially hydrogenated fats are listed in Table 5-4 and 5-5.[81-83]

Table 5-5. Trans-fatty acid content of common foodstuffs

Food Sources	Trans-Fatty Acids(grams)
Animal Products	
Beef (5 oz)	0.9
Butter (1 tsp)	0.1
Chicken (5 oz)	0.1
Pork (5 oz)	0.1
Vegetable Fats	
Reduced-calorie mayonnaise (1 tsp)	0.01
Soft margarine (1 tsp)	0.27[a]
Stick margarine (1 tsp)	0.62[a]
Vegetable oil (1 tsp)	0.02[a]
Vegetable shortening	0.63
Commercial and Fast-Food products	
Cake (1 piece)	1.04[a]
Cookie (1)	0.86[a]
Corn chips (1 oz)	1.42[a]
Cracker (1)	0.12[a]
Danish pastry (1)	3.03[a]
Doughnut (1)	3.19
Deep-fat french fries	
Large order (4 oz)	5.5
Small order (2.5 oz)	3.6
Muffin	0.09[a]
Pie (1 piece)	1.00[a]
Pizza (1 slice)	0.13[a]
Potato chips (1 oz)	0.11[a]

Source: *New England Journal of Medicine* [81,89]
[a]The grams listed represent the average of several brands.

Consumption of foods high in trans-fats have four major negative health effects (Figure 5-7): They elevate the levels of artery-clogging LDL cholesterol and triglycerides; they reduce the levels of artery-clearing HDL cholesterol; and to make matters worse, they also raise the level of an aggressive type of artery-clogging cholesterol found in lipoprotein(a).[84-87]

Professor Walter Willet and colleagues from Harvard showed from the Nurses' Health Study, that women with the highest intake of trans-fats exhibited the highest rate of heart attacks:[88]

> In the Nurses' Health Study, women with the highest intake of *trans*-fatty acids from processed vegetable fats assessed in 1980 experienced the highest risk of MI (myocardial infarction or heart attack) during the next eight years. When those women whose intake of margarine had greatly increased or decreased over the previous 10 years were excluded, the risk was nearly 80 percent higher for those in the highest 20 percent of intake compared to those with the lowest 20 percent.

Kathleen Koehler Ph.D. of the Food and Drug Administration (FDA) estimated that removing all the trans-fats from margarine and reducing, by 3 percent, the current levels of trans-fats in baked foods could prevent more than 17,000 heart attacks and in excess of 5,000 deaths annually. Prevention of heart attacks could save between 3 billion and 8 billion dollars annually."[90]

Although proposals have been forwarded to declare foods as "free of trans-fats" or the specific trans-fatty acids content of foods, manufacturers are still not required by law to do so. Updates on this evolving debate can be monitored at the Food Labeling and Nutrition page of the U.S. Food and Drug Administration's Center for Food Safety and Applied Nutrition: http://vm.cfsan.fda.gov/~dms/lab-cat.html.

The call is for better alternatives to trans-fats. The case for tropical oils has already been issued a guilty verdict in North America and Europe, but there is great need to re-examine the evidence. A recent Netherlands's study has resurrected the claim of many in the tropics who are adamant that tropical oils have been given a bad rap.

Tropical Oils (coconut and palm oils):
Are they as bad as some believe?

Populations in the tropics have subsisted on heavy intakes of coconut products for centuries *without* suffering high rates heart disease as their European and American counterparts.
The traditional production of tropical oils is far different from the harsh industrial production methods used to extract, refine, and deodorize tropical oils.
African red palm oil is one of the richest sources of beta-carotene (preformed vitamin A)—about 15 times that found in carrots.[91]

The kernel of coconuts and other nut-bearing palms contain a lot of fat. Fifty years ago, copra (the fatty dried kernel of coconuts) and copra oils was a major industry in many Caribbean and Pacific countries. These used to be the prime source of oils for the soap industry. Copra production has since plummeted due to competition from cheaper oils. But there has been resurgence in the export of these oils from the tropics as manufacturers found that they possessed properties that are desirable in the food processing industry.

Tropical oils used in the industry in the United States and Europe are not the same as tropical oils made at home or in simple cottage industries. The tropical oils that are demonized as "bad saturated fat" in the North America are arguably very different from tropical oils made using simple traditional methods. Traditionally-made coconut oil possesses a characteristic smell and a distinctive taste. These oils extracted from the kernel of various palms (coconut, palm, cohune) are made using the simple extraction method of grating and boiling. There is an even simpler method to extract the cream (coconut cream). Coconut cream (containing the emulsified, water soluble oil) is extracted by grating the hard kernel of the coconut and squeezing out the cream with nothing but a good pair of hands, a cloth strainer, and water.

People use coconut and its oils in so many dishes, very similar to the way the Greeks use their olive oil—they consumed lots of it ... until the verdict from North America declared that it was "bad." Its consumption has consequently declined—quite markedly. Ironically, these populations that historically exhibited relatively low rates of cardiovascular diseases (while indulging in coconut oil and coconut products), now find themselves with an oil-change, and a new burden of chronic diseases.

Coconut oils possess a unique composition and are among nature's richest sources of medium- and short-chained fatty acids. The major fatty acids in coconut oil are lauric (12:0) acid (45-50%), myristic (14:0) acid (15%), palmitic (16:0) acids (10%), capric (10:0) acid (7%) and caprylic (8:0) acid (8%). The details of these numbers (14:0 and 10:0 etc.) are outside the scope of this book, but they refer to the length of the chain-link or backbone of carbon atoms found in every fatty acid.[92] The smaller the number (e.g. 12:0) the shorter the chain and the more water-soluble it is. This is why the fats in a coconut can be extracted from the grated kernel using only water (coconut milk).

What is the significance of this? As a general rule, the fatty acids of plants are of the polyunsaturated or monounsaturated variety. These are heart healthy as they lower the bad LDL cholesterol (Figure 5-7). Uniquely among plants, and for reasons unknown to me, the oils of coconuts are of the saturated variety, but they behave very differently from the long-chain saturated fatty acids found in animal fats. Saturated fats from animals elevate blood levels of LDL-cholesterol and triglycerides (Figure 5-7). The question is—does coconut oil do the same?

Medium- and short-chained fatty acids (MCTs for short) are water soluble and handled very differently than animal fats. After absorption MCTs enter directly into the blood stream (and not via the special lymph channels designed for the transport of water-insoluble animal fats), and are immediately available as a source of energy. They do not place the same stresses on our metabolism like animal fats.[93-97] MCTs are, for these same reasons, used in those intravenous feeding solutions.

In 1987, the FDA submitted a bill to the U.S. House of Representatives to label all foods containing coconut oil (tropical oil) as "saturated fat" (meaning "bad: fat). The bill was opposed because the special committee (that was appointed to investigate) emphasized that the potential effect of any single fat source must be viewed within the context of the total diet. In fact, they showed that coconut oil in the normal diet had a neutral effect. It neither lowered nor raised blood cholesterol levels. According to a 1988 report (in *Cajanus*—a respected Caribbean publication) by Professor George L. Blackburn M.D. from Harvard, There is a noteworthy twist to the coconut oil debate:[98]

> How did the vendetta against coconut oil started? Coconut oil was known as pure saturated oil. It was cheap, and easy to use in animal experiments to investigate the basic science of atherosclerosis (narrowing of the arteries). While such experiments were helpful in these investigations, they bear no relationships to the topic of a healthy heart diet.

Whenever I discuss this subject with my colleagues in the UK or the U.S, they quote studies done in mice. It is true that these show clogging of the arteries, but there is enough grounds to say, not only were these studies different from the real picture in humans, but the oils that masquerade as coconut oil in laboratories and factories are not the same as home-made coconut oil. Home-made coconut oil cannot be stored for any long period, it goes rancid rather quickly. A recent study (2001) by a group from the Netherlands even considered coconut and palm oils as better substitutes than the commonly used shortenings in the food processing industry:[99]

> Consumption of a solid fat rich in lauric acid [from coconut or palm kernel oils] gives a more favorable serum lipoprotein [cholesterol] pattern than consumption of partially hydrogenated soybean oil rich in *trans*-fatty acids. Thus, solid fats rich in lauric acids, such as tropical fats, appear to be preferable to *trans*-fats in food manufacturing, where hard fats are indispensable.

The closing argument is this: Coconut oil is not the healthiest oil, but it is nowhere near the villain that it has been purported to be. Therefore coconut oil deserves an apology, or at least a new trial (using humans, not mice; and using the peculiar-smelling, home-made coconut oil, not the generic-refined-deodorized-industrial or laboratory version).

Another maligned tropical produce is the avocado (*Persea gratissima* or *P. americana*). This native of Mexico and Central America is becoming increasing popular in North America for use in salads and guacamole recipes. In Latin America, there is a rumor that it is high in cholesterol. Nothing could be further from the truth. Avocadoes have a high fat content that gives its smooth and sometimes buttery texture, giving rise to the nickname "butter-pear". No fruit has a fat profile closer to that found in olives. The major fat in avocados is oleic acid, a monosaturated fat; 60 percent of its oils are in this form compared to 72 percent in olives (Figure 5-7).[77]

Meaty Matters

Meats have been considered as the best source of protein, but high meat consumption has been linked to a variety of chronic diseases. It is best to obtain protein from plants, sea food, and lean poultry.

There are those who are quick to point to the sins of the modern food industry, the health concerns over saturated fat, and the use and abuse of hormones (and antibiotics) as grounds on which to discourage meat consumption altogether. Many justifiably decry the use of minced animal parts and entrails (bone meal) to feed livestock and its connection to mad cow disease or bovine spongiform encephalopathy (BSE, see Chapter 7, "Organic Foods, Alarm over Mad Cow Disease)[100]

Are our bodies designed to handle animal products? To put it another way, does the way we consume meat help or hurt our health? Historically, many societies embrace the belief that meat makes us stronger. Deep inside our psyche, we associate strength and dominance with the meat-eaters. Lions and the tigers are the kings of the jungle as sharks and the barracudas are the captains of the seas. They are dominant, and they are all meat eaters.

In many societies, meat consumption has important historical and socio-economic significance. As people moved up the socio-economic ladder, it was reflected in the type of foods they consumed. In tribal cultures, higher status is given to those who possess more cattle. The "fatted calf" was a sign of blessing in Mesopotamian and Judaic cultures. Meat consumption remains a luxury in many countries. In such societies, only the rich eat meat on a daily basis. To compensate for this desire for meat, meat-like vegetarian cuisines made from lentils, egg plant, tomatoes and avocados serve as the "poor man's meat." The premium placed on meat consumption in Western and some traditional societies has been heavily influenced by social, cultural, and religious perspectives.

How much meat should we eat? The USDA pyramid recommends two to three servings of meat per day but critics of the pyramid say the scientific evidence supporting this is misplaced.[101]

> The USDA Pyramid serves up as equals, red meat, poultry, fish, eggs, beans, and nuts. All are excellent sources of protein. But red meat is a poor protein package because of all the saturated fat and cholesterol that come along. Red meat may give you too much iron in a form you absorb whether you need it or not. Chicken and turkey give you less saturated fat

The average person needs only between 21 and 65 grams of protein daily, or an average of 50 grams daily to maintain bodily requirement.[102] This equates to hardly more than a single chicken breast to meet the entire daily protein requirement. Americans consume 250 to 450 grams of protein daily, several times above the average daily requirement.[102]

Dr. Russell Chittenden (1909) at Yale University argued that excess protein intake above the body's needs means extra work for the liver and the kidneys to rid the body of the excess protein breakdown products.[103] The German scientist Rubner advised his countrymen to invest in large herds of cattle and sheep in place of cereal production in the years leading up to World War I. Rubner believed that a high meat protein promoted physical superiority and increased vigor. This mistake led to serious food shortages during the Allied blockade of 1917. An acre of farmland produces six times more energy if cereals are grown instead of grazing cattle.[104]

Not all protein sources are the same. They vary in grade and quality. A higher protein quantity in a food does not necessarily mean that it is of a better quality. Many erroneously believe that animal proteins are complete and plant and vegetable protein are incomplete. This has led to the belief that animal sources are superior to plant sources. Generally speaking, animal protein provides higher levels of essential amino acids than plant sources, but all foods, both plant and animal, have protein. Vegetarians can easily get their complete daily protein requirements of high grade proteins by consuming a wide variety of legumes, cereals, and grains. High meat consumption concomitantly increases the intake of saturated fat which is a known contributor to high blood LDL cholesterol levels[105] (Figure 5-7 and Table 5-6).

High protein intakes of both animal and vegetable origin can lead to significant losses of calcium from the body. With every gram of protein consumed in adults, there is a 1 milligram increase in urinary losses of calcium. A similar effect is seen following consuming high-sodium foods. High meat (animal protein) and dairy product consumption increase losses of calcium from the bones and the urine. Calcium losses increase by 50 percent when dietary protein intake is doubled. This has implications for osteoporosis (thinning of the bones), an important public health problem in the elderly, especially in the industrialized world. It is important to note that the highest rates of osteoporosis are found in high meat eating and dairy consuming countries, i.e. industrialized western societies.[106-109]

Table 5-6. Typical Composition of Some Meats (raw)
per 3.5 oz. (100 grams) of Edible Material

Meat		Calories	Fat (grams)	Protein (grams)
Beef	Lean	123	4.6	20.3
	Fat	637	66.9	8.8
Lamb	Lean	162	8.8	20.8
	Fat	671	71.8	6.2
Pork	Lean	147	7.1	20.7
	Fat	670	71.4	6.8
Chicken Meat only		121	4.3	20.5
Meat & Skin		230	17.7	17.6
Turkey Meat only		107	2.2	1.9
Meat & Skin		145	6.9	20.6

Source: D.A. T Southgate. Human Nutrition and Dietetics (1993).[105]

Concerns over the safety of meat will continue to spur debate. Many have responded by becoming vegetarians, citing health, philosophical, or religious objections. Others have opted for organic meats which employ traditional animal rearing methods. The choice is yours, but the balance is clearly in favor of eating less meat protein and using plant-based substitutes. The Western diet is guilty of consuming too much meat at the expense of healthier alternatives.

Poultry

Most of the fats in poultry are located in their skins and the bone marrow, so the practice of eating chicken skins and chewing their bones are significant contributors of high blood cholesterol and triglyceride levels.

Poultry products (chicken, turkeys, ducks, geese, and ostrich) have less fat in their muscles compared to beef, lamb and pork (Table 5-6). Ducks and geese have more fat than chicken. Because chicken is the number one meat consumed in many countries, the way chicken is prepared for consumption has important health complications. In the commercial preparation of fried chicken, the use of the re-heated oils (see Chapter 7) and vegetable shortening can raise blood cholesterol and triglyceride levels.[105] Consuming chicken skin and the popular use of high-fat batters for baking and frying are not recommended.

Many are at odds with the poultry industry citing the same food safety concerns (rearing practices, the use of hormones and antibiotics) voiced about the meat industry.

Seafood

Seafoods are a good source of low-fat protein. Fatty fish (salmon, sardines, mackerel, and herring) have a special kind of fat called omega-3 or (n-3) fat that protects against heart disease, blood clots, inflammation, and age related diseases. Shellfish (shrimp, lobster, and mollusks) are the lowest in fat, despite their relatively higher cholesterol content.

Fish and marine products tend to be low in fat. Fatty fish, whose oils consist largely of omega-3 fats called docosahexanoic acid (DHA) and eicosapentanoic acid (EPA), have both been shown to protect against heart disease. Fatty fish are easily identified by their darker colored flesh. The list includes sardines, salmon, herring, mackerel, ocean jack, and tuna (Table 5-7). White fish are so called because of the appearance of the flesh which contains very little fat.   They include the bulk of commonly consumed fish. [110-112]

Table 5-7. Composition of Some Fish (White and Fatty Varieties)
per 3.5 oz. (100 grams) Edible Matter

Fish	Calories	Fat (grams)	Protein (grams)
Cod (white fish)	76	0.7	17.4
Haddock (white fish)	73	0.6	16.8
Catfish (white fish)	90	2.7	16.1
Perch (white fish)	84	1.3	18.1
Herring (fatty fish)	234	16.8	16.8
Mackerel (fatty fish)	223	19.0	19.0
Salmon (fatty fish)	182	18.8	18.8

Source: D.A. T Southgate. Human Nutrition and Dietetics (1993).[105]

The percentage of fat found in these fish vary widely depending on their breeding cycles and the method of preparation. Canned tuna, for example, is a poor source of fish oils (0.5 g per 100 mg portion) compared to fresh tuna (9.9 g per 100 mg portion). Much of the healthy fish oil is lost during preparation. The Western diet is also guilty of insufficient fish consumption. Regular fish consumption has been associated with lower rates of heart disease.[113]

A popular misconception is that shellfish (shrimp, lobster, crayfish, oysters, and conch) consumption is a major culprit for elevating blood cholesterol levels. Shellfish, as a rule, are characteristically low in total fat content and saturated fat. Shellfish contain relatively higher levels of cholesterol (Table 5-8), but the relationship between dietary cholesterol intake and its influence on blood cholesterol level is an often misunderstood story.

Concern exists over the accumulation of trace elements and heavy metal contaminants in fish. These issues have become more relevant as our oceans and waterways have become more polluted as a direct result of increasing industrialization and population pressures. A recent report from the Physician's Health Study did not support the fears over mercury intake, fish consumption, and heart disease.[114,115]

Table 5-8. Content of 3.5 oz (100 g) portions of raw shellfish

Shellfish	Calories	Saturated Fat	Cholesterol
Mollusks			
Clams	74	.09	34
Octopus	82	.23	48
Oysters (Eastern)	69	.63	55
Scallops	88	.08	33
Squid	92	.36	233
Crustaceans			
Dungeness Crab	86	.13	59
Lobster (Spiny)	112	.24	70
Shrimp	106	.33	152

Source: D.A. T Southgate. Human Nutrition and Dietetics (1993).[105]

Misunderstandings about Dietary Cholesterol

It is not cholesterol in food that elevates blood cholesterol. It is the saturated (animal) fats, and the trans-fats (margarines, shortenings, and processed foods) that are chiefly responsible. Therefore … Do not be fooled by food labels which yell, "No Cholesterol!"

Dietary cholesterol is strictly an animal product. You will not find cholesterol in plant products except when these products are prepared using animal fats. It is important to understand that the biggest contributor to blood cholesterol is the consumption of saturated fats and trans- or partially -hydrogenated fats.[116]

At the current levels of intake (200 to 500 mg daily), dietary cholesterol has minimal effect on raising blood cholesterol levels. This is especially true if saturated fat intake is also low. Based on dietary studies, there is only a 2.2 mg per deciliter rise in blood cholesterol levels for every 100-mg rise in dietary cholesterol. At higher levels of cholesterol intake (more than 800 mg daily), especially if the diet is also high in saturated fat, blood cholesterol levels rise proportionally.[78,79] The current recommendation by the National Cholesterol Education Program (NCEP)) is that Americans should consume less than 300 mg of cholesterol daily.[117]

Since cholesterol is found only in animal products, and since high meat intakes are linked to cardiovascular diseases and cancer, it is recommended to reduce the intake of high cholesterol-containing foods. Questions on high blood cholesterol often arise over eggs, crustaceans (shrimp, lobster, crayfish, crab), and mollusks (conch, squid, oyster). The flesh of crustaceans and mollusks are characteristically very low in fat (Table 5-8). Although some of these foods are relatively high in cholesterol, they are not as heart-unhealthy as many have been led to believe.

There is a small group of people, whose cholesterol levels respond markedly to dietary cholesterol (the hyper-responders). Such individuals are best advised to avoid high cholesterol foods, especially if they suffer from high blood cholesterol levels, even if they have no cardiovascular complications.[78]

Milk and Dairy Products

Man is the only creature that insists on drinking milk beyond the age of infancy. We have been led to believe we will be worse off if we don't get our calcium from milk/dairy products, but *half* of all hip fractures resulting from osteoporosis occur in North America and Europe—the very countries where people consume the most meat, milk, and dairy products.[109]

Cooper C, Campion G, Melton LJ 3rd. Hip fractures in the elderly: a world-wide projection.
Osteoporosis International. 1992 Nov;2(6):285-9.

Most of us grew up believing that milk is the perfect food. After all, it (breast milk) is the only food needed until we are about six months old. Milk packs all the nutrients that mammals need for growth and development. However, breast milk as a food for infants and growing children, and cow's milk as food for fully-grown adults, are two different scenarios.

The dairy industry piggybacks on our infantile rendezvous with milk and takes it even further. The "Got Milk?" campaign is in full swing. If you believe certain sources, even adults cannot survive well without milk. This of course is not true, as well as the widely held impression that the best and healthiest source of calcium is milk and dairy products.

The scare in the industrialized West over calcium and osteoporosis has caused leading experts like Walter Willett, M.D. of the Harvard School of Public Health to declare, "Calcium: No Emergency." The thinning of the bones (osteoporosis) is related to factors that have little to do with calcium intake. According to Dr. Willett, increased dairy product consumption have never convincingly led to increased bone mass in adults.[118] Studies on increasing milk and dairy consumption have shown no benefit, and sometimes, even a paradoxical increase in osteoporosis.[119]

> Some populations have low fracture rates despite minimal dairy product consumption and low overall calcium intake by adults. Milk and other dairy products may not be directly equivalent to calcium from supplements as these foods contain a substantial amount of protein, which can enhance renal [kidney] calcium losses.

Casual observation has triggered a commonsense question, "From where do herbivores (cows, horses etc.) get calcium for their strong bones and teeth? It is obvious that they get it from plants. They are herbivores. It is true that our digestive systems differ from theirs, but then how do you explain why half the fractures resulting from osteoporosis, occur in North America and Europe—known for their higher intakes of milk and dairy products? Please do not blame it on their genetics or some other obscure reason. Furthermore, the most recent studies actually show that the rates of osteoporosis have begun to rise in China and Japan. This new trend has nothing to do with milk or dairy products, and everything to do with Westernization of their diets and their lifestyles. Therefore, if you want strong bones, follow those diets and lifestyle patterns that have a proven track record of low osteoporosis rates (see Chapter 8 and Chapter 9). You will be better off consuming plenty of greens (mustard, kale, bok choy, broccoli, almonds, and collard) and getting much needed resistance exercises.[109, 120-128]

The composition of milk, with its high calcium and high fat concentrations is designed with babies in mind. Milk is the only food they need until they are weaned. It is packed with much calcium because this is precisely what is needed for growing bones and teeth. The extra fat provides much needed calories during this phase of rapid growth. None of the aforementioned applies to fully grown adults. The fat, and possibly calcium, can do harm. There are scientific grounds to link high calcium and high protein intakes to increased risk of prostate cancer, and quite possibly, osteoporosis (see under "Milk, Dairy Products, and Prostate Cancer, and "Meaty Matters"). Excess dairy fat also elevates blood cholesterol and triglyceride levels.

Fresh cow's milk averages 4 percent fat by weight. Milk-fat gives milk its creamy texture. The amount of fat in milk varies according to the species as shown in Table 5-9, but milk-fat is predominantly of the saturated variety. This is what gives us butter. Low fat alternatives to full-cream milk have become increasing popular with increasing consumer demand. Semi-skimmed milk is 2 percent fat and skimmed milk is virtually fat-free (0.1 percent fat).[129]

Table 5-9. Composition of Milks of different species (per 100 mg)

Constituent	Human	Cow	Goat	Sheep	Camel	Buffalo
Water (g)	88.2	87.8	88.9	83.0	88.8	83.3
Energy	.	.	.	.	.	.
Calories	69	66	60	95	63	92
Kilojoules	289	276	253	396	264	385
Protein (g)	1.3	3.2	3.1	5.4	2.0	4.1
Fat (g)	4.1	3.9	3.5	6.0	4.1	5.9
Lactose (g)	7.2	4.6	4.4	5.1	4.7	5.9
Calcium (g)	34	115	100	170	94	175

Adapted from FAO (1972); Paul and Southgate (1978); Holland et al. (1989).

Milk, Dairy Products, and Prostate Cancer

When New York mayor Rudy Giuliani was diagnosed with prostate cancer, a row erupted over anti-milk billboards showing the mayor with a "milk moustache." The words "Got Prostate Cancer?" was emblazoned over these ads. The billboard was in poor taste with no "milk of human kindness," but it may have served to highlight a debate that has been all but ignored by the mainstream scientific community and the public in general.[130]

In an article titled, "Calcium and milk and prostate cancer: a review of the evidence," that appeared in the journal *Prostate*, Edward Giovannucci, M.D. and colleagues of the Harvard School of Public Health, presented data on the connection between milk and dairy consumption, and the risk of developing prostate cancer:[131]

> Milk consumption was associated with a 5-fold increase in the relative risk of prostate cancer … Epidemiologic studies, based on inter- or intranational comparisons, and case-control and cohort designs tend to support a positive association between milk or diary consumption and a

higher risk of total, advanced, or fatal prostate cancer. This relatively consistent finding in diverse settings, the use of a variety of study designs, and the lack of other confounding factors indicate that this association is causally attributable to milk or dairy product consumption.

Prostate cancer is the commonest cancer in men. The strongest dietary link to prostate cancer is the consumption milk and dairy products. The Health Professionals Follow-up Study looked at the relationship between diet, lifestyle, and health in more than 50,000 male health professionals between ages 40 to 75. In this study, milk drinkers exhibited almost twice the rate of advanced prostate cancer compared to non-milk drinkers. Although these studies do not "prove that altering milk or dairy consumption would change a man's risk of prostate cancer," some researchers express fears that high levels of calcium in milk (especially at intakes exceeding 2,000 milligram per day) can suppress 1,25-dihydroxy-vitamin D levels—the active form of circulating vitamin D. This form of vitamin D normally exerts a protective effect against prostate cancer. If its levels are reduced, this may lower the body's ability to protect against prostate cancer. This issue is of public health concern, especially in the light of the "Got Milk?" campaign that trumpets milk as the best source of dietary calcium.[132-137]

Cured, Smoked, and Charcoal-Grilled Meats

Cured meats and meats prepared by smoking, barbecuing, or grilling are high in nitrites, polycyclic aromatic hydrocarbons (PAHs), and heterocyclic amines (HCAs).
These are all potent carcinogens.

Concerns have been expressed over a group of naturally-occurring nitrogen compounds called nitrates, nitrites, and N-nitrosodimethylamine (NDMA). Their chief sources are plant foods, water, air, cigarette smoke, alcoholic beverages (dark beer), pesticides, car interiors, and cosmetics. More than 80 percent of all dietary nitrates come from vegetables, including potatoes. Nitrites are mainly from cured meat products (bacon, ham, sausages), and NDMA are obtained from cured meats, smoked, and salted fish. Dietary nitrates, nitrites and NDMA can be converted in the stomach to N-nitroso compounds (e.g. nitrosamines) that are potent carcinogens (cancer-causing substances).[69-72]

In the food industry, sodium nitrite is an important preservative for preventing botulism, a deadly form of food poisoning (see this chapter under "Too Many Highly Processed Foods." Population studies on the role of nitrosamines in stomach cancer reported a high incidence in Japan, the Korean peninsula, and Costa Rica where volcanic agricultural soils are rich in nitrates. Consumption of large amounts of smoked or grilled meats may lead to significantly higher levels of stomach cancer.

Charcoal grilling, broiling, and cooking meats at high temperatures impart flavor, but unfortunately causes the formation of heterocyclic amines (HCAs). These are generated from the scorching of proteins in the meat. HCA production is greatest within the burnt or charred areas—the more charring that occurs, the greater the development of HCAs.[66-67]

There is another process that takes place during barbecuing. When fatty portions of meat (including skins) are used, the fat melts and then drips unto the hot coals. Combustion of this fat creates polyaromatic hydrocarbons (PAHs). The newly generated PAHs get vaporized and then are absorbed unto the surface of the meat. Therefore, eating the charred outer areas can spell double trouble—increased levels of both HCAs and PAHs. It is said that an 8-ounce charred steak can contain as much HCAs and PAHs as you can get from smoking two packs of cigarettes. Even the smoke arising from such barbecues are not without their hazards, vaporized PAHs are said to be plentiful in smoke that arises from a barbecue.

Excess Sodium; Reduced Potassium and Magnesium

Small amounts of sodium occur naturally in foods. Almost 80 percent of sodium is added to food during commercial processing or preparation either at home or in a restaurant.

U.S. Dietary Guidelines (1995)

There was a time when salt (table salt/sodium chloride) used to dominate the nutrition debate. This stemmed from its relationship to hypertension—a major risk factor for heart attack and stroke. Almost 1 in 4 U.S. adults are hypertensive. The figure is higher in minority groups, immigrant populations and people of lower socioeconomic status.

In the average Western diet, there is a gross imbalance in the intake of sodium compared to a similar, but competing mineral called potassium. Higher intakes of processed foods at the expense of fresh fruits and vegetables are the primary cause of this imbalance. Salt that is added during processing (hidden salt) can tremendously increase the intake of sodium, leading to a disturbance of the sodium/potassium ratio.[138] Fruits and vegetables contain relatively little sodium, but are rich in potassium. We say that these foods have a low sodium-high potassium ratio. On the contrary, processed foods with added sodium can have a disturbingly higher sodium/potassium ratio. The recommendation is to eat more foods with low sodium-high potassium ratios. To do this you don't need to shop with a sodium-potassium checker in hand, all you need is to eat more fresh fruits and vegetables, and minimize your intake of highly processed foods. This is what will deliver the best sodium-potassium intake (see Chapter 7).

Consuming fresh plant based foods provides you with much more potassium than sodium. A fresh 5-ounce tomato can provide 10 milligrams of sodium, but processed tomato paste (5 oz) may contain 800 mg of sodium or a can of tomato juice 1200 mg of sodium (see Chapter 7, "Processing and the Nutritional Value of Foods"). Popular foods like cornflakes do great injustice to the sodium/potassium ratio. In fresh corn, the ratio of potassium to sodium is about 9 to 1; in corn flakes, the ratio is completely reversed. Higher sodium intakes also lead to increased urinary losses of calcium. This may be yet another contributor to the higher rates of osteoporosis in Western societies.[107-109]

Hypertension is, in part, a disease of civilization. Many societies throughout the world, as exemplified by the Yi farmers of southwestern China, exhibit little or no change in blood pressure as they age. However, when they migrated to urban environments, it was accompanied by a steep rise in their blood pressures. The so-called primitive diet with little or no processed foods, along with high levels of physical activity was their insurance against the health ravages of civilization.[139]

Magnesium is an important but often overlooked mineral that is plentiful in green leafy vegetables. Plants are green because of the green pigment chlorophyll, and you can't have chlorophyll without magnesium. Therefore, plentiful intakes of such foods deliver plenty of magnesium. This mineral contributes to lower blood pressure and reduced insulin requirements.[140]

Many societies indulge in salted foods, especially salt-cured or brine-preserved meats (beef, pork tails, etc.), salted fish, and pickled vegetables. Animal experiments show that excessive salt can promote stomach cancer. Japan, Korea, parts of China, and Latin America consume more pickled foods and suffer higher rates of stomach cancer and stroke than their counterparts in the United States.[141-145]

Too Much Alcohol: Weighing Risks and Benefits

The French Paradox and a Paradox

The French Paradox refers to the observation of low rates of heart disease in France, compared to Northern and Eastern Europe where there exist some of the highest rates of heart disease in the world.

> The French custom of wines with meals, extra virgin olive oil, and generous servings of vegetables, has led to far less deaths from heart disease in France, compared to the Britain.
> However, If premature deaths (from alcohol) in France were considered, It cancels out the gains from the prevention of heart attacks.

Moderate consumption of one to two alcoholic drinks per day can reduce the risk of a heart attack by 30 to 50 percent.[120] This, however, is not the end of the story.

Alcohol can make you gain weight. The average drink contains 14 grams of ethanol or about 100 calories. The ethanol in alcoholic beverages packs a hefty 7 calories per gram.[146-151] Compare this to 3.75 calories per gram for carbohydrates, 4 calories per gram for protein, and 9 calories per gram for fat and it becomes clear that (at the proposed preventive level of 1 to 2 drinks per day) it would add an extra 1,400 calories per week to amount an already overweight population. That can translate into a weight gain of 20 pounds over a year.

On the medical front, a clear association exists between alcohol intake and cancer of the oral cavity, pharynx, larynx, esophagus, and liver. There are also suggestive associations with breast and colon cancer. The organs of the digestive system are directly exposed to the negative effects of alcohol. Excess alcohol can damage the liver, leading to cirrhosis and other complications. Heavy drinking (three or more alcoholic drinks per day) raises blood pressure and increases the risk of stroke. Alcohol excess raises blood cholesterol and triglycerides. It is not uncommon to see triglyceride levels exceeding 1000 mg/dl in heavy drinkers. These can fall dramatically following complete cessation of alcohol.

Chronic alcohol abuse increases the risk of abnormal heart rhythms and sudden cardiac death. Heavy drinkers generally exhibit other unhealthy lifestyle patterns compared to non-drinkers. Those who progress to alcoholism typically exhibit multiple nutrient deficiencies, especially that of thiamine (vitamin B_1), that can lead to heart failure and irreversible brain damage (Wernicke-Korsakoff's syndrome).

Alcohol abuse has also given rise to enormous social, financial, and medico-legal problems. Any recommendation to increase alcohol consumption with the aim of preventing new heart attacks must take into account not only these problems listed above, but also the fact that alcohol caused 750,000 more deaths globally than it prevented.[152-158]

Having spelt out the positives in the midst of so many negatives, it then becomes a question of balance. We should salute the French Paradox of low heart disease rates that accompany the French custom of wine with meals, olive oils, and wonderful salads. However, to ignore the social and public health costs associated with alcohol excess would be irresponsible. The facts are that, even in France, alcohol excess has led to premature deaths that cancel out any gains made from its prevention of heart attacks. A scientific case can be perfectly made for an individual to partake in the benefits of drinking a glass of wine with meals, or at social occasions. However, public health advice on alcohol needs to be qualified, and advice on reducing heart disease should look at the entire lifestyle. We do not want to save a heart on one hand, and create a killer on the other. That is a zero-sum game.[159-162]

Reduced Fruits, Vegetables, Greens, Grains, and Fiber

It is not a mystery why many people don't consume sufficient fruits, vegetables, nuts, and grains. The answer is simple …
They are consuming something else.
Many opt for artificially-flavored drinks in place of fresh-squeezed juices; pastries for dessert rather than fresh fruit; cole slaw and creamy salads in exchange for green salads and olive oil; and too much meat that substitutes for nuts, legumes, and whole grains.

Americans have been encouraged to eat at least five or more servings of fruit and vegetables daily. However, less than 20 percent of the populace have heeded this "Five-a-Day" call. This is the major failing of the Western diet. Many are unified in their dislike for vegetables, and even those vegetables that are consumed are either too highly processed, or are improperly prepared. The grains consumed in most popular breads, cereals, baked products, and pastries are primarily of the highly refined variety.[163,164]

Missing out on fruits and vegetables means being short-changed on the very ingredients in the diet that are consistently linked to reduced rates of chronic diseases. Increased fresh fruit and vegetable intakes are linked to lower prevalence of cardiovascular diseases, stroke, high blood pressure, and cancer. The consumption of whole grains and seeds can exert the same benefits. On the other hand, people who eat less fruits, vegetables, and whole grains exhibit higher levels of cardiovascular diseases, cancer, and type II diabetes. Low intakes of fruits and vegetables translate to less protective antioxidant vitamins, minerals, and a myriad of other health promoting ingredients. [165-171]

History and climate have skewed Western tastes towards a well-rehearsed list of fruits and vegetables from which to choose. These pale in comparison to the rich and interesting varieties bestowed to regions with warmer climates. There is not a strong historical "culture of greens and salads" in most Western countries. This is why this book advocates a Cosmopolitan Diet (see Chapter 8). The exceeding wealth of choices in fruits and vegetables around the world can be brought together into a tasty salad which we can all enjoy. The choices of fruit and salads on offer in North American supermarkets are often unimaginative, and the more interesting varieties are relatively expensive. These, together with cheap and tasty options, have led to the continuing failure of the masses to heed the call for increased fresh fruit and vegetable consumption. One thing is certain, if there are to be changes in health outcomes, things on the fruit-and-vegetable front must change. If we persist in the current patterns of consumption—this Western diet, we should expect more of the same.

Risk Charts and Tables

When you read books, magazines, or surf the Internet, you are bound to encounter charts, questionnaires, or tables that invite you to measure your risk of having a heart attack, stroke, diabetes, or cancer. These charts attempt to quantify your risk of developing these diseases over time. They do so by asking for personal information about known risk factors for these diseases, and this information is used to calculate individual risks (as percentages) for developing these diseases over time.

Some risk factors are stronger predictors of future heart attack than others. The degree of risk is multiplied when other risk factors are present. If you smoke 40 cigarettes daily, and have high cholesterol and hypertension, you have a far greater risk than a similar individual who smokes less, and has lower cholesterol and blood pressure. When the specific numbers are entered into the risk chart or table, it then quantifies your risk of developing heart disease over the next 10 years

Examples of such risk charts include the Texas Heart Institute Heart-Health Test, the American Heart Association's "My Heart Watch." These all attempt to quantify and predict (based on studies like the Framingham Study), the likelihood of developing a heart attack.[172]

Despite differences in their appearance and complexity, risk charts and tables have a number of things in common. They request information on your family history, personal history, lifestyle information, physical examination findings, and laboratory examinations. Family history gives an indication of the possible genetic tendency to have a heart attack or a stroke. Personal and lifestyle histories provide information on physical activity, smoking, and previous or current medical problems such as high blood pressure, diabetes, stroke, or heart attacks. Laboratory examinations include total blood cholesterol, HDL or good cholesterol, and LDL or bad cholesterol levels. This information completes the picture and your risk score can then be calculated.

The score given is an estimate of your future risk of having an attack over the next 10 years. Your 10-year risk can be categorized as very high (over 40 percent), high (20-40 percent), moderate (10-20 percent), mild (5-10 percent), or low (less than 5 percent). On the American Heart Association's website, "My Heart Watch" (http://www.myheartwatch.org, see "Health Tools"), the respondent is asked to enter information into the "Risk Assessment Tool" that estimates your risk of having a heart attack or dying of coronary artery disease over the next 10 years. This applies only to individuals without a previous history of diabetes or heart disease.

Interactive charts (e.g. Coronary Heart Disease Risk Charts or the Joint British Societies CHD Risk Charts) permit the user to enter personal information. Clicking on the appropriate option will lead to another window where requested information must be entered. Color-coded sections refer to different categories of risk (Figure 5-8).[173, 174] To understand how they work, log on to these websites and explore.

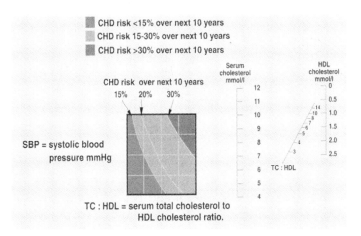

Figure 5-8. The Coronary Risk Prediction Charts 1998

from the British Cardiac Society, British Hyperlipidaemia Association, British Hypertension Society and Diabetes UK.[173] http://www.diabetes.org.uk/infocentre/inform/heart.htm

The Metabolic Syndrome
—the Insulin Resistance Syndrome

The cover of this book highlights the metabolic syndrome that affects 50 million Americans
(and multiplied millions more worldwide).
The main trigger is abdominal obesity.
People with this syndrome are prone to develop type II diabetes, lipid abnormalities, and are at increased risk of having hypertension, or dying from a heart attack or stroke.

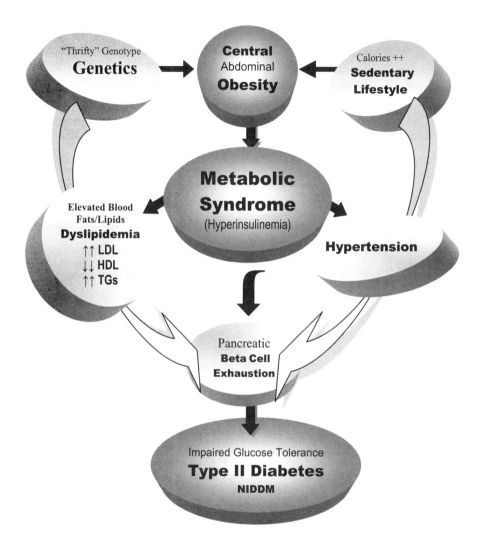

Figure 5-9. Genetics, Lifestyle, and Central Obesity leading to the Metabolic Syndrome
HDL—High Density Lipoprotein Cholesterol; LDL—Low Density Lipoprotein Cholesterol;
Lp(a)—Lipoprotein (a) cholesterol; TGs—Triglycerides.

This important syndrome was introduced at the beginning of this book (Introduction and Chapter 2). Researchers involved in the care of people with diabetes and heart disease have noted that several risk factors cluster together in the same individual. This connection between these risk factors has been named the insulin resistance syndrome or the metabolic syndrome. It was first described in 1966 by J.P. Camus[175] and coined as a syndrome (1988) by Professor Gerald Reaven, M.D. and his colleagues from Stanford University. They described a cluster of physical findings and blood test abnormalities that lead to the development of type II diabetes, and premature deaths from heart attacks and stroke.[176-198]

The metabolic syndrome has reached epidemic proportions and affects 50 million Americans. Genetic factors, abdominal obesity, the Western diet, and sedentary lifestyle are central to its development (Figures: 2-4, 5-6, and 5-9, and Table 5-10). Central or abdominal obesity results in resistance to the action of insulin. This leads to major metabolic disturbances that affect how the body handles food and virtually every bodily function. The hyperinsulinemia of the metabolic syndrome eventually leads not only to pancreatic exhaustion and type II diabetes, but also to changes within blood vessels leading to hypertension and increased risk of heart attack and stroke.

Table 5-10. Major features of the Metabolic Syndrome

Risk factors	Features
Central / abdominal obesity (Ch. 8)	"Apple-shaped," BMI ≥ 25; Waist Circumference>40 inches (men); >35 inches (women)
Elevated blood pressure	Hypertension > 130/85 mmHg
High circulating insulin levels (hyperinsulinemia)	Impaired Glucose Tolerance (IGT); Fasting Glucose > 110 mg/dl, but < 126 mg/dl; or Random Glucose > 140 mg/dl (frank Type II Diabetes)
Abnormal blood lipids (Dyslipidemia)	Low HDL-cholesterol < 40 mg/dl, (elevated LDL) Elevated Triglycerides ≥ 150 mg/dl
Elevated blood clotting factors	Fibrinogen and Plasminogen Activator Inhibitor
Elevated uric acid	Gout
Microalbuminuria (elevated protein in urine)	Increased risk of Hypertension and Kidney Failure

Purists draw a distinction between the insulin resistance syndrome and the metabolic effects of obesity, or the metabolic syndrome. They point to cases of the insulin resistance that occurs in the absence of obesity. For public health purposes, however, drawing a distinction between the two is a trifle matter. The overwhelming majority of individuals who develop the insulin resistance syndrome are obese. Obesity is the fastest-growing preventable public health problem in America and around the entire globe. This "globesity" epidemic will not be contained by doctors and hospitals. It will be arrested when we recognize that the solutions to this silent epidemic rest largely within our hands.

Beyond Risk—Towards Maximized Health

Tackling risks can add years to your life...
Going beyond risk aims to add life to your years.

Preventive medicine is not just about preventing disease. Quitting smoking, improving nutrition, and becoming physically active should not merely attempt to minimize the risk of developing cancer, heart attack or diabetes. Many people are settling just for early detection and prompt treatment when diseases arise, but there is more to prevention than this. Despite the abundance of hype and exaggerated claims for perpetual youth, good preventive measures can lead to the regain of lost health and improved quality of life.

Increased physical activity, good nutrition, and weight reduction also carry other benefits. They can relieve stress, improve body-image, improve sexual performance, and reduce your medical bills. Correcting risk factors should not only add years to your life but it can realistically improve the quality of your years (Table 5-11).[199-201]

Table 5-11. Years You May Gain By Caring For Your Heart

Risk Factor Controlled	Potential Added Years	
	Men	Women
Weight	0.7 – 1.7	0.5 – 1.1
Smoking and tobacco use	1.2 – 2.3	1.5 – 2.8
Blood Pressure	1.1 – 5.3	0.9 – 5.7
Total Cholesterol	0.5 – 4.2	0.4 – 6.3

Source: Tsevat J et al. Expected gains in life expectancy from various coronary heart disease risk factor modifications. Circulation 83, no. 4 (1991), pp. 1194- 2001. Copyright (c) 1991 American Heart Association [202]

Towards Aggressive Prevention

Simply knowing the risk factors that lead to chronic lifestyle diseases is not the goal. The real challenge is to make choices that will lead to optimal health.

Arteries never become clogged overnight. The heart is never perfect one minute and suffers a massive heart attack the next moment; the clogging of the arteries is incremental and progressive. It actually begins in childhood.

This process continues throughout subsequent decades until the clogging becomes clinically evident.[203,204] This means that by the time you read this book, you are bound to have some degree of atherosclerosis or clogging of your arteries. You don't need an angiogram to tell you this. Aggressive prevention aims not merely to reduce the risk of developing overt disease that requires hospitalization. It also involves adopting a mindset that focuses on prevention and quality of life at every stage of your life.

Summary

Risk factors increase the likelihood of developing diseases. The chronic diseases cause 7 out of every 10 deaths and more than 60 percent of all medical care costs in America. A similar pattern is developing worldwide. The major risk factors for these diseases are rooted in behavior—smoking, obesity, and physical inactivity.

The Western diet plays a major role in the genesis of all these diseases. Its major failings stem from the excessive intake of highly processed, high-calorie, high-protein, high-fat foods at the expense of fresh fruits and vegetables, nuts, and whole grains. The metabolic syndrome is the link between unhealthy lifestyles and the global epidemic of cardiovascular diseases, type II diabetes, and cancer.

The future challenge is to fix what went wrong, and to chart a new course premised on prevention and the desire for optimal health.

******

Chapter 6

Growing Older and Aging
...When the Rust Steps In

Chapter Outline

Introduction: Aging Does Not Start At 50................................211
Aging: Perceptions and Misconceptions. 212
Perceptions of Youth and Aging 213
A New Paradigm on Aging 215
Definitions of Aging...215
Aging: Chronology and Biology.......................................215
Chronological Aging..216
An Aging Society...218
Why We Age: Theories on Aging......................................219
Integrated Theories...220
The Onslaught of Free Radical Damage 220
Free Radicals and Cellular Function.................................221
Free Radicals and Cellular DNA 223
Free Radicals and Cell Membranes...................................224
Free Radicals and the Immune System 225
Free Radicals and the Cardiovascular System 226
 Blood Vessels and Cholesterol Effects 226
 The Heart, Brain, and Male Sexual Function....................229
 Smoking, Free Radicals, andthe Circulation....................230
Free Radicals and Cancer...231
The Aging Skin: Effects of Sun, Sex, and Race 231
 Sun Exposure 232
 Skin Aging and Race...232
 Skin Aging and Sex...233
Lifestyle Aging Accelerators 233
Stress and Modern Living:...234
 Killing Ourselves Trying To Make a Living......................234
Words to the Workaholic 235

Doctors in Distress 235
Personal Reflections 236
Chronic Sleep Debt: Sleep Deprivation 238
How to Know if You Have Not Slept Enough 239
The Medical Ravages of Sleep Deprivation 240
Never Too Late 241
Stop Smoking! It's Never Too late To Benefit 241
Good Nutrition Choices 242
Strengthen Those Muscles and Keep Active 243
Don't Let Your Mind Go to Waste 243
The Okinawa Formula 244
Longevity 245
Summary 247
An Ode to All Who Age 248

Although the risk of disease and disability clearly increases with advancing age, poor health is not an inevitable consequence of aging.[1]

National Center of Chronic Disease Prevention and Health Promotion
Center for Disease Control (CDC), 2001

Our culture medicalizes age, as though growing older is a disease.[2]

Bernard Lown, M.D., Professor Emeritus, Cardiology (Harvard).
Author: *The Lost Art of Healing*

"Important factors that are under people's control that they can use to live a longer, happier and physically comfortable life are not (to) smoke, not (to) abuse alcohol, (to) be in a warm and stable marriage, (to) have mature and adult coping mechanisms, (to) maintain an appropriate weight and (to) get some exercise."[3]

Kenneth Mukamal, M.D., Instructor in Medicine, Harvard Medical School.
Co-author: *Successful Aging*

§§§§§§§§

Introduction: Aging Does Not Start At 50

How we live determines how we age
Getting older is one thing, *how* we get older is another.

The words "old" or "aged" are seen by many as a distant stage in life—far off events that lie several years down the road. Such notions miss an important point if they ignore that daily choices determine future health. Paying attention to the present rather than being preoccupied with the future can have a profound impact on the way we age.

The daily decisions we make have a significant impact on our health. These daily patterns and habits are what constitute lifestyle. We grow older by the day, and getting older needs to be seen in the context of these day-to-day decisions. Added together, these processes influence how we age. They can either hasten or hinder the inevitable process of getting older. Therefore, when we speak of aging, we must remember the big picture that commences the very day we exit the womb.

Staying healthy throughout one's entire lifetime is a reasonable and achievable goal, but it is heavily contingent on choices. People can get away with reckless living during youth, but persistent neglect comes back to haunt many during their later years. What separates those who enjoy robust health in the advancing years has more to do with what was done, or not done, during the earlier years than perhaps anything else.

Successful Aging is really about Successful Living

Successful aging is not a futuristic pursuit. It is about making daily choices for better health, day by day.

No one just arrives at a destination; there is a journey that must be made. How you arrive at that destination has much to do with the nature of your preparation and the course of your journey. If you pay attention to the preparation and the course of the journey to optimum health, barring happenstance, you are slated for a successful arrival.

This view is not wishful thinking. The elderly can remain attractive and lead active and productive lives. A study done by Harvard Medical School researchers examined the physical and mental health of more than 700 men over a sixty-year period. They noted that those men who kept physically and mentally fit beyond age 50 reaped similar health dividends in their later years.[4]

Most people are not long-term planners when it comes to their health. Many are content to settle for a future that resigns its fate to Medicare and nursing homes. A mindset that entrusts its future in a healthcare system plagued by special interests and cash-strapped economies is bound to be dogged by great uncertainty. The golden years are not the time to be plagued by anxiety, depression, and worries over poor health and healthcare systems.

Aging: Perceptions and Misconceptions

Aging is often seen as an unwelcome event. Much of this is fueled by the familiar images of poor health, loss of attractiveness, and functional independence. These need not be.

When life is seen in its entirety, people are more than mere physical beings. Aging well has as much to do with outlook and attitude, as it has to do with physical health and lifestyle. Getting a good night's sleep and having a clear conscience are as important as good nutrition and regular exercise. In this chapter, the discussion will be limited to physical health with some discussion about stress, sleep deprivation, and premature aging.

There is an old riddle that describes man as having four legs in the morning, two at noon, and three at night. The three legs signify the additional need for a cane to assist with the expected physical and postural decline that frequently accompanies advanced age. This picture persists in the minds of many about the aging process.

Although it is inevitable that structures and materials corrode with time (including our bodies), becoming debilitated and diseased are not inevitable with aging.

These depressing associations with aging have lead many to dread the thought of ever becoming old. Many see aging as the loss of one's ability to make a meaningful contribution to society, the inability to enjoy life, and the loss of functional independence (Table 6-1). This has led many to overindulge during the prime of life "before the evil days draw nigh."

An encounter with an old family friend exemplified this point. Bert was known for his great sense of humor and his love of spirituous liquors. He was sorely distressed during an office visit following being diagnosed with diabetes. He had just turned fifty and said that he spent all day in bed, depressed. The cause of his depression was that 50 meant one thing—the inevitable downhill slide when everything starts going wrong.

Table 6-1. Positive and Negative Perceptions of the Aging Process

Positives	Negatives
• Experience	• Change in looks (External aging)
• Wisdom & maturity	• Change in feelings(Internal aging)
• Financial independence	• Functional changes (Loss of strength, endurance, and sexual function)
• Influence/power	• Loss of functional independence
• Maturity	• Onset of disease

Perceptions of Youth and Aging

In often subtle yet powerful ways, our culture still sends the message that growing older is a failure, something to be avoided at all costs.
Aging Gracefully[5]

Western societies have a hard time coming to terms with the process of aging. Part of this has to do with the observation that as societies become more affluent, people aspire to enjoy the fruits of their labor for as long as possible. This is a perfectly rational pursuit. With increased spending power comes the ability to have more disposable income for leisure, travel, and pampering the outward appearance. The aspiration to remain physically attractive in later years is a perfectly reasonable pursuit.

The problem begins when we lose our sense of perspective. This happens when chronological aging is scorned rather than embraced, or when undue emphasis is placed on external appearance at the expense of inward character, or when the ability to get a job rests more on how we look, rather than on who we are. When *how we look on the outside* becomes more important than *how we are on the inside*, self-deprecation and susceptibility to exploitation are likely to follow.

Today's culture adores youth and good looks. An unblemished skin and the absence of wrinkles have universal appeal, and modern societies place a high premium on such characteristics (Table 6-2). There is no shortage of products and services to treat wrinkles, cellulite, graying and balding hair, and other familiar hallmarks of aging. In an era when Hollywood and the media set the agenda in America and the world, anti-aging therapies have become a multi-billion dollar industry. People may go to great lengths and spare no expense to rejuvenate the outward appearance. Certain branches of dermatology and plastic surgery cater almost exclusively to cosmetic procedures. Pseudo-scientific claims, that peddle products purporting the reversal of aging or remaining "forty-something forever," abound. These claims typically promise far more than they can ever deliver, but as the saying goes, you can sell almost anything if you can package it well.

Many people abuse their bodies and then blame it on aging. Healthy aging is not wishful thinking. Healthy aging is heavily dependent on lifestyles. People should be able to live long and productive lives, but much of this is contingent on simple choices. In our quest for healthy aging and longevity, the challenge is to understand those aspects of aging that are amenable to behavior and lifestyle. Unfortunately, modernity and capital-driven economies have introduced unprecedented demands on the way people live. Stress and chronic sleep deprivation wreak havoc on millions. If we continue at the current trend, we are guaranteed an unwelcome harvest of an aging-sick population that will consume a disproportionate slice of the healthcare dollar. It is already a major contributor to the rising cost of healthcare in Western societies.

Table 6-2. Perceptions on Youth and Aging in Modern Culture

Desirable	Undesirable
• Youth, beauty and good looks	• Loss of attractiveness
• Attractiveness and fashion	• Frailty, debility, feebleness
• Potency	• Senility, dementias, Alzheimer's
• Peak physical performance	• Cancer and chronic diseases
• Fecundity	• Age discrimination
• Employability	• Medicare

A New Paradigm on Aging

Diseases Are Not Inevitable Consequences of Aging

A few decades ago, old age was described as "severe debilitation after age 65" and "old-old" was beyond the age of 80 or 85. The CDC has coined a new term—"healthy aging"—preventing disease and improving quality of life among older Americans.[6]

Definitions of Aging
Aging: chronology and biology

Aging begins in childhood. Pediatric cardiologists consider the first streak of fatty deposits (the fatty streak) detected on the walls of the arteries during childhood as the earliest stage of cardiovascular disease.[7] This is useful because it underscores the need to pay attention to those primary nutrition habits that begin in childhood. Tastes and preferences are acquired early in life and behavior patterns become progressively ingrained.

Others consider aging to start somewhere between 20 and 30 years old, when the body begins its gradual decline. A receding hairline or the appearance of wrinkles and grey hair are held by such proponents as a sign of the commencement of aging.

Aging can also be defined in terms of functional ability. Old age is said to have arrived when established functional deficits occur. These include a diminution in physical and reproductive capacities. If aging ensues unchecked, there arise those familiar sights (e.g. the need for a cane or a wheel chair) that predictably culminate in the loss of functional independence and the need for assisted care.

"Old" means different things in different cultures. In societies where life expectancy is low, over age 40 may be considered as old. Judeo-Christian traditions consider three score-and-ten years as old.[8] Modern western culture, which places emphasis on prolonging life, has developed specialized medical and geriatric care for the over 65s. The age bar has been raised to 78 years and above in some European countries, but prevailing attitudes largely determine what care is available in institutions.

If you live like Britain's late Queen Mother, you could get your hip replacement surgery when you are almost 100, but other prevailing norms and practices exist in other countries. In some of these, you are expressly ineligible for certain medical services such as admission to the intensive care unit if you are over age 65, or a do-not-resuscitate (DNR) order for a cardiac arrest, if you have exceeded a certain age.

Chronological Aging

As we move from infancy through childhood, adolescence, and unto adulthood, bodily functions mature and peak around ages of 20 to 25 years. Thereafter, a subtle decline in body function begins. This effect is largely unnoticed as their impact on our bodily functions is not easily measured. Normal aging (summarized in Table 6-3), can be hastened by a number of lifestyle, behavioral, and environmental factors.[9] This we can call accelerated or premature aging.

Table 6-3. Changes associated with normal aging

Gerontology:
The study of
normal aging

*studies on normal aging may be difficult, because as most people age, healthy subjects become harder to find

Gradual Decline in Body Systems

- **Skin**: loss of a elastic and supporting tissues
- **Eyes**: loss of flexibility of lens
- **Immune System**: reduced immunity
- **Cardiovascular**: reduced heart output
- **Lungs**: loss of capacity and elasticity
- **Muscular**: loss of muscle mass
- **Skeletal**: reduced bone mass and joint wear
- **Digestive**: general slowing, loss of teeth
- **Liver**: generally well preserved
- **Endocrine**: (hormones) general reduction in output
- **Metabolic**: slowed metabolic rate
- **Kidney**: reduced blood flow and elimination
- **Nervous System**: Slowed reflexes and response time

Chronic diseases most commonly manifest themselves after decades of wear and tear that occur behind the scenes. If you wait for the classic definition of hypertension laid down by the World Health Organization (blood pressure exceeding 160/90 mm Hg) before thinking about the problem, you may be decades too late. There is an incremental progression in blood pressure that took place long before it became problematic.

The same principle applies to all the chronic diseases. Type II diabetes, heart attack, and stroke become manifest only after years of underlying metabolic stresses. The metabolic syndrome, insulin resistance, and the pre-diabetic state are forerunners of the full-blown disease (see Chapter 2, "The Root of the Matter" and Chapter 5, "The Metabolic Syndrome—Insulin Resistance Syndrome"). A scheme highlighting the need for prevention and early detection of these diseases appear in Figures 6-1, 6-2 and Table 6-4.[10] These diseases do not suddenly appear out of nowhere. The trick is to look after your health long before your doctor has to look after your disease.

Progression of Diseases with Aging

Sub-Clinical
Behind-the-scenes changes
Undetectable
Detectable using special tests
Aim: **Primary Prevention** (preventing or delaying the onset of disease)

Clinical
Obvious detectable changes
Medically treatable
Aim: **Secondary Prevention** (early diagnosis and preventing complications)

Advanced Disease
Established complications & disability
Aim: **Tertiary Prevention** (damage control and rehabilitation)

Figure 6-1. A Schema for the Progression of Disease with Aging

Table 6-4: Advanced Age is a Risk Factor for Several Medical Conditions

Diseases Associated with Aging

1. **Skin:** wrinkles, sun damage, skin spots, and skin cancer
2. **Eyes:** presbyopia (reading glasses),cataracts, glaucoma, and age-related macular degeneration(AMD)
3. **Teeth:** loss of dentition and reduced fiber intake
4. **Immune System:** increased frequency and severity of infections and cancer
5. **Cardiovascular Diseases**: coronary heart disease, angina, heart attacks, high blood pressure, transient ischemic attack (TIA), stroke, and erectile dysfunction (impotence in men)
6. **Respiratory Disease:** pulmonary embolism, emphysema, lung cancer
7. **Neurological**: stroke, dementia, Alzheimer's, Parkinson's disease, and depression
8. **Musculo-Skeletal:** osteoarthritis, degenerative joint disease, osteoporosis, and fractures
9. **Endocrine:** type II diabetes, decreased sex hormones (loss of libido and impotence), and thyroid dysfunction

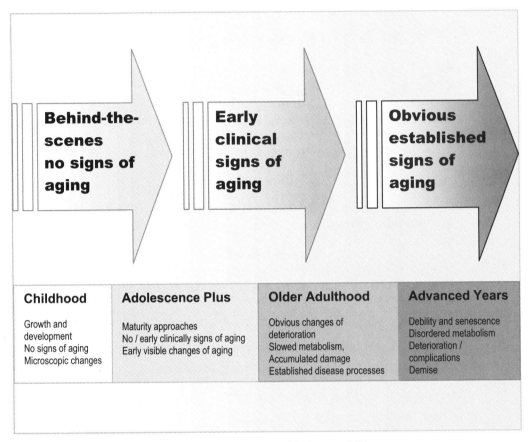

Figure 6-2. The Spectrum of Aging and Disease

An Aging Society

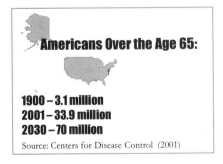

Figure 6-3. Projections for an Aging Population (United States)

According to the Center for Disease Control (CDC) in Atlanta, the demographics of the U.S. population is changing. Americans now live longer (Figure 6-3), and as the population ages, so does the cost of medical care.[11]

The United States is on the brink of a longevity revolution. Life expectancy has increased dramatically, from 47 years in 1900 to 76 years in 1990. Since 1900, the U.S. population has tripled, but the number of older adults (those aged 65 years or older) has increased 11-fold, from 3.1 million in 1900 to 33 million currently. By 2030, the number of [elderly] Americans will have more than doubled to 70 million, or one in every five Americans.

This growing elderly population now consumes a disproportionate share of the healthcare dollar (Figures 6-4 and 6-5).[12] Falling birth rates in many Western countries, concomitant with an aging-sick population, is creating a nightmarish scenario for health and financial planners. Future generations are bound to be saddled with an unbearable financial burden if the current trends persist.

Americans Over 65: Health-Related Costs

- Comprise 12% of population
- Account for 40% of acute hospital bed days
- Consume 30% of all prescriptions
- Purchase 40% of over-the-counter drugs
- Use 30% of health budget (> 65% of federal health budget)
- Nursing home beds outnumber acute hospital beds since 1972
- 40 % of those over 65 spend time in nursing home before they die
- Survivors beyond age 80, > 50% will die in nursing home

Figure 6-4. The Elderly Consume a Disproportionate Share of Healthcare Resources[10]

Snippets on aging and chronic disease

> 65% of Americans >65 years have some form of cardiovascular disease
> 50 % of all men and > 65% of all women > 70 years have arthritis
~ 40% of older adults not living in institutions, were limited by chronic conditions

Source: Center for Disease Control and Prevention (2001)

Figure 6-5. Prevalence of Chronic Disease in the Elderly:[11]

Why We Age: Theories on Aging

... Before the days of trouble come and the years approach when you will say, "I find no pleasure in them."—before the sun and the light and the moon and the stars grow dark, and the clouds return after the rain; when the keepers of the house tremble and strong men stoop ... (The Teacher) [13]

Mankind is programmed to age. The exact reasons for this have defied explanation. Even the brightest of minds and the greatest of scientists are yet to discover scientifically, why we are programmed to age. A sample of the more noteworthy explanations (theories) among their number is tabled below (Table 6-5).[14-17]

Table. 6-5 Theories on Aging

	Major Theories on Aging
Cellular	Free radical damage Changes in DNA and genetic material Interference in protein synthesis Limited cell division
Organ Systems	Progressive loss of immune (repair and defence) function Nervous system and hormone changes
Population	Simple wear and tear Rate of living and life span programming

Source: Weindruch RH, Walford RL: The Retardation of Aging and Disease by Dietary Restriction. [14]

Integrated Theories

Our bodies face numerous assaults. Free radicals continuously attack our DNA. Though our genes possess a near flawless capacity for self-repair, tiny errors invariably creep in over time and exert their negative effects on our nervous system and hormonal processes. They also interfere with our immune systems, which when weakened, invite further damage to our biochemical systems. These damages then accumulate, deterioration sets in, and the aging process hastened.

Because there is no way to completely eliminate these onslaughts (in the same way we cannot completely stop iron from rusting), let us turn our attention to how we can slow the aging process, or at least, not accelerate it. We can slow down the aging process by daily lifestyle choices. This we will investigate by looking at the most popular theory of aging—the free radical story.[18-21]

The Onslaught of Free Radical Damage

Our bodies have many enemies that continually wage war against us. Chief among them are the free radicals. It is a war that we did not ask for, but one that has to be fought.

Our ability to wage war successfully against these determined enemies depends on whether we are equipped for the battles that lie ahead. The most effective weaponry in our arsenal to defend against free radicals is the antioxidants.

In 1954, an American researcher at the University of Nebraska, Denham Harman M.D., Ph.D., coined the free radical theory of aging. In short, it states that our bodies and tissues face continual onslaughts by chemically active substances called free radicals. They chip away at our bodies and cause the changes and diseases we associate with aging. Dr. Harman based his theory on experiments that showed animals lived longer when fed antioxidants. In 1970, he founded the American Aging Association (AGE), a research organization aimed at understanding and slowing the aging process.[22]

Linus Pauling, the scientist who gained the rare distinction of winning two Nobel prizes (Chemistry and the Peace Prize), published *Vitamin C and the Common Cold and the Flu* (1976) after being personally impressed with its effects. He considered vitamin C an important agent for fighting infections by boosting the immune system.[23,24]

Today the evidence is indisputable: cardiovascular diseases, cancer, and many of the age-related diseases are mediated or aggravated by free radical damage (Table 6-6).

Free Radicals and Cellular Function

Antioxidants are to our bodies, what lemon juice is to a cut apple, or rust inhibitors are to metals.
They protect body tissues against free radicals.
Antioxidants are our security forces.
They protect against continuous attacks from both foreign and home-grown free radicals.

Every living cell in our bodies produces free radicals.[25] They emerge when the cells generate energy from the food we eat. These radicals exert what is known as oxidant stress. Oxidant stress is also called free-radical stress. Such stresses generate reactive oxygen species—radicalized forms of oxygen—that are unstable and destructive in their behavior. The commonest free radicals within our bodies include superoxide, singlet oxygen, hydroxide, nitric oxide, and peroxide (similar to the hydrogen peroxide used in mouthwash and disinfectants).[26]

Table 6-6. Free Radicals, Sources and Disease

Major Free Radicals, their Sources, and Associated Diseases

Types	superoxide, peroxide, hydroxyl radical, nitric oxide Oxidized forms of cholesterol, carbohydrates, fats, proteins, and genetic material
Sources	Cigarette smoke Atmospheric pollution, toxins Pesticides, herbicides, additives Prolonged sun exposure Endogenous (produced by normal cells) Exercise
Associated Diseases*	Atherosclerosis ("clogging" of the arteries) Cardiovascular diseases (CVD)(coronary artery disease, heart attack, high blood pressure, stroke, peripheral vascular disease (PVD, claudication), erectile dysfunction (ED) Cancer Diabetes mellitus Alzheimer's disease and dementias Arthritis

*Many researchers believe that almost every disease is somehow mediated or aggravated by free radical damage or oxidant stress. This can be likened to the ubiquitous corrosion (oxidation / rusting) of metals.

Free radical occurrence is a natural inescapable phenomenon that affects all systems on earth, both living and non-living. Free radical stress is the same stress that causes iron and metals to corrode (oxidation) or a cut apple to turn brown. Our bodies are equipped with innate protective devices against free radicals. Without these, bodily functions would speedily deteriorate under the merciless onslaught of the free radicals. The health of body tissues depend on free radicals being kept in check by the anti-oxidant protective mechanisms.[27]

Free radicals do not keep to themselves; they have a great appetite for mischief. They molest and interfere with literally everything. They can radicalize or oxidize every tissue they encounter, or they can recruit converts (newly generated free radicals) that wreak progressive damage to the body. If these radicals are not neutralized or kept in check by the antioxidants, they can disrupt normal cellular function and propagate a vicious cycle that results in disease.

In fairness to the free radicals, they are not all mischievous; they can be as helpful as they can be destructive. Free radicals play important roles in our body's fight against infections. Their destructive energies are daily harnessed to kill bacteria and other infective agents that invade our bodies. The same principle is used when bleach and peroxide are used to kill germs. This principle is also harnessed in the chlorination of drinking water and swimming pools. Bleach and peroxide are potent oxidizing agents that generate enormous amounts of free radicals that kill bacteria and viruses lurking in our drinking water and your swimming pool. Free radicals are kind when helping us fight bacteria, but they are totally unkind when it comes to their effects on the aging process.[28]

If our bodies come under a repeated barrage of free radical artillery (e.g. smoking) they can overwhelm the body's antioxidant defenses (Table 6-7). Under this scenario, free-radicals may have free reign, and in anarchic fashion, wreak mischief on our cellular components. Unless antioxidant re-enforcements are provided (in the form of plenty of fresh fruits and vegetables +/- a supplement) to arrest and neutralize the situation, damage and disease will result. Major antioxidant agents in our bodies include Vitamin C (ascorbic acid), Vitamin E (d-alpha tocopherol), superoxide dismutase (SOD), catalase, and glutathione peroxidase, which contains the important mineral called selenium. Vitamin C is water-soluble and is the chief antioxidant patrolling our body fluids and secretions, including tears, lung fluids, and semen. Vitamin E is an oily substance that predominates in the cell membrane which envelops every cell in the body.[29,30]

Table 6-7. Major Antioxidants Present in Body Fluids and Tissues

Major Antioxidants in Body Tissues and Fluids

Vitamin C (ascorbic acid)
Vitamin E (the tocopherols, e.g. d-alpha tocopherol)
Flavonoids
Carotenoids, including beta-carotene
Superoxide dismutase (contains copper)
Catalase (contains heme iron)
Glutathione peroxidase (contains selenium)
Urate, bilirubin, and plasma proteins

Free Radicals and Cellular DNA

Free radicals are like terrorists, they target and attack the command and control centers of our cells—our DNA.

A primary target of free radical attack is the command-and-control center of the cell, called the nucleus. The nucleus houses the chromosomes and the genetic material called DNA (deoxyribonucleic acid). The major function of DNA is to propagate and express the genetic code. Translation of this code forms the proteins that control body structure and function. Damage to DNA can therefore lead to infidelity of translation and defective protein structure and function. The long-term result of free radical attack is that normal cellular function can be spun completely out of control. It is estimated that the DNA in each cell of our bodies receives ten thousand free radical attacks per day. Clones of these abnormal cells can then proliferate in an anarchistic fashion—a law unto themselves.[31]

This is what we mean by cancer—abnormal and uncontrolled growth of cells that arise from normal body tissues, but subsequently disobey all protocols of growth and normal behavior. The result is a predictable breakdown in the way tissues grow and function. If not halted, it leads to the familiar form of death (cancer) that kills more than 500,000 Americans every year.

Sharon Begley and Mary Hager in *Newsweek* (1990) gave a vivid description of the action of free radical attack on DNA and the impact on the aging process:[32]

> The first [theory] holds that the changes that accompany aging are the inevitable result of life itself. DNA, the molecule of heredity, occasionally makes mistakes as it goes about its business of synthesizing proteins; metabolism produces toxic avengers (free radicals) that turn lipids in our cells rancid and protein rusty. This damage accumulates until the organism falls apart like an old jalopy . . .

Free Radicals and Cell Membranes

Vitamin E protects cell membranes by neutralizing free radical attacks.
In so doing, it prevents the fat-filled cell membrane
from becoming oxidized or rancid.
Vitamin E, in this sense, extends the shelf-life of cells.

Free radicals spare no tissues. They corrupt carbohydrate, fat, and protein structures as they seek to radicalize them.[33] Each cell in our bodies is encased in a protective covering that works in a way akin to how our skin protects our internal structures. Damage to the cell membrane leads to a predictable loss of normal cell function due to leakage and loss of important cell components. The end results of these insults can manifest in increased susceptibility to infections and premature death of the cell.

The cell membrane is essentially two microscopically-thin layers of special fats called phospholipids. They are reinforced by protein elements that span both layers. When free radicals attack the cell membrane, they oxidize the fatty layer. Oxidized fats become rancid in the same way that air exposure turns oils rancid. This is the same process that causes whiteheads on the face to become blackheads (comedones). Exposure to air causes the oily contents of whiteheads to become dark (blackhaead) and develop a characteristic (rancid) smell. This is the oxidation of fats.

Antioxidants counteract this oxidation (rusting), and hence their name. This is why antioxidants are added to cooking oils—to improve their shelf-life. Vitamin E, which resides in the cell membrane, acts by neutralizing free radicals that attack the cell membrane and prevents it from becoming oxidized or rancid. In this manner, vitamin E plays an important antioxidant role by extending the shelf-life of cells. This is the basis of the argument for using vitamin E to protect against diseases where free-radicals play important roles (see Chapter 8, pp. 319-322).[34-36]

Free Radicals and the Immune System

Our immune systems are like the armed forces: the army, the air force, and the marines. They are a vital defense against the onslaughts that lead to disease. Our immune systems are high on the target list of the free radicals.

A striking feature of aging is a reduction in the function of the T-cells, so named because of their relationship to the thymus, which is a gland positioned in the upper chest, just behind the breastplate. This is where T-cells mature, and are equipped for their important job of ridding our bodies of viruses, bacteria, fungi, and cancer cells. The thymus normally shrinks and disappears by adulthood.[37-40]

People with impaired immune function are prone to infections. Infections further generate free radicals, and this serves only to worsen an already precarious situation. A prime example of this is the person with badly controlled type II diabetes. High blood sugars not only attract infections, but the hyperglycemic condition reduces the ability of white blood cells to tackle infections. To worsen matters even further, free radical (or oxidative) stress haunts the diabetic state. Consequently, people with diabetes are prone to infections, which can be both limb- and life-threatening.[41-44]

Just as free radical stress can overwhelm the immune system, so can antioxidants deliver a much needed boost. Linus Pauling highlighted vitamin C (an antioxidant) in the fight against viral infections. He was so impressed by its effects that he ended up writing a book. During attacks by viruses that cause the common cold, vitamin C levels fall below normal. These levels can be restored only by taking mega-doses of vitamin C. Vitamin C levels are measured in laboratories by checking the levels in the foot soldiers of the immune system, the white blood cells (leukocytes). This reflects the close connection between vitamin C status and the body's ability to fight infections successfully.[23] This is not a strange concept; vitamin C is a well-known immune booster. The example of its effectiveness in fighting herpes simplex infections was discussed in Chapter 2 (see "How Pharmaceuticals Work").

This effectiveness extends into the realm of aging. Vitamins and minerals, either in food or as supplements, improve immune function especially as we grow older. Antioxidants are a good way to improve immune function as we age.[45-52]

Free Radicals and the Cardiovascular System: Blood Vessel and Cholesterol Effects

> Cardiovascular diseases are the leading causes of death. Free radical damage plays a central role in the genesis, the progression, and the complications of cardiovascular diseases.[53-63]

Blood vessels endure constant free radical insults as they fulfill their vital role of delivering oxygen and nutrition to body tissues. The narrowing or clogging of the arteries is the process of atherosclerosis. This affects mainly the arteries—the high pressure system that delivers blood to body tissues, throughout the entire circulatory system, with some areas being affected more than others.

Depending on the predominant area of involvement, they are given different names. When significant clogging occurs in the coronary arteries that supply the heart, it is called coronary artery (or coronary heart) disease. When it occurs in the cerebral arteries that supply the brain, it is called cerebrovascular disease. When it occurs outside of these systems, especially within the longest arteries that supply the extremities, it is known as peripheral vascular disease.

Symptoms vary according to the extent of narrowing of these arteries. Atherosclerotic narrowing must be quite advanced (over 60 percent stenosis) before symptoms manifest. So a person with heart disease may have absolutely no complaints, or they may be plagued by recurrent chest pains or angina pectoris that occur with exertion. People with cerebrovascular disease may experience symptoms that range from unnoticeable memory loss to the more ominous TIA (transient ischemic attack)—a warning sign of a stroke. Peripheral vascular disease or arterial claudication is the name given to advanced clogging of the arteries to the legs, but many people are unaware that Pfizer's best selling drug (Viagra) is actually a billboard for peripheral vascular disease. It highlights that no part of the circulation is spared, including those to the masculine extremity.

These events are not mutually exclusive. Clogging is not confined to a single area of the body. It occurs throughout the cardiovascular system as will be discussed in the next section (Table 6-8). From a prevention perspective, it is crucially important to understand that if you wait for symptoms to appear before taking action, you are off to a very late start.

Table 6-8. The Spectrum of Cardiovascular Disease

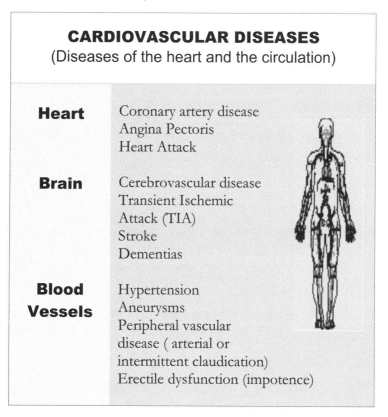

CARDIOVASCULAR DISEASES
(Diseases of the heart and the circulation)

Heart	Coronary artery disease Angina Pectoris Heart Attack
Brain	Cerebrovascular disease Transient Ischemic Attack (TIA) Stroke Dementias
Blood Vessels	Hypertension Aneurysms Peripheral vascular disease (arterial or intermittent claudication) Erectile dysfunction (impotence)

Blood vessels are very sensitive to free radical damage. Free radical injury begins quite insidiously in a manner similar to how rust spots develop. Free radicals trigger a series of events that occur in the endothelial lining (endothelium) of blood vessels. The earliest visible sign of atherosclerosis is called the fatty streak. These streaks form when certain types of circulating white blood cells called foam cells (monocytes and macrophages) become radicalized during the body's attempt to rid the blood of rancid (oxidized) LDL-cholesterol particles.[64-71]

Free radicals injure the delicate endothelium and attract foam cells that accumulate at the site of the fatty streak. These foam cells in turn attract a host of different white blood cells to create a more organized entity called the fibrous plaque. Fibrous plaques occur throughout the circulatory system. They can enlarge into complex lesions that resemble clogged pipes. These complex lesions contain a core of central oxidized LDL-cholesterol particles. Complex lesions behave unpredictably. They can remain the same, or they may enlarge, rupture, and release their undesirable contents into the bloodstream. This complication can manifest itself in the form of a heart attack, a stroke, or other circulatory problems. Complex lesions can also regress. This is an important point to remember for the prevention of cardiovascular diseases (see Chapter 8, "Lifestyle Heart Trial")

At the American Heart Association's 70th Scientific Session in 1997, a team from the University of Georgia presented their findings on free radicals and the cardiovascular system. They blamed increased free radical production for the greater incidence of cardiovascular disease among African Americans compared to their Caucasian counterparts. A two-fold increased free radical production in the former group led to one third higher incidence of cardiovascular disease:[72]

> The body produces free radicals, which are highly reactive molecules that circulate in the bloodstream and can attack body tissues such as the blood vessels and damage them … Some free radicals, including one called superoxide, have been shown to interfere with the ability of blood vessels to vasodilate or relax. Constricted blood vessels reduce the flow of blood and raise blood pressure. When vessels in the heart are severely constricted or totally blocked, they can cause a heart attack … Free radicals also may play a role in the development of plaques such as occurs in atherosclerosis, or hardening of the arteries, by attacking the blood vessel walls, damaging them so they can't relax.

Blood vessels can suffer negative effects from even a single fatty meal. These effects are worse if animal fats are consumed, especially if it is at the expense of fresh fruits, fresh vegetables, and nuts (foods high in antioxidants). A University of Maryland study of twenty healthy hospital employees, ages 24 to 54, demonstrated negative short-term effects of a single high-fat meal. Study participants given meals high in fat exhibited constriction of the arteries that lasted up to four hours. This constriction, triggered by free radicals generated by the fatty meal, was eliminated if pretreatment with antioxidants—vitamins C (1000 mg) and vitamin E (800 I.U.)—was given along with the fatty meal.[73]

Such findings support the contention that even people on unhealthy high-fat diets can minimize their negative effects by also consuming foods rich in antioxidants. Healthy foods and supplements have redeeming value when combined with less healthy food choices.[74,75] This is of practical significance, because even those diets that are considered healthy actually have their share of unhealthy ingredients. The highly recommended Mediterranean diet has its share of unhealthy animal fats in the form of cheeses, red meats, and dairy products, but heavy fruit and vegetable intake along with virgin olive oils and wine with meals have lead to comparatively low rates of cardiovascular diseases (see Chapter 8). Therefore antioxidant-rich foods can neutralize the harmful effects of foods that generate free-radical stresses.

This further highlights the need to look at the whole diet rather than a single component (Chapter 8, "The Medicalization of Nutrition"). The major problem with the Western diet discussed in the previous chapter is that there is an overwhelming intake of unhealthy foods at the exclusion of healthier alternatives.

The Heart, the Brain, and Male Sexual Function

What is bad for the heart is also bad for the brain and sexual function. Although the heart and the brain are more noticeably affected, atherosclerosis ("clogging") affects the entire circulation—penile arteries included.

The entire body is a single integrated unit. This simply gets lost in this era of medical super-specialties. The cardiovascular system is one unit with several components and extensions. What is bad for the heart is also bad for the brain, but good for Pfizer (the drug company that makes Viagra).

The endothelial cells (that line blood vessels) play active roles in maintaining the circulation. One such role is the production of nitric oxide, a short-lived agent that relaxes blood vessels and increases blood flow. This is the same substance that is produced when angina sufferers place nitroglycerin under the tongue to increase blood flow to the heart.[76] Viagra (sildenafil citrate) mimics nitroglycerin, but acts preferentially on the arteries that supply the penis. This leads to increased nitric oxide production and the resultant increased blood flow to the penis in the same way that nitroglycerin improves blood flow to the heart. Therefore you can be excused for saying that sildenafil relieves "penile angina."

The risk factors for heart attack and stroke are the same risk factors for the clogging of the arteries that supply the penis. Men who suffer from coronary heart disease, stroke, and arterial claudication are at increased risk for erectile dysfunction (ED). The risk factors for heart disease (e.g. smoking, hypertension, diabetes, and lipid disorders) are also the same risk factors for ED. The Massachusetts Male Aging Study revealed that 40 percent of 40-year old men suffer varying degrees of ED. Atherosclerosis is responsible for more than 50 percent of ED. Reduced blood flow to the penis, therefore, is the major underlying cause of ED or secondary impotence in men ("secondary" indicates these males were previously capable of attaining normal erections).[77-81]

Erection occurs when more blood enters the penis than actually leaves. Loss of "hardness" of penile erections may be a sensitive indicator of cardiovascular disease. Penile erections are under mental and nervous control, but penile rigidity depends on having good blood flow to the penis. The prelude to ED is often quite subtle, and frequently manifests as a gradual loss of penile "hardness" during sexual intercourse.

Most men consider this a part of normal aging, but it may be a reflection of the progressive clogging of the penile arteries, rather than aging itself. This may be the prime reason why millions of otherwise normal men, dissatisfied with the firmness of their erections, have experimented with Viagra, with the hope of a return to form (as in their twenties). My advice to such men is this: Think more above the belt … Use your head and get to the root of the matter. Stop smoking, get active, eat right (and take good care of your beloved). ED, or the signs that suggest early ED, should serve as a wake-up-call to prevent what is happening above your belt—clogging to your heart, and clogging to your head.

Smoking, Free Radicals, and the Circulation

Cigarette smoking is easily the most damaging lifestyle habit that kills almost half a million Americans annually. It unleashes a heavy free radical attack on the cardiovascular system.

Cigarette smoking is a major source of free radicals (oxidative stress). Smoking attacks the cardiovascular system. Cigarette smoke consists of a gaseous phase and a tar phase (stains the teeth and fingers). It is profoundly irritating to blood vessels. Free radicals from smoke attack the cardiovascular system via a variety of mechanisms (Figure 6-6).[82-86]

The free radical onslaught from smoking depletes vitamin C levels, the antioxidant found in highest concentration in body fluids. The resultant lower vitamin C status is a major reason why heavy smokers are more susceptible to infections, cancers, and chronic diseases (Figure 5-4). Reduction or loss of antioxidant defense system in body fluids and tissues leaves our bodies more vulnerable to attack.

Just 20 minutes in a room filled with cigarette smoke is enough to a cause measurable increase platelet activity in the blood of non-smokers. Platelets are cell fragments that increase the stickiness and the ability of the blood to clot. These are the targets of anti-platelet drugs (e.g. aspirin, ticlopidine, and clopidogrel) that are used to prevent heart attacks. A single cigarette is enough to dramatically reduce blood flow to the heart of smokers. Smoking is still the number one cause of preventable death in the United States, Europe, and an increasing number of countries around the world.

**Smoking, Free Radicals,
and the Cardiovascular System**

Mechanism

- Reduces the blood's ability to deliver oxygen to the heart
- Reduces the ability of the heart to effectively use the oxygen it receives
- Reduces the ability of the heart muscle to convert oxygen to energy (ATP)
- Damages blood vessel lining (endothelium)
- Increased activity and stickiness of blood platelets
- Increased levels of fibrinogen (increased tendency to clot)
- Lowers "good" HDL-cholesterol

**Clinical
Effects**

- Higher resting heart rate
- Elevates blood pressure (hypertension)
- Increased strokes (cerebrovascular accidents)
- Increased heart attacks (acute myocardial infarction)
- Increased irregular heartbeat (arrhythmias and palpitations)
- Increased sudden death
- Increased risk of type II diabetes
- Increased impotence (erectile dysfunction)

Figure 6-6. Smoking and its impact on cardiovascular system.

Free Radicals and Cancer

Free radicals attack DNA, the immune system, and a number of actions discussed earlier. These can result in the loss of normal cellular controls and the risk of disordered growth. Such growths we call cancer.
Cigarette smoke and unhealthy diets are potent generator of free radicals. Both increase the risks of many cancers.

The Aging Skin

The aging skin is perhaps the most obvious sign of aging. This is not necessarily a reflection of internal aging, because skin appearance is influenced by a number of genetic and environmental factors.

The Effects of Sun, Smoke, Race, and Sex

As we age, progressive loss of supportive tissues leads to the appearance of wrinkles. The supporting collagen and elastic fibers normally keep the skin looking youthful. Unfortunately, time and various onslaughts cause these supports to weaken, and wrinkles and sagging gradually develop. A number of factors hasten the development of wrinkles. They include sun exposure, cigarette smoke (including second-hand smoke), stress (of all kinds), environmental factors, a poor diet, and racial factors.

Vitamin C is now famous for its antioxidant health benefits. However, its past claim-to-fame is based on its biochemical action of promoting cross linkages within collagen, the major structural protein that gives strength to the skin and supportive tissues. Scurvy, a vitamin C deficiency disease, historically killed many sea-farers who lacked fresh fruit. Collagen is also damaged by free radicals, and when this occurs, leads to loss of integrity and flexibility in those connective tissues where it normally abounds. Antioxidants, especially vitamin C, beta-carotene (precursor to vitamin A), vitamin E, and alpha lipoic acid all play major roles in maintaining healthy skin. They protect against free radical damage.[87]

Sun Exposure

The sun's ultraviolet rays cause sun damage or photo-aging by generating free radicals that destroy collagen. Skin damage is more obvious following direct exposure to sunlight. The effect is cumulative and the wrinkles and sun spots visible at age 40 are a reflection of sun exposure that occurred much earlier. The tan that many light-skinned individuals seek can lead to irreversible skin damage that accumulates with repeated exposure. These negative results may be minimized but not completely eliminated by sunscreen. The major risk posed by cumulative sun exposure is the development of skin cancer—the commonest of all types of cancer in Caucasian populations. The most frequent type of skin cancer is basal cell cancer (rodent ulcer). More than 400,000 new cases are diagnosed annually in the United States, predominantly in fair-skinned individuals.[88-90]

Skin Aging and Race

Normal skin contains melanin pigment that protects against the sun's ultraviolet rays. People of African ancestry rarely develop skin cancer, thanks to melanin. Albinos, who are genetically unable to produce melanin, are at highest risk for skin cancer. Negroid skin is thicker than the skin of Caucasoid races due to thicker layers of supporting tissues. There are two sides to this coin. On one side of the coin, Negroid skin wrinkles less and suffers far less skin cancer than Caucasoid skin, and this effect becomes more manifest as people age. The flipside is that Negroid races are more prone to develop a more robust scar tissue reaction to injury, leading sometimes to bigger scars (hypertrophic scars or keloids) and increased pigmentation (post-inflammatory hyperpigmentation).[91] The thing about this coin, though, is that you cannot choose.

My first real appreciation for the differences in skin thickness occurred while assisting at gynecologic surgery. The chief gynecologist, Peter Morris M.D. had just made his first stroke with the scalpel to the patient's abdomen, but no blood was seen. He looked me in the eyes and whispered, "I can tell you a patient's race with my eyes closed." Of course, he was urged to keep his eyes open.

Skin Aging and Sex

Women have thinner skins than men. Women's skins appear to age more quickly than those of men. Women have less muscle, less supporting tissues, and more fat than men. For these reasons, cellulite is suffered mainly by women. A man in his seventies may exhibit shrunken muscles but no cellulite. For women who think this is not fair, take comfort in the fact that women live longer than men. External aging does not necessarily equate with internal aging.

There is another twist to aging of the skin. Its appearance can be affected by sexual activity. Dr. David Weeks, clinical neuropsychologist at the Royal Edinburgh Hospital in Scotland, discussed the effects of sex on aging in his book, *Secrets of the Superyoung*. In it he reported that sexual activity at least three times a week made people looked ten years younger! These findings apparently applied only to those in stable committed unions and not to those involved in trysts and casual sex. Perhaps, it had to do more with matters of quality, commitment, and contentment in relationships (see Chapter 9, pp 373 - 374).[92]

Lifestyle Aging Accelerators

> Much of what we call aging
> is actually premature or accelerated aging.
> The aging process is hastened by several factors.

There are behaviors that hasten the rate at which people age. These we can call aging accelerators. Some of these are completely outside our control (e.g. diseases and accidents), but some relate directly to the challenges of modern living (e.g. stress and chronic sleep deprivation). Many of these cluster in people who exhibit unhealthy lifestyle patterns (Table 6-9). Therefore, in our quest for successful aging, the downsides of modern living will have to be somehow tamed. This is something for you to decide.

Table 6-9. Five Major Aging Accelerators

Major Lifestyle Aging Accelerators	1. Cigarette Smoking
	2. Unbalanced Nutrition
	3. Sedentary Lifestyle
	4. Stress
	5. Chronic Sleep Deprivation

Stress and Modern Living: Killing Ourselves Trying To Make a Living

"… in the worry and strain of modern life, arterial degeneration (hardening and narrowing of the arteries) is not only very common but develops at a relatively early age.
For this I believe that the high pressure at which men live and the habit of working the machine to its maximum are responsible."[93]

Sir William Osler, 1897

The person who coined the saying, "The surest thing about life is death and taxes," left out an important word, "stress." This word has its origins in the word *estresse,* meaning "oppression." Dorland's medical dictionary defines stress as "a state of physiological strain caused by adverse stimuli, physical, mental, or emotional that tend to disturb the functioning of an organism and which the organism naturally desires to avoid." We can paraphrase it this way … Stress is a disturbance, we all want to avoid it, but we all keep getting it. Stress is normal and inevitable.

Doctors frequently ignore the important role stress plays on people's medical problems. Much of this could be blamed on the short times allotted for medical consultations. Real people face real issues, and most of these, doctors don't really want to hear (unless they are paid); because they are over-stressed with their own issues (see the cover story, *Time Magazine,* June 9, 2003).

The person who sits in the doctor's surgery is far more than a diabetic or a heart patient. Even this book's primary focus on nutrition and physical activity is really only part of this bigger picture. People faced with pressing financial, relationship or other stresses can be so weighed down, that it relegates even the primary focus of this book into near irrelevance, at least in the short term.

Stress is necessary for survival, but prolonged unresolved stresses can exact a heavy toll on health. Stress kills. It elevates blood pressure and is a known trigger for heart attack and stroke. Stress can hasten or aggravate almost any disease.[94-100]

Well known to cardiologists are the many high-strung high-achievers who exhibit the type A behavior pattern. The label is not as important as the behavior itself. Individuals who lead such lives are at higher risk for heart attacks. Friedman and Rosenman define the type A behavior pattern as follows: [101,102]

> Type A behavior pattern is an action-emotion complex that can be observed in any person who is aggressively involved in a chronic, incessant struggle to achieve more and more in less and less time, and if required to do so, against the opposing efforts of other things or persons. It is not a psychosis or a complex of worries or fears or phobias or obsessions, but a socially acceptable—indeed often praised—form of conflict.

There is little dispute that this is the price many must pay to gain material success. It is worth your heart to pay attention to the maxim, "Work smarter, not harder."

Words to the Workaholic

Few things in life are achieved without sacrifice. However, working too hard is a great disservice to the body. Overworked and sleep-deprived people are more likely to eat poorly, get insufficient exercise, and indulge in other bad habits.

The issue is not whether you cannot afford to look after yourself now; it is whether you can afford not to. This is a simple matter of setting priorities.
If you are a workaholic, you can either choose to pay the price of prevention today, or end up paying too high a price later.

Just in case you are one of those people who believe that the job cannot be done without you, it is a sobering reminder that
the world will keep on spinning long after you leave.

Doctors in Distress

Life can be like a never-ending treadmill,
but it is up to you
to know when to get off!

Today's medical schools and residency programs are guilty of making mockery of their claims to be the guardians of health. This verdict can be issued on the basis of how young doctors are trained. The training of medical interns, residents and junior doctors (UK) obscures a sad irony. The training and lifestyles that many doctors have to endure is the anti-thesis of healthy lifestyles. Additional hassles, stresses, and growing disillusionment, further expose major contradictions within the practice of the profession. This is the direction to where many people turn for advice on healthy living.

Personal Reflections

The verdict: messed up!

What I found ironic was how messed up we doctors were during our training. … Sickening ourselves, practicing a lot of wrong habits: eating lousy food, working ungodly and inhumane hours, guzzling cup after cup of coffee… literally killing ourselves trying to make others well!

Not many of my then colleagues could lay claim to being as motivated as I was, especially after winning a scholarship to attend medical school. I was consumed with near evangelical zeal. I had to stay on top of things—I had to have all the books, I could not afford to miss a day, and I would not sleep until the day's work was done. My study habits were intense, to put it mildly. Anatomy was my pet subject; I was keen on knowing all the structures that comprise the human body. This is not an exaggeration. The books were always open—sometimes exceeding fifteen different books—all at once. Not to be short-changed, I did not settle for the recommended box of disjointed bones containing only half a human skeleton—I needed all those bones, fully assembled, at all times—not in my closet, but by my bedside.

Medical school was akin to the military; it meant serious discipline and training. Great sacrifices had to be made. Social relationships were largely confined to medical colleagues because there was little time to socialize with anyone else (misery loves company). Many doctors leave medical school and residency feeling disillusioned, questioning whether the rewards were really worth the sacrifices, especially when they discover how better off their former high school and college colleagues were, and with less sacrifice. A number of television documentaries have documented the ordeal doctors endure during training (Table 6-10. and Figure 6-7.) [103]

I observed a sort of madness in the medical profession. Most doctors and medical students lead rather unhealthy lifestyles. The respect you get from your colleagues seems proportional to the hardships and stresses you endure. These vibes were evident following emergency on-calls. The less sleep you got, the more demanding your on-call was, and the more sleep-deprived you appeared led to more accolades and respect from your teachers and colleagues.

Table 6-10.Chief Stressors for Physicians:

Stressors for Physicians	• Volume of work • Sleep deprivation • Teaching and research demands • Potential for litigation (malpractice) • Increased demands of the public • Interference with social life • Delayed marriage and family plans

Modified from Canadian Medical Association Code of Ethics[104]

Earning the respect of your peers is one of the best feelings in medical school and residency training. It was as if to say, "Welcome to the club, thou good and battered colleague!" Doctors-in-training study hard, work long shifts, suffer chronic sleep-deprivation, get little exercise, eat poorly (subsisting on cafeteria food, energy bars and snacks along with lots of coffee), and are then supposed to teach patients about healthy lifestyles. Hats off to our teachers and our noble profession! In some ways, things have changed for the better, but medical students and doctors remain as stressed out as they have ever been (Table 6-10 and Figure 6-7).

Doctors in Distress

• Physicians and the systems in which they train and work, are encouraged to remember the essential elements of well-being—such as rest, exercise, family activities, and healthy nutrition. (*CMA Code of Ethics*)[104]

• After 24 hours of wakefulness, cognitive function deteriorates to a level equivalent to having a 0.1% blood alcohol level. Such doctors would be considered too unsafe to drive, but they are still allowed to treat patients for 12 more hours.[105] (*Nature*)

• 41% of resident physicians attribute their most serious mistake in the previous year to exhaustion.[106] (*Journal of the American Medical Association*)

Figure 6-7. Concerns over Physicians Stresses

Chronic Sleep Debt: Sleep Deprivation

Military strategists are familiar with the effects of sleep deprivation during warfare. If you prevent the enemy from sleeping, you can win the war. Days of sleeplessness leave people befuddled—unable to think, act, and function properly.

There is a cycle or rhythm in nature. There is night, and there is day. There is a time for leaves to appear, and there is a time for them to fall. Even machines and motors are built with switches that turn them on, and turn them off. Remaining in any one mode for too long can lead to damage or demise.

The same principle applies to the daily human cycle. We work during the day, and we sleep during the night (most of us, that is). There are important reasons for sleep: rest, recovery, and repair. Sleep is when we rest our bodies as well as our minds; it provides both physical and mental refreshment. Sleep is necessary for survival. It is sad to see how our sleep-deprived culture rushes to prescribe drugs for a legion of ailments—ranging from headaches to chest pains—when the best therapy is nothing more than getting some badly needed sleep.

Substituting Caffeine for Sleep

Rather than making those changes that can lead to increased efficiency and productivity, many have opted for stimulants— inadvertently substituting one bad habit for another.

Many make it a habit of routinely using stimulants to remain alert and awake. It has become so acceptable to use stimulants that many routinely drink caffeinated beverages with little appreciation of the abuse (Table 6-11).[107]

A poll taken by the National Sleep Foundation indicated that America is a sleep-deprived nation. The average American adult gets 6 hours and 54 minutes of sleep per day. This is one hour less than the eight hours recommended by sleep experts. Perhaps here is a good place for many of us to pause and make a confession. One-third of the adults surveyed, confessed to sleeping less than six and a half hours nightly, and 50 percent expressed no hesitation that they would sleep less to get more work done.[108]

Insufficient sleep exacts a heavy toll on many fronts. Cornell University psychologist and sleep expert Professor James Maas reported that an estimated 100,000 traffic accidents are caused by sleepy drivers. This claims an average of 1,500 American lives per year. Sleep deprivation and sleep disorders cost the U.S. economy at least

150 billion dollars annually. Professor Maas described the "sleep debt" as the difference between the hours of restorative rest people need for optimal physical and mental well-being, minus the number of hours they actually get.[109] If we do our own arithmetic, we can easily see many of us needing one complete day off each week from work—just to sleep. The problem is that most of us don't pay, at least not yet.

Table 6-11. Caffeine in the Diet.

Common Sources of Caffeine	Caffeine (mg)
COFFEE (5 oz.)	
Drip, automatic	137
Drip, non-automatic	124
Percolated, automatic	117
Percolated, non-automatic	108
Instant, regular	6
Instant, decaffeinated	3
TEA	
Black, imported, brewed 5 minutes (6 oz.)	65
Black, U.S., brewed 5 minutes (5 oz.)	46
Green, brewed 5 minutes (5 oz.)	31
Decaffeinated, brewed 5 minutes (5 oz.)	1
CHOCOLATE	
Baker's brand baking chocolate (1 oz.)	25
Sweet dark chocolate candy (I oz.)	20
Milk chocolate candy (1 oz.)	6
Chocolate milk (8 oz. glass)	5
Cocoa (6 oz. cup)	5
SOFT DRINKS	
Coca-cola	45
Pepsi-cola	38
Mountain Dew	54
NON-PRESCRIPTION DRUGS (standard dose)	
Weight-control aids	168
Certain diuretics (water pills)	167
Alertness/ Pick-me-up tablets	150
Some Painkillers	41
Some Cold and allergy medicines	27

Adapted from "Caffeine: How little, How Much for You and Your Family?"
American Dietetic Association, (booklet) 1998.[107]

How to Know if You Have Not Slept Enough

Some individuals, especially older people, can function well on less than six hours of sleep. Our bodies have a good way of telling us when they need more rest. The trouble is this: Many of us don't listen! When our bodies demand sleep, we interrupt with alarm clocks, stimulants, and other activities that interfere with the natural rhythm of sleep. It pays to heed the familiar indicators of insufficient sleep listed in Table 6-12.

Table 6-12. Simple Indicators of Sleep Deprivation

Insufficient Sleep
(failure to secure restorative rest)

- Wake up feeling tired and un-refreshed
- Difficulty getting up for work
- Falling asleep on the job
- Moodiness
- Lack of concentration
- Irritability
- Failure to heed the alarm clock
- Need coffee to stay alert or awake

Conspicuously absent from this table is the way you look (your appearance). No one needs to tell you when you have not slept enough. Don't let someone have to say to you, "You look like you need to get yourself some sleep!" Your general response is, "... I know." What they are actually trying to tell you is that you appear "less than good," or quite bluntly, "bad." That itself should be enough motivation to sleep.

The Medical Ravages of Sleep Deprivation

Cutting back from the standard eight down to four hours of sleep each night produced striking changes in glucose tolerance and endocrine function—changes that resembled the effects of advanced age or the early stages of diabetes—after less than one week. *The Lancet*[110]

Until recently, most of the concerns about sleep deprivation centered on the mental and psychological consequences. But in 1999, Dr. Eve Van Cauter and colleagues published a landmark study on the medical consequences of sleep deprivation. They showed that just one week of sleep deprivation caused healthy young men not only to feel, but also to function, like people in their sixties. Highlights of the study appear in Figure 6-8.[110]

Figure 6-8. The Medical Ravages of Sleep Deprivation in Healthy Young Men

The Medical Ravages of Sleep Deprivation

Up until this landmark study, most scientists did not believe that sleep deprivation caused any significant medical problems.

Findings of the Study
- May hasten the onset and severity of diabetes, high blood pressure and memory loss
- Causes profound changes in insulin and stress hormone levels (cortisol, thyroid hormone.
- Can cause the pre-diabetic state in healthy young men with no risk factors for diabetes, after just one week of cutting down to 4 hours of sleep daily.

- Changes in metabolism in healthy young men in their early 20's resembled the changes typically seen with men in their 60's.
- Changes reversed quickly after fully resting
- Young adults may function best after 8 hours sleep

Other Effects

- Memory loss (short term effect)
- Delayed thinking and delayed reflexes: impairs judgment and performance
- Weakened immune system: increased tendency for infections

(Source: The Lancet: Dr. Eve Van Cauter and Colleagues, University of Chicago)

Never Too Late

At any time you decide
to improve your behaviour and make lifestyle changes,
they make a difference from that point on.

Dr. Jeffrey Koplan
Former director of the Centers for Disease Control and Prevention (CDC)

Now then, what hope is there for those who awake to the prevention message in the twilight of life? Can healthy changes make a difference if you are already diagnosed with the complications of obesity, cardiovascular diseases, or type II diabetes? The answer is an emphatic "yes!"

Even those who now suffer the ravages of a previously indulgent lifestyle can reap benefits by embarking on positive lifestyle changes. It is never too late.[111] Most people can expect some benefit however late they start. Some benefits occur quickly like those that occur following smoking cessation (Figure 6-9). Change and benefits occur incrementally. Certain habits such as smoking can be stopped "cold turkey," but for most people, old habits die hard.

Stop Smoking! It's Never Too Late to Benefit

Smoking cessation is the healthiest act that a smoker can do. It kills almost half a million Americans annually. It is never too late. Once a smoker quits, blood levels of carbon monoxide (a colorless odorless gas in cigarette smoke) fall rapidly. The stickiness of the blood (with attendant increased risks of heart attack and stroke) in smokers can be reversed after less than a week. The very day a smoker quits is the day his or her risk of cardiovascular disease begins to decline. The risk of suffering a heart attack in a previously heavy smoker approximates that of a non-smoker after 10 to 15 years of a smoke-free existence (Figure 6-9).[111-115] Make up your mind to quit the habit and do whatever is necessary to succeed. This includes avoiding exposure to second-hand smoke and smoke-filled environments. Parents ... please remember the children. They can suffer irreparable damage from living in one smoke-filled environment that the anti-smoking laws can't reach, your home.

When a Smoker Quits

Within 20 minutes of smoking that last cigarette, the body begins a series of changes that continues for years:

20 Minutes
Blood pressure returns to normal
Pulse rate returns to normal
Temperature of extremities: (hands and feet) returns to normal

8 Hours
Carbon monoxide (harmful gas) level in blood returns to normal
Blood oxygenation returns to normal

24 Hours
Risk of a heart attack falls

48 Hours
Enhanced repair of nerve endings
Improvements in smell and taste

2 Weeks to 3 Months
Improvement in blood circulation
Walking becomes easier, less pains in the calf if history of claudication
Lung function improves by up to 30%

1 to 9 Months
Coughing, sinus congestion, fatigue, and shortness of breath decrease
Cilia regenerate in lungs, increasing ability to handle mucus, clean the lungs, and reduce infection

1 Year
Excess risk of coronary heart disease is reduced by 50%

5 Years
Lung cancer death rate for average smoker (one pack a day) is reduced by 50%
Stroke risk is reduced to that of a nonsmoker 5-15 years after quitting
Risk of cancer of the mouth, throat, and esophagus is reduced by 50 %

10 Years
Lung cancer death rate almost that of a nonsmoker
Risk of cancer of the mouth, throat, esophagus, bladder, kidney and pancreas all fall

15 years
Risk of coronary heart disease returns to that of a nonsmoker

Sources: American Cancer Society, The Centers for Disease Control and Prevention and American Cancer Society, Cancer Response System, 1-800-ACS-2345 Number 2656

Figure 6-9. The Health Benefits of Smoking Cessation

Good Nutrition Choices

A healthy diet can be similar to getting a good night's rest. This is the subject of the two chapters that follow. A big glass of freshly-squeezed juice with a sumptuous fruit-and-nut breakfast can provide a much needed boost, but saying goodbye to unhealthy foods and moving in the direction of health provides more than a short-term high. Much benefit can be gained from making changes even during your advanced years. The damage to your health can be repaired. It is never too late to give up excess alcohol, lose weight, and start eating right.[116-123] But the sooner you start, the better.

Strengthen Those Muscles and Keep Active

It can make you younger

Regular physical activity can rejuvenate the elderly
by 10 to 15 years.

The great benefits of exercise can be quite striking, especially as people age. Aging is accompanied by loss of cardiovascular fitness, loss of muscle mass, and a reduction in bone density. Deciding to remain physically active is one of the most important choices people can make as they age. Physical activity pays great dividends. The greatest benefits occur in men and women who begin weight training in their thirties and forties. Cardiovascular exercises and aerobic activity are most beneficial, if engaged in at least three times weekly, to the point of breaking into a sweat.[129-130]

Weight training can reverse some of the effects of aging. Tufts University researchers showed that elderly nursing home residents (ages 86 to 96) experienced dramatic improvements in strength and balance following an 8-week supervised weight-training program. Being physically active rejuvenates physical capacity in the elderly by 10 to 15 years. According to Dr. Maria Fiaratone M.D., who headed the research, these frail residents (most of whom had arthritis and heart disease) benefited not just from physical improvements, but also in terms of their mental and social capacities after the program.[131,132]

Physical activity can provide a host of benefits including the prevention of type II diabetes and cardiovascular disease (see Chapter 9).[133,134]

Don't Let Your Mind Go To Waste

The mind: a terrible thing to waste

People who put their minds to good use
and remain active following retirement
lead happier, longer, and more productive lives.

There is an oft-ignored unease that has accompanied modernity in the Western world. The enormous brain power and experience invested in our elderly is customarily carted off to retirement communities and other less-than-glamorous environs. Prevalent attitudes in our increasingly materialistic world frequently discriminate against the elderly and retire many to pasture after outliving their usefulness. This interpretation may seem insensitive, but it reflects the way many elderly feel. The elderly treasure their independence, but many harbor feelings that society treats them with veiled ingratitude and disrespect.

Many traditional societies have adopted a completely different attitude toward their elderly population. Metellus Cimber of Julius Caesar's fame made mention of the elderly Cicero in flattering fashion, "O, Let us have him! For his silver hairs will purchase us a good opinion, and buy men's voices to commend our deeds." Patriarchal societies hold their elderly in high esteem. In these and other traditional societies, the elders continue to shape public policy for as long as they are mentally capable. Here, the aged represent experience, wisdom, and stability. However, as societies worldwide become more modernized, these traditions gradually erode.

The Western practice or retiring the elderly has no scientific basis. Studies have demonstrated that there is little basis for retiring or refusing to hire older employees. Employment does wonders to maintain dignity and self-esteem in the elderly. People die more quickly when they feel worthless and isolated. Retirees who continue to work are happier, have higher morale, are better adjusted, and live longer. People who remain mentally active, not only enjoy longer lives, but they also suffer less cognitive brain diseases. The mind is a terrible thing to waste. Many elderly have gone on to prove their critics wrong—they are early to work, late to leave, no maternity benefits, and easy to please.[135-138]

The Okinawa Formula

Great interest and efforts have been made to study those populations that exhibit longevity. One such group is the elderly population on the Japanese island of Okinawa, home to a large U.S. military base. Okinawa endured one of the bloodiest campaigns of the Second World War. Despite its turbulent past and its controversial present, Okinawans enjoy better health, lead more healthy independent lives, and live longer than Americans and their fellow Japanese. Okinawan centenarians number about 34 per 100,000 of the population compared to less than 10 centenarians per 100,000 in the United States who, in contrast, are far more likely to spend their final years in poor health and in a nursing home.[139]

A book based on twenty-five years of research, *The Okinawa Program*, written by Bradley J. Willcox M.D., Craig Willcox Ph.D., and Makoto Suzuki M.D. is the first book that introduces the Okinanwans secrets for better health and longevity. The

Okinawa formula is not a strange one—diet, exercise (including martial arts), stress management, social and family ties, and spirituality, all play important roles.

On the dietary front, Okinawan elders ate an average of seven servings of vegetables and fruits, seven servings of grain and two servings of soy products daily along with fish rich in omega-3 fatty acids. Dairy products and meat intake were minimal. Low-temperature stir-frying with canola oil was the preferred method of cooking food. In addition, they consumed far less food. They practiced a self-imposed habit of calorie restriction, referred to as *hara hachi bu*—eating 8 out of 10 parts full. Okinawan elders seemed to have also mastered the art of hassle-free living. Concerns have been expressed whether the new generation of Okinawans will be able to escape the tentacles of globalization. Some are pessimistic, but others hope to the contrary.

Longevity

Important Steps to Aging Well

Good Nutrition
Physical Fitness
Mental Fitness
Healthy Social, Family, Community Relationships
Financial Health
Spiritual Value System

Good nutrition and physical activity play major roles in health, but life is more than a matter of diet and exercise. Other parameters, though not the easiest to scientifically quantify, also play very important roles. The quality of a person's marriage, family, and social relationships can make an important difference. These can have an overriding impact on an individual's outlook and motivation in life. Financial health may be just as important as physical health. Life is more than the physical, therefore life and health must be seen in its entirety—man does not live by bread alone, but man needs bread to live. A number of Harvard-based studies, looking at the determinants of health and disease in later life, revealed that education and social status were major determinants of better health and longevity, even among inner city participants.[140-142]

Social isolation is a major problem for many elderly. As you age, you progressively outlive your peers and there is then an ever dwindling circle of contemporaries with whom to ruminate. Older people live longer if they are married and die sooner if they are widowed, divorced, or single. Many lonely elderly patients, starved of social interaction, sometimes visit their doctor just to engage in conversation or to hear a re-assuring voice. Doctors can score very high marks with their elderly patients if they only take time to listen. Pay them a home visit, they will feel on top of the world![143-145]

A positive aspect of getting older is the anticipation of achieving financial independence. However, a sad reality is that chronic illness can wipe out the entire savings of so many. The single most important factor, outside of physical diseases that affects health and longevity is a person's financial status. Number two on the list is their nutritional status, and number three is their educational level. People who live in richer countries live longer.

Countries with per capita incomes of less than seven thousand dollars are less likely to have life expectancies exceeding 70 years. Even within individual countries, poorer people live less healthy lives and die younger. Socioeconomic status is a key determinant of longevity. How much money you make can determine how long you live, but be careful, as many have killed themselves prematurely while trying to earn this money. The watchword, therefore, is balance.[146-153]

In the midst of our quest for longevity, one thing is certain. Life, as we know it, is but for a moment, and all mankind must one day make an exit. As the journey of aging nears its inevitable end, mankind is forced to grapple with some of life's most unseating questions. Aging is a reminder that we are mere mortals, and this generally fuels the quest for deeper meaning and purpose.[13] Sam Quick Ph.D. and colleagues from the University of Kentucky, could not have summed it up better:[5]

> Some adventurous older people, as part of their spiritual perspective, have chosen to view aging as an advanced curriculum for the soul. They see later life as an unusually challenging time—a time for which all their previous experiences have prepared them. The physical decline that is a part of aging reminds them that who they are is far more than their bodies. As death approaches, they keenly realize that each moment is a gift.

Doctors are generally not comfortable or equipped to deal with these issues, because they invariably delve into culture and belief systems. These are largely impenetrable to medicinal infusions and surgical knives.

However, even hard-core medical institutions have come to terms with the idea that good medicine is not just about saving lives, or the cold application of technological science.
It can inject doses of warmth and compassion for patients and their families, even during those times when our own helplessness and our own mortality have been laid bare.

Summary

Growing older is a must. The diseases and ailments so prevalent in the elderly, however, are not the inevitable consequences of aging. There is a normal deterioration of our bodies over time, but these changes are not in themselves diseases. This is normal aging.

Our bodies are programmed to age, but our bodies face daily onslaughts from free radicals that attack our physical bodies. Added to these, are onslaughts that can accelerate the aging process. Chief among them are cigarette smoking, poor nutrition, the stresses of modern living, chronic sleep debt, and physical inactivity.

Our bodies will inevitably fade. For those in the advancing years, all is not lost. It is never too late to make better choices. Embarking on healthy lifestyles can lead to great benefits at every stage in life. As we age, it is a helpful reminder that aging is not just a physical matter. Interpersonal relationships, our attitudes, cultures, and belief systems exert profound influences on how we age, and how we bid farewell.

*****

An Ode to All Who Age

We grow older with each passing day
We grow older; no one is here to stay
What's best to do along life's way?
In the book 'tis to make the most of each and every day

But take care not to take things too seriously
For in the end we need tranquility
No money, fame, or fraternity
Could surpass the love of God and family

So in food, in drink, in work and society
All these must flow in perfect unity
Mixed together with internal piety
Will bring peace, long life, and eternity.

beb

******

PART IV

All That Enters
Your Mouth

The reasons for our food choices are complex.
Individual, cultural, socioeconomic, and political factors
all play important roles.
Let us take a closer look at these factors, as well as what the
modern food revolution has meant to the quality of our foods.

Chapter 7

Food and Choices
The "Dynamix" of Why We Eat What We Eat

Chapter Outline

Life and Choices in the Real World 253
Doctors and Governments Cannot Legislate Food Choices 255
The Complexities of Food Choices 257
Hierarchy of Food Choices 258
Socialization and Food Choices..260
Targeting the Children 262
"Ameri-sizing"...265
Economics and Food Choices...265
Politics and Food Choices..268
The USDA Food Guide Pyramid...268
The Media and Food Choices...271
Globalization and Food Choices..272
Individual Issues and Food Choices 273
Introduction to Food Processing 275
Industrial Food Processing Methods 277
Spectrum of Food Processing Methods 278
Newer Food Processing Methods 280
Processing and the Nutritional Value of Foods 280
Hidden Salt (Sodium) 283
Hidden Sugars 284
Impact of Processing on Vitamins 285
Raw or Natural Can Be Dangerous..287
Enrichment and Fortification of Foods 290
Reducing Nutrient Losses While Cooking...290
Health Concerns over Some Cooking Methods 291
Food Toxins Produced during Grilling and Barbecuing........................291

Irradiated and Microwaved Foods 292
On Aluminum Pots and Alzheimer's Disease 292
Deep Fat Frying and the Reheating of Oils...............................293
Concerns over Technology and Agricultural Practices 294
Organic Foods; Alarm over Mad Cow Disease..........................294
Organic Foods—Definitions 296
"Certified Organic" 296
Genetically Modified (GM) Foods 298
Is The American Food Supply Too Clean?.................................299
The Need for Balance 301
Food Labels 301
The New Food Label 303
Dissecting Food Labels...305
Deciphering "Labelese" 306
Food Labels—A Personal View 308
A Question of Balance 309
Summary..309

Once upon a time, life was rather simple. People did not have to worry much about choices. There was no confusion from television ads ... in fact there was no television, no radios, no cars, and no supermarkets (as we know it). Today, all that has changed. As choices have increased, so have those who seek to influence them.

An important inhibitory factor in the exclusion of nutrition from medical practice is the low expectation of compliance. ... Even after we learned how to deliver nutrition information in a way that makes it possible for a patient to comply, the number of those who do so seems low. Even if teaching is carried out properly, changing eating habits is , as you know, very difficult, and inhibited by cultural concepts of "normal" nutrition, lack of education, economic barriers to buying proper foods, a frantically overworked and hurried society that doesn't take the time to cook or eat correctly, etc. etc.

Commentary by David Singer, M.D.
Harvard Medical School

§§§§§§§

Life and Choices in the Real World

Chronic diseases are a vexing issue in medical practice, chiefly because results frequently prove elusive.
For obesity and related disorders, the easiest part is to hand out diet sheets, or tell patients to lose weight.
The reality, however, is that people face competing challenges that influence what they eat. These go far beyond anything that a doctor can prescribe.

Perhaps no other area of life forces us so frequently to make as many choices as what we put into our mouths. For some, this is their major occupation; for many, it is their major pre-occupation. It can be a source of delight and great pleasure and a toasty prescription for family, friendship, and fraternity. Sadly, it has also led to fusses, fights, and fetish. Housewives are known to complain that the only communication they ever receive is, "What's for breakfast, what's for lunch, and what's for dinner?"

The medical profession, for reasons mentioned in the third chapter, prefers not to get involved in people's kitchens and their culinary choices (and understandably so). However, if we fail to appreciate why people choose the foods they do, then we have failed to grasp one of the most important determinants of health and disease. All this takes place *outside* of a doctor's office, a hospital, or a healthcare system. The reasons people choose the foods they do are complex (Figure 7-1).[1]

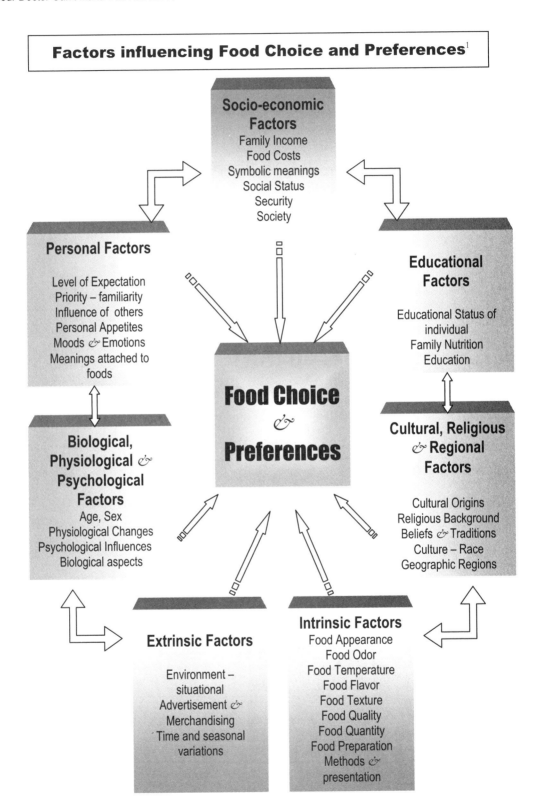

Figure 7-1. Factors Influencing Food Choice and Preferences.

Nutrition books give much information, but remain largely silent on the reasons people choose the foods they do. There is a notion that this is the job of the dietician or the behavioral psychologist. Choices, however, are the bottom line. This is where the execution of knowledge in nutrition and lifestyle takes place. This is where at first glance, the reasons for choices may appear simple, but is more complex than is often realized.

Several factors influence food choices (Figure 7-1). What we eventually choose depend on conscious and unconscious influences that are deeply rooted in our culture, up-bringing, and our socioeconomic realities. The exact transaction varies from individual to individual, but the payback can, over time, affect the outcome of your quality of life. Any effort to promote health and prevent diseases cannot escape a discussion on why people choose the foods they do.

Nowhere is this more evident than when dealing with the global epidemic of obesity. The typical scenario is one in which the majority of obese patients continue with the same weight struggles, despite repeated attempts to lose weight. It is not politically correct to say so, but doctors would prefer not to treat severely obese patients. A major reason is that this category of patients makes doctors feel impotent, as success rates are dismally low. Obesity is not a disease that can simply be zapped with a pill or a tumor that can be surgically removed.

Doctors and Governments Cannot Legislate Food Choices

To be unmindful of the fact that food policies are heavily influenced by powerful food industry forces to which many politicians are subject, and often indebted, is to be downright naïve.

My first thoughts on this subject began to coalesce almost ten years ago during my Nutrition program at King's College, University of London. I had chosen to write an essay on the role of governments in the nutrition choices of their populations. My views at that time were idealistic, overly enthusiastic, and heavily bureaucratic. ...The problems of the world were easy to solve. All that was needed was good governments, problems solved. Time and reality, however, have taught me otherwise.

There are two influential, but opposing views on human behavior and choices. On one extreme are those who adopt a defeatist view that individuals are at the mercy of their environments. The other camp believes that even in the midst of an unhealthy environment, knowledgeable and motivated individuals can make healthy choices. The first view is exemplified by comments made in the *British Medical Journal* on the subject of preventing obesity and type II diabetes. According to this view, it is futile to pursue lasting lifestyle changes to prevent and manage diseases like diabetes without changing the environment. This was the stance adopted by Dr. Colin Guthrie in his letter "Health promotion helps no one." His views are based on experience garnered while working as a physician in Scotland. He summed up his prevention efforts as well-intended, time-consuming, but a waste of time and resources:[2-3]

> In the end I realized that it is not patients who don't understand but we doctors who don't. For how we behave, what we eat, what opportunities we have to exercise, are all shaped by what confronts us in our environment. If our environment is unhealthy then we are unhealthy. ... I also learnt that the poorer you are then the more you are adversely affected by your environment; the richer you are the more easily you can manipulate your environment to create a health advantage. This is called having lifestyle choices. The poor are simply stuck with their usual foul environment.

Dr. Guthrie[3] further challenged a Finnish report[4] that promoted an individual-level, lifestyle approach to diabetes prevention. He considered any such efforts as futile unless they were accompanied by changes in the "obesogenic" environment.

> Our increasingly "obesogenic" environments are the driving forces for weight gain and diabetes. ... Until the obesogenic environments take center stage in a broader public health approach, the prevalence of obesity and type II diabetes will continue to rise, especially in populations with a low income and in disadvantaged populations.

Not only would doctors' attempts to make patients healthy prove futile, but also the efforts of governments to do the same. This is not to say that legislation and policies directed at changing food environments are unimportant. To the contrary, they are of tremendous importance. For certainty we need legislation and policies to encourage health-friendly environments. However, to be oblivious to the fact that food policies are heavily influenced by powerful food industry forces to which many politicians are subject, and often indebted, is to be downright naïve.

Although it is noble to lobby for changes in the food environment, the evidence is that you will receive better dividends by taking responsibility for your own health, regardless of your environment. Such attitudes will see you through whether you are in New York or Nairobi, Adelaide or Antananarivo. You are not an absolute victim of your environment. Indeed, history has shown that environments change when people demand change. Fast-food outlets have changed the composition of their oils in response to consumer demand. Supermarkets have stocked more produce, even organic varieties, again in response to consumer demand. The food industry, the Goliath that dictates what is available on the supermarket shelves, arguably pays more attention to what people buy than what governments legislate.

There is a disappointing shift towards fast-food culture in much of the globe. Many people in developing countries are marching headlong into duplicating lifestyles prevalent in much of the industrialized world. One consequence of this is that many developing countries (with third world healthcare budgets) have caught up with, and now surpass, lifestyle disease rates once typical of the industrialized West. For many people in the developing world, Western lifestyles carry potent desirable symbolisms, such as upward social mobility and liberal thinking. But imitating certain lifestyle patterns prevalent in the industrialized world, has led many in developing countries to secure themselves a future laden with obesity, cardiovascular and related diseases. We are witnessing an epidemic of heart disease and type II diabetes in the Indian subcontinent and most countries around the world.[5]

Even in these countries, market forces, not governments, will ultimately have the last say. Supply will always rise to meet the demand. Let us educate and empower individuals to make good choices, and encourage them spend their money on what promotes health, rather than on what causes disease. The food industry and the food environment will to follow suit. Politicians and governments should assist in creating a healthy environment, but even if such were created, it is ultimately up to the consumer to choose. As the saying goes—you can take a mule to water, but you cannot make him drink it.

The Complexities of Food Choices

Despite many hurdles, individuals need to make the best of their environment and make better choices.

Although there are many factors influencing food choices, it goes without say that people can only eat what is available. Furthermore, the choices are limited by physical as well as economic access. Although we live in an age of unprecedented globalization, many people are still limited in their choice of foods, especially if the items in question are decidedly rare, exotic, or ethnic:[6]

> The answer to the question 'why does one eat what one eats?' is indeed a complex one. Most people would probably feel that they are free to choose their own diets—and most would be surprised to learn the constraints that are in fact operating in limiting their choices. Various models of food choice processes have been proposed over the years. Some have emphasized environment, others have concentrated internal motivation. Each has contributed to an understanding of the factors which shape our food choices, whilst at the same time leaving many questions unanswered. Indeed, it seems unlikely that the plethora of factors which impinge on food choice can be codified in a single paradigm.

Consider the real-life example of the well-educated cleric in his forties who is a loving family man, with clear features of the metabolic syndrome discussed in Chapter 5. He recognizes the need to make dietary and lifestyle changes, but he does not. For him, knowledge is not the problem. Neither is it the home environment, for his wife, more than most women, has embarked on pursuing a healthy lifestyle. What is it that causes an otherwise intelligent human being to ignore advice on prevention?

Look at a completely different real-life scenario—that of a troubled teenager who is kicked out of school, home and unemployed. He struggles to survive, subscribes to Rastafarianism, becomes a vegetarian and avoids salt, processed foods, and dietary patterns associated with what he refers to as "Babylon system." The latter is a Rastafarian term for rampant commercialism.

Yet still, there is the scenario of the grossly overweight, middle-aged, hypertensive patient with type II diabetes and heart disease. Despite her physician's pleadings to lose weight, she confesses that she hates cooking, and she hates vegetables. She had resigned to her daily cocktail of prescription drugs. Her desire was simply to feel okay. Others like Mike Milken, financier, prostate-cancer survivor, and patron of cancer research, took charge and became a soy fanatic. His cancer-fighting recipes appear in his book, *The Taste for Living Cookbook*. The reasons people choose the foods they do are complex—not merely an educational or a socioeconomic matter.

Hierarchy of Food Choices

"Look, I am about to die," Esau said. "What good is the birthright to me?"
But Jacob said, "Swear to me first." So he swore an oath to him, selling his birthright to Jacob.
Then Jacob gave Esau some bread and some lentil stew.
The Book of Beginnings [7]

For the man who is extremely and dangerously hungry,
no other interests exist, but food.
He dreams food, he remembers food, he thinks food,
he emotes only of food, he perceives only food. [8]

A Theory of Human Motivation.—AH Maslow

Amidst the choices we make, what is it that makes people choose one type of food over another? For most people, the first thing that comes to mind when they are hungry is to satisfy that hunger. When on emergency call or when working in a busy hospital clinic, hunger sends one message—it demands to be satisfied. What to satisfy this craving with depends largely on what is available, unless you decide to fast or go on a hunger strike. This is what Maslow's hierarchy of needs calls the survival mode. When people are hungry, they want food, any food. Quality of food is then dismissed as an unimportant trivia. At this stage, hardly anything else matters (Figure 7-2).[8]

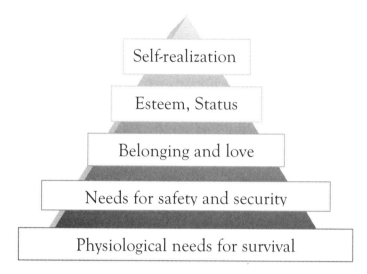

Figure 7-2. Functions of Food: Maslow's Hierarchy, as Applied to Food Habits[9]
(Eckstein, 1980)

Only after hunger is satisfied can rational thinking can take place. People who are preoccupied with food insecurity can easily remain trapped in the survival mode. They simply have no choice but to take what is on offer. Those with higher incomes and a greater degree of food security can progressively make more room for the finer functions of food (e.g. for status, or for health). These are they who have gained a greater degree of control over their food choices and their environment (Figure 7-2). Without question, which room you occupy in the pyramid, can determine how much room you can make for healthy choices.

People who have demanding jobs and those whose jobs require frequent travel are far more likely to rely on convenience foods. Traditional nuclear families with one parent working at home generally have a greater proportion of home-cooked meals. Major demographic shifts including an increase in working-women have led an increased consumption of convenience foods. As more food is consumed outside the home, there is the accompanying loss of control over the quality of food eaten. A prime example of this is what takes place during air travel. Airport food is generally of the unhealthy variety, but according to an *Airwise News* report, there is some hope for the future:[10]

> Plane changes and layovers can be frustrating enough without being limited to mystery-meat chili dogs and greasy hamburgers. Unfortunately, less than 60 percent of the airport restaurants we surveyed offer healthy, vegetarian meals. LAX, for example, is home to no fewer than four McDonald's and

four Burger Kings, and Las Vegas is overrun with barbecue joints and sausage stands. The good news is that healthy food is everywhere if you just know where to look, and some restaurants are getting creative with delicious-sounding choices like portabello mushroom sandwiches and linguine with garlic and vegetables. Even in the worst airports, you can usually find a bean burrito or veggie burger.

As people demand healthier choices, consumer products arise to fill the demand. Unfortunately, this trend does not manifest itself everywhere. This may be true in the United States, but in many countries in the developing world, people are preoccupied with more mundane priorities—that of mere survival. Where healthier choices are less available, consumers must be highly motivated to make healthy choices. Healthy food choices are difficult, if not impossible, where such choices are simply not available, affordable, or accessible (Table 7-1).

Table 7-1. Important Issues Influencing Food Choices

Core Issues Influencing Food Choices

1. Availability
2. Affordability
3. Accessibility (physical and economic)
4. Other: Socio-cultural, ideology, motivational etc.

Socialization and Food Choices

Humans are social beings. We grow up in homes, cultures, and countries. We are all subject to these social influences that sway our choices. To what extent do these dominate? … And to what extent does society influence the food choices we make?

Food habits, by definition, are patterns that are learned and have become entrenched over time. They arise in infancy and become established at a rather early age. Infants and toddlers have no choice in what they eat, apart from refusal. They simply have to consume what is provided by the adults who feed them. Certain tastes become ingrained early in life. Most people eat like their parents; people generally choose the foods that they are used to. As children grow older and as they become exposed to ever-widening spheres of influence, they find themselves facing new challenges that influence their tastes and choices (Figure 7-3).[11-14]

Socialization is a lifelong process by which those culturally valued norms of behavior are passed from generation to generation. Cultures tend to resist change, but they are not impregnable. Despite the early entrenchment of tastes and habits, food choices are amenable to change. The history of man has been a history of shared knowledge and experiences. The cross-pollination of diets is a subset of this phenomenon. The historical spice trade between Europe and the East was an early example of the globalization of foods and flavors. Therefore, East-meets-West is not a new phenomenon. Mankind has constantly interacted with his environment and has adopted foreign tastes and flavors. The "Westernization of diets" is not so much a Western phenomenon, as it is a response to the demands of modern living. The constant drive towards increased efficiency and productivity as well as the emergence of cities has fueled the development of today's food consumption patterns.

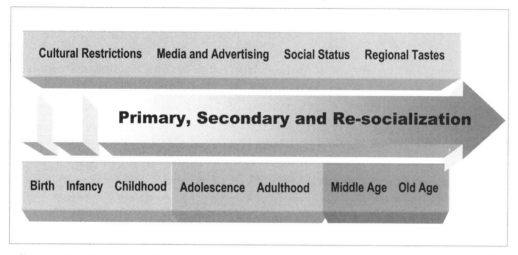

Figure 7-3. The Acquisition of Food Habits and Socialization continues throughout life.
Source: Fieldhouse P., Food and Nutrition, Customs and Culture [12]

Anti-Americanism has become disturbingly popular, and America-bashing for the export of its fast-food culture seems to be the order of the day. While it may be true that America does a better job at marketing food and lifestyles than any other country on the planet, the fast food culture and its contribution to the global obesity epidemic is more a product of modern urban lifestyles and capitalism, than it is an innately American ideology.

This pattern has been adopted overseas because it works well in the modern environment. People around the world, in their pursuit of material success, have been quick to both adopt and adapt the American model. The global export of "The American Way" has been facilitated in an unprecedented way by satellite television, the Internet, and the ease of international travel. Great symbolism and significance is placed by many (in the developing world) on choosing American-styled foods. Drinking Coca-Cola and eating at McDonald's can make powerful political and social statements abroad. In some cultures, it may be seen as being progressive and open-minded on one hand, or branded as rebellious and Westernized on the other.[12]

The impact of the Macdonald's and Coca Cola culture is evident, but the charges have been taken to ridiculous extremes, as exemplified in the recent class action lawsuit that sought damages from McDonald's for causing obesity. The sober judgment (in January 2003) of U.S. district judge Robert Sweet declared that nobody was forced to eat at McDonald's. It takes two to tango. There will always be sellers so long as there are buyers.

Alcohol consumption and certain types of foods carry social dividends that enable partakers to feel a sense of belonging. The stage of adolescence heralds the start of independence in social habits and food and drinking patterns. Children, however, are the most vulnerable and impressionable age group. They are the premier targets of the food, beverage, and fashion industries. These industries exert a tremendous impact on the food and drink choices of children. Social and peer pressures in children aggravate the situation further. Not many children can withstand peer pressures and follow the advice of their parents. There are reports of parents, quite happy that their child always ate their home-prepared lunches (as judged from the empty lunchbox), only to be devastated to discover that the fruit and vegetables ended up in the waste-basket. It is not an easy thing for children to endure being labeled as a horse or a rabbit (for their love of greens). It is easier for most, to endure the wrath of their parents, than to endure the verbal wrath of their peers.[15]

Targeting the Children

> There will be no victory in the public health arena without victory in instilling healthy lifestyles at an early age.
> The stakes are extremely high. Failure to aggressively tackle food choices of youth are already resulting in worrying trends, which if ignored, can become a public health nightmare.

Herein lies a tragedy in the making—the wanton assault on the children of America (and the world) by the food and beverage industries that incessantly explore ways and means of spreading their influence and garnering a faithful following. The marketing of foods to children has been a very effective strategy for the food industry. One aspect of this was introduced in Chapter 2 on the subject of "pester power"—the ability of children to nag their parents into purchasing foods and other items they would otherwise not buy.[16] Winning the hearts and minds of children can provide industry with an important and a growing market.

We decry strategies and devices that attempt to market tobacco and alcohol to children, but a similar effort to protect the food and beverage choices of our children does not seem to be a priority. It will be a crucial mistake to gloss over the continuing threats to healthy food choices in children (Table 7-2).[17-19]

The CBS program, *60 Minutes,* recently aired a disturbing program on the commercial exploitation of schools.[20] Cash-strapped schools were eager to accept help from any sector willing to provide them with much needed funds for academic and sporting amenities. The food industry came to their rescue. Some sectors in the industry, in their strategy to tap into this lucrative market, had recruited psychologists to assist them in targeting American youth in schools. Advocacy groups were outraged that the very people who should be protecting the youth, were instead, recruited to manipulate them into developing unhealthy food (and drink) choices. Advocates claimed that children could not defend themselves against such onslaughts. School nutritionists felt that they were fighting a losing battle.

High schools across America are being increasingly subjected to food franchises that have set the nutrition agenda. Competition can become vicious with companies vying for lucrative profits and brand loyalties among youth. Among the most profitable franchises are those for soft drinks, where profits have been reported to exceed 90 percent. Participating schools in return receive lots of perks for these "pouring rights" and other rights to sell franchised-foods. The report aptly concluded, "Grease has won the battle over greens."

Table 7-2. Important Factors Influencing Food Choices In American Children and Adolescents

Factors Influencing Food Choices In American Youth

- **Peer Pressure**
- **Media**—influence over food choices, plethora of food commercials, especially snacks, candy, fast foods, and cereals, disordered perception of body image and eating disorders
- **Family**—primary socialization, what they are taught at home
- **Social realities**—fewer meals at home
- **Economic status**

An in-depth look at this phenomenon is contained in Professor Marion Nestlé's excellent book, *Food Politics—How the Food Industry Influences Nutrition and Health.* The section on "Exploiting Kids, Corrupting Schools—Starting early: Underage consumers and pushing soft drink,"[21] is one of the best references on this subject. The stakes are extremely high. The 900-billion-dollars-a-year food industry will not be easily deterred, and they are unlikely to make changes without pressure from lawmakers and market forces. This will be an enormous struggle, but consider the alternative of doing nothing. Failure to address the food choices of American youth can balloon into frightening medical price tag too big for any singular institution to contain.

The full consequences of this fallout are yet to be seen. The term "adult-onset diabetes" (the epidemic that is now sweeping America and the world), has become somewhat of a misnomer. An increasing proportion of youth are now developing adult onset or type II diabetes. Type II diabetes has now surpassed type I or juvenile onset diabetes as the major form of diabetes in American youth. This striking shift is the direct result of increasing calorie intake and low levels of physical activity. Almost 25 percent of all American children are, to some degree, overweight, and the tendency is for them to remain overweight throughout adolescence. In the rest of the world, obese (very overweight) children number more than 35 million. Obese children are twice as likely to become obese adults with all the attendant risks of medical complications.[22,23]

There appears to be a fundamental disconnect between what children are taught compared to what they do. A study done by researchers in the United Kingdom examined how children understood the "Five A Day" (five fruits and vegetable servings daily) health message.[22] They interviewed 68 children between the ages of 5 to 6, and 71 children between the ages of 10 to 11. These children were asked to categorize photographs of fruits, vegetables, and other food groupings. They concluded that even though 60 percent of them knew that orange juice, carrots, apples, grapes, and bananas were good for them, about half that number did not know if they should also eat more snacks, sweets, and soft drinks. Some children even consider such choices consistent with being a vegetarian. Many define the term "vegetarian" in terms of what you don't eat, vis-à-vis, no meat. Therefore, children believed that consuming lots of potato chips, snacks, and soft drinks was consistent with being a good vegetarian.

We must not forget the devastating impact of poverty and social deprivation on children.[25] This is the other end of the spectrum of nutrition, not the prime concern of this book, but we must pause to remember that these ills have a major impact on children. Indeed, infants and children bear the brunt of these scourges. The food choices of children are largely the responsibilities of adults, both at home and at school. We must protect them. Serious consequences are likely to follow if we shirk from this responsibility. Children need to have good choices made for them until they learn to fend for themselves.

Children need all the help that they can get, not only from their core families, but also from school, interest groups, the media, and legislators. Preventive cardiologists will tell you that heart disease begins in childhood. Failure to intervene early on behalf of our children can result in massive additional healthcare expenditures in the future.[26-28] A future without healthy children is a future without healthy adults.

"Ameri-sizing"

The words "portions" and "serving sizes" have no uniform definitions in America. Super-sized portions have become increasingly popular as food outlets compete for consumer dollars.
The portion sizes printed on food labels are much smaller than the serving sizes Americans actually eat.[29]

Americans now consume 500 calories more (per day) than they did in the 1970s.[30] Convenience foods now dominate the American landscape and have been bolstered by the entry of 60 percent of women into the workforce. One result of this demographic trend is that more food is eaten away from home. Just over a generation ago, 75 percent of the money spent on food went into preparing home-cooked meals. Today, 50 percent of the money spent on food is spent on food away from home, mainly at restaurants and fast-food outlets.

As competition increases in this multibillion dollar market, so do the portion sizes (see Chapter 5, "Excess Food, Excess Calories"). The words "portions" and "serving sizes" are being re-defined. Super sized portions are fast becoming the order of the day—everything big is becoming the norm. What is certain is that the food and portion sizes listed on the USDA's Food Guide Pyramid and on food labels are much smaller than the serving sizes that Americans actually eat. In a practical sense, this renders much of the dietary advice given on food labels as potentially misleading. This may be one reason why obesity rates continue to escalate in the midst of the current USDA food pyramid guidelines. Large sizes and servings mean value-for-money in America. Unfortunately, this is filling more than just stomachs and the coffers of companies, but it is fueling the American obesity epidemic and filling our hospitals.

A study done by the Department of Nutrition and Food Studies at New York University clearly demonstrated that the obesity epidemic in America had at its root, an increase in portion sizes. Researchers noted a 700 percent increase in the size of cookies, a 200 to 500 percent increase in foodstuff portion sizes (e.g. bagels and pasta) that went far beyond USDA-recommended levels. This trend was directly attributed to marketing tactics brought on by increasing competition within this massive multibillion dollar industry.[31]

Economics and Food Choices

People with more money have more choices. It is as simple as that. This does not mean that people with more money make healthier choices, but money clearly influences the ability to choose. Most people around the world are preoccupied with survival issues—putting food on the table and paying the bills with the hope that things will be better some day. Such populations occupy the bottom two rungs of Maslow's hierarchy of needs pyramid (Figure 7-2). The poor are limited in their choices; most are trapped in the survival mode. With more money comes status and prestige. Its impact on choices is quite striking in countries where wide socioeconomic disparities are entrenched.

I had an opportunity to speak with Harvard's Walter Willett, Professor of Epidemiology and Nutrition at the Harvard School of Public Health. He gave me a few personal insights into the whole issue of health and nutrition in America. I interpreted his views to mean that healthy living had become "a tale of two Americas." There is one group of Americans who presently enjoy excellent health and doing all the right things, but on the other hand, there is a large group that is painting a less than promising picture, with socioeconomics at its core. Such views coming from a scientist of Dr. Willett's stature deserve much consideration.

Table 7-3. Food Choices and Socioeconomic Status in the UK
Differences in Vegetable, Fruit and Bread Consumption

Foods Consumed	Low-Income Group (D and E2) oz per person per week	High-Income Group (A) oz per person per week
Fresh green vegetables	4.35	7.81
Other fresh vegetables	7.03	15.46
Processed vegetables	18.90	14.99
Potatoes	43.38	23.21
Fresh fruit	6.21	24.41
Other fruit and fruit products	2.23	15.22

Modified from source: Household Food Consumption and Expenditure 1990, HMSO (UK)[32]

Surveys done in the United Kingdom clearly show the impact of income on food choices. Whether this is the result of less disposable income by the economically disadvantaged to invest in fresh food and greens or whether it is a reflection of educational status, ignorance, or simply taste preferences is yet to be determined (Table 7-3).[33] The impact of disposable income on food choices, however, is not in dispute:

> One thing that most clearly distinguishes the diets of poor consumers from the better-off is consumption of fresh fruit and vegetables. The *National Food Survey* also shows marked differences between social groups. The richest fifth consumes 20 percent more fresh green vegetables, 70 percent more fresh fruit, and over 400 percent more fruit juice than the poorest fifth.

A paradox may exist here. Poverty has different implications in different communities. Being poor in America has a completely different meaning from being poor in India, or being poor in Belize (see insert: *When low per capita income can lead to better choices).* I was taught in London that urban populations are socio-economically better off than rural populations. Such realities may be true in England, but not in Belize.

Poor rural communities around the world grow their own food, and are better off (nutritionally speaking), than those held hostage in the city. Rural populations may lack the cash to purchase commodities and hardware items, but they may follow good nutrition guidelines simply because their choices are restricted to foods that are simple, but nutritionally superior. They may not be able to afford meat, but they subsist on vegetables and ground provisions, with less purchasing power to buy highly processed and imported foodstuffs.

When low per capita income can lead to better choices

Let me illustrate a point from my native Belize (formerly British Honduras), that may be misjudged as poor according to per capita income figures, but is wealthy in many ways, especially in terms of access to healthy lifestyle choices. It is a sparsely populated country of some 250,000 inhabitants in an area the size of Massachusetts. From a nutrition standpoint, you can buy 100 fresh oranges for less than US$3.00 or 20 bananas for US$1.00—extremely cheap, even by local standards. Better still, you may not need to buy these at all. The climate supports a variety of fruit trees that bear fruit throughout the year. Edible tubers and vines easily grow with minimal attention. No shortage of meats exists and there is plenty of game. Fish is everywhere—in ponds, rivers, lagoons and the sea. Rufus X (a well-known local personality) says you have to work hard to starve in Belize.

Herein lies an unfortunate paradox. There is a lingering vestige of colonialism and global influences that has wreaked havoc with local attitudes and eating practices. Fast food is now everywhere, and eating "well" means eating like Americans or the British—the stuff that is advertised on television. Upward social mobility is reflected in one's ability to fill up supermarket carts with fancy U.S. and European imports. Many locals still despise their birthright. "Poverty" means that you can't afford all things American.

As time passes and as consumer awareness grows, many now realize that reduced income, although it may denote reduced ability to buy fancy imports, does not condemn you to poor health. Here, reduced income may actually mean reduced ability to indulge in less healthy choices. Many natives are now discovering that the things they once despised, like organically-grown traditional farm products, are prime commodities that can fetch, not only handsome prices overseas, but can also deliver better health.

The Food and Consumer Service (FCS) runs the U.S. Food Stamp Program whose primary mission is to ensure access to nutritious and healthy diets for all Americans. Its assistance and education efforts encourage consumers to make healthu food choices. According to their survey, "Few low-income households meet the twin objectives of using foods that provide a healthful diet and spending less than the thrifty food plan (TFP) amount." Very few low-income households use foods from home supplies that meet the dietary guidelines for total and saturated fat. These are summarized in Table 7-4.[32,33]

Table 7-4 Major Findings of the Report on *Understanding the Food Choices of Low Income Americans*

**Findings of Focus Group Discussions of
Food Stamp Recipients (U.S.)**

1. Food stamp recipients are generally well-informed.
2. Food price is the most important determinant of food choices.
3. There is great reliance on convenience foods.
4. Children's food preferences are very strong determinants of family choice.
5. Ethnic and cultural traditions play very important roles in food choices.
6. Awareness of the healthy eating guidelines exists, but changes will be difficult.

There are other socioeconomic factors must be taken into account when considering the food choices. People who live in isolated or impoverished neighborhoods with little access to fresh foods are often forced to shop for non-perishable items, resulting in little intake of fresh fruits and vegetables. Access to private transportation is usually nonexistent. These are the so-called "food deserts" that can plague socio-economically deprived neighborhoods, and lead to undesirable food choice patterns along with all its negative health implications.[34,35]

Politics and Food Choices

Next to the U.S. Congress, the food industry probably exerts more influence over nutrition policy than any other segment of American society. Much of what Congress does is influenced heavily by the food industry lobby.

One important role of government and lawmakers is to legislate and implement food safety, security, and quality. The key players involved in establishing nutrition policy in the United States are shown in Figure 7-4.[36]

The USDA Food Guide Pyramid

One of the most influential federal agencies that influence the food choices issues of American is the USDA. The *Dietary Guidelines for Americans* comes under its jurisdiction. Their Food Guide Pyramid: a guide to healthy food choices was developed in 1992 with the help of a special committee of nutrition experts in the Departments of Health and Human Services (DHSS) and the USDA (Figure 7-5)[37]

Key Players involved in U.S. National Nutrition Policy

- **The Congress:** authorizes, appropriates, and oversees nutrition policy
- **The White House:** through three main components of the Office of the President; reviews and regulates policy.
- **Department of Health and Human Services (DHHS):** consists of multiple agencies.
- **The National Institutes of Health (NIH):** the most important federal entity influencing nutrition policy.
- **The Food and Drug Administration (FDA):** involved in the Nutrition Labeling and Education Act of 1990.
- **Centers for Disease Control (CDC):** major player involved in scientific aspects of nutrition policy.
- **U.S. Department of Agriculture (USDA):** plays a major role in policy and research
- **The Food Industry:** major influence over nutrition policy; major food lobbying of Congress
- **The Federal Trade Commission:** regulates food advertising
- **Other Federal Agencies**
- **Advisory Institutions**
- **Scientific Societies and Organizations:** e.g., the American Medical Association (AMA)
- **International Organizations:** World Health Organization (WHO), Food and Agricultural Organization (FAO).
- **State and Local Organizations**
- **Consumer Organizations**
- **The Media**

Figure 7-4. The Key Players Involved in Establishing U.S. Food Policy

Carbohydrate-rich foods are lumped together at the base of the pyramid and command the biggest share of the recommendations (6 to 11 servings daily). Fruits and vegetables (at least 5 servings daily) are on the next level. Dairy products and protein sources, regardless of whether they are from meat, poultry, or eggs, are huddled together as one group. All fats, oils, and sweets are placed in one basket at the summit of the pyramid with the warning label "Use Sparingly," giving rise to the popular American notion that "fat is fat, and all fats are bad." Critics have argued that the food-industry lobby groups (e.g. the Milk Board, the Beef Council, and the Wheat Foods Council) have exerted too much influence on the committee's decisions.[38-39]

The USDA pyramid has some supporters like Miriam Nelson, Ph.D., associate professor of the School of Nutrition Science and Policy at Tufts University. She considers the pyramid an important step towards developing nutrition guidelines because of its focus on the whole diet, and because all foods fit in the pyramid regardless of food preferences, religious beliefs, or heritage.[40]

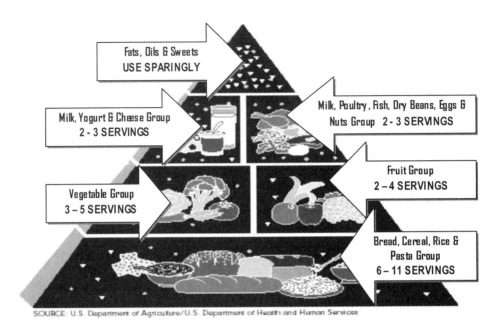

Figure 7-5. The popular USDA Food Guide Pyramid (daily recommended intakes)

A leading critic of the pyramid is Walter Willett, M.D., professor and chair of the Department of Nutrition at the Harvard School of Public Health. In his book *Eat, Drink, and Be Healthy,* he declared that USDA Food Guide Pyramid was built on shaky scientific ground. According to Dr. Willett, the pyramid "has been steadily eroded by new research from all parts of the globe … that have chipped away at the foundation (carbohydrates), the middle (meat and milk), and the apex (fats)."

Dr. Willet insists that the USDA pyramid has to be rebuilt to maintain scientific credibility. Special interest groups that have agendas other than the health of the American public helped to engineer its foundations:[38]

> The thing to keep in mind about the USDA pyramid is that it comes from the Department of Agriculture, the agency responsible for promoting American agriculture, *not* from agencies established to monitor and protect our health...And there's the root of the problem—what's good for some agricultural interests isn't necessarily good for the people who eat their products. Serving two masters is tricky business, especially when one of them includes persuasive and well-connected representatives of the formidable meat, dairy, and sugar industries. The end result of their tug and war is a set of positive, feel-good, all-inclusive recommendations that completely distort what could be the single most important tool [the food guide pyramid] for improving your health and the health of the nation.

According to this leading expert, the footprints of politics were to be found all over the pyramid. The dairy industry's "milk moustache" ads were a prime example of this. "No calcium emergency" exists in the United States, declares Dr. Willett. In his view, the USDA pyramid's call for two to three servings of dairy products daily are scientifically unjustified.[40] But Dr. Willett and colleagues did not stop at just diagnosing of the ills of the USDA pyramid. He prescribed an alternative—the Healthy Eating Pyramid. This was the cover story of Newsweek (January 20, 2003), and can be accessed from "The Nutrition Source" section of the Harvard School of Public Health website: http://www.hsph.harvard.edu/nutritionsource/.

Professor Marion Nestlé's book, *Food Politics, How the Food Industry Influences Nutrition and Health,* is a must-read for those who seek an in-depth look at the enormous grip of the food industry over politics and food policies.[21] In this award-winning book, she reveals the dynamics of the American food supply and its impact on public health. She reveals how the American food industry co-opted the government's dietary guidelines, and paved the way for the corruption and the exploitation of American schoolchildren. Nestlé's book, in the words of one reviewer, is "a devastating analysis of how the naked self-interest of America's largest industry, influences and compromises nutrition policy and government regulation of food safety." The fattening of America and the ensuing medical fallout are heavily intertwined with the politics and economics of this 900-billion dollar industry.[21,41] There is, without question, an insatiable craving by industry for an ever bigger slice of this lucrative American pie.

> "No system for nutrition policy exists per se, nor is there likely to be one in the foreseeable future. What one has to learn, often the hard way, is that if you want to play the game, you have to touch a lot of bases"[36]
>
> Allan L. Forbes
> Former Director of Office of Nutrition and Food Sciences
> Center for Safety and Applied Nutrition, Food and Drug Administration (FDA)

The Media and Food Choices

The "mother-of-all-bombs" that is mobilized early in the food war is the media. Its design is not so much about winning hearts and minds, as it is about conquest by any means necessary. The technologies employed are not the least bit concerned about collateral damage, indeed this is the primary purpose for its existence. It spares no medium (television, radio, print, the Internet), it respects no age (indeed it targets them all), and it spares no home. Advertisements for food and drinks gobble up more television time than any other product line. Food advertising is a multibillion dollar industry.

Television dominates with the powerful impact of its images that cleverly market to people of all sizes, shapes, colors, customs, and creeds. Targeting children is especially effective because they are so good at influencing the food choices of their parents—the "pester power" or the child-perpetrated blackmail introduced in Chapter 2. Children are especially vulnerable. They are largely unable to discern the difference between programs versus advertisements, and they are certainly unaware of the motives behind television ads. The media and food choices are a book by itself, but the strategies that they employ fall into broad categories that are summarized in Table 7-5.[42-45]

Table 7-5. Marketing Appeals in Food Advertising

The Food Itself	• Convenience • Newness • Naturalness • Traditional or cultural • Nutritional value
Economics	• Cost • Value for money • Specials • Economy packs
Symbolism (food as a means to something else)	• Status value • Endorsement by personalities • Popularity • Ideal mother/wife • Sexual attraction • Fitness and slimness • Reward • Success

Globalization and Food Choices

It is "cool" to blame America for exporting junk food and fattening the world. Urbanization and the fast-food culture are part-payment for modernity and capitalism, but the pursuit of capital is not the preserve of the United States. They are simply the leaders of the pack, and there is no shortage of wolves trying to catch up.

A seemingly unstoppable phenomenon is the impact of rapid changes brought about by the ease of international travel, transportation, and communications that will continue to define this new millennium. The spice trade is long gone, and so are the days of the steamships. For opportunists and prospectors, globalization symbolizes unprecedented opportunities. For traditionalists and those on the receiving end, moves towards globalization are met with suspicion and resentment because it invades previously impregnable traditions and customs, and empowers largely those who have financial clout. Globalization enthusiasts have welcomed it as an unparalleled way of keeping in step with the forward-thinking global community.

In the context of health, we cannot separate the trends toward globalization from the economics, the politics, and the symbolisms. There are the haves and the have-nots. The have-nots aspire for the spoils of the haves, and in betwixt them both are the want-to-be's. The peoples of the developing world want to have the trappings (food and all) of the industrialized world.

It is not fair to accuse the United States and the industrialized countries of deliberately exporting their ideals. Rather, it is more a matter of the developing world craving to live like Americans and the West. You cannot have a sale without a buyer. Therefore, when you see the big Coca Cola sign in the slums of Zambia, it is because some Zambian makes money by selling an American product.

Examine the global trends. Many cities share more commonalities than differences. The design of the malls and public buildings and the fashion trends are often indistinguishable. This same applies to food. Many around the world prefer Coke, Pepsi, and McDonald's to traditional beverages and foods. It is easy for people to blame America for exporting junk food and fattening the world. Urbanization and the fast-food culture are part-payment for modernity and capitalism, but the pursuit of capital is not the preserve of the United States. They are simply the leaders of the pack, and there is no shortage of wolves trying to catch up.

There is a thing called choice. People in the developing world need to acknowledge their own roles and culpability in all of this. Whether justifiable or not, much of the worlds have-nots are bent on acquiring the lifestyles of the haves. There are many positive lifestyle changes occurring in the West, such as the ban on cigarette ads and smoking in public places, the mandatory labeling of food, and moves towards healthier food choices. If more people in the developing world would pursue these positive trends with the same vigor they pursued the negative trends they blame on America, it would go a long way to demonstrate that positive benefits can also result from living in a global village.

Individual Issues and Food Choices

Can we legislate healthy eating? The answer is an emphatic "No!" No amount of policies, plans, and government regulations can prevent people in a democratic society from killing themselves if they so choose.

The findings of a National Cancer Institute Survey concluded that individual-personal-internal factors were the most important factor influencing food choices and dietary behavior.[46]

The charge continues to be made that people are simply at the mercy of politics and the economics of food. This may be true, but only to a limited extent. Time and experience have shown that there are so many individuals who have the gumption to go against the grain. An individual is not at the mercy of the prevailing trends that are taking place. What is it that motivates an individual to make healthy choices? In a sense this gets to the heart of what this book is all about—helping the individual to make those choices that promote health and prevent disease. But this book can only go as far as providing knowledge and insight; the actions that follow must be an individual decision.

The National Cancer Institute conducted a survey on factors influencing the recommended daily intake of fruits and vegetables. More than 2,500 adults aged 18 years and older were asked questions based on their knowledge, personal, and other variables that influenced why they chose to eat more fruits and vegetables. They concluded that individual-personal-internal factors were the most important determinants influencing food choices and dietary behavior.[46]

A number of other studies have supported these findings. Dietary changes do not occur overnight. They occur in stages, moving from mental contemplation to the stage of implementation and maintenance of these changes (see Chapter 10). Knowledge of the Five-A-Day (at least 5 daily servings of fruits and vegetables) message for better health was the most important predictor of fruit and vegetable consumption. A noteworthy barrier to increased vegetable consumption was the lack of time needed to prepare vegetables compared to fruit that can be eaten raw.[47]

Another study that highlighted the primacy of individual responsibility, over institutional measures to promote healthy lifestyles, was the Cardiovascular Health Awareness Program (CHAP). This study looked at 278 hospital employees in Connecticut that enrolled in a program aimed at preventing heart disease. One group participated in a highly structured exercise, nutrition, and weight-management program. The other group opted not to engage in the structured program. Both groups exhibited improvement in risk factors, but the greatest improvement was seen in those who opted out of the structured program. At first glance, this appears contrary to expectations, but it does reflect, among other things, that self-motivated individuals will exhibit healthy lifestyles when no one else is looking.[48] These people needed little in the way of external motivation. They made the right choices for reasons other that a mere structured externally motivated system. Have you ever wondered how a person can spend 12 years in the military and still end up undisciplined?

People who are keen on making good choices and maximizing their health will go beyond what is simply prescribed. They are more likely to take the initiative and explore ways and means of achieving better health. But choices must be based on knowledge. Health-conscious individuals will make time and effort to learn about betters ways and means of achieving nutrition knowledge, they will read up about this and related matters. A British study revealed just that. It had studied the nutrition practices of 1,630 participants and showed that health enthusiasts were willing to supplement an already healthy diet with other healthy practices. Nutrition-savvy consumers prefer foods with more natural health benefits, and tend to avoid highly processed foods.[49]

Can we legislate healthy eating? The answer is an emphatic "No!" No amount of government policies, plans, or regulations can prevent people in a democratic society from killing themselves if they so choose. Highly-motivated individuals will not wait for government, or institutions, or their doctor to make decisions to improve their health. They are keenly aware that they have no real control over government policies or medical priorities. They recognize that their energies will be far better spent on doing those things that no one else can do for you. … That is the gift of choice.

******

Introduction to Food Processing

Our Food Supply Has Changed.

Ninety percent of the foods North Americans eat are of the processed variety. The greatest change ever in the history of the human diet has occurred over the past 75 years.
If you compare what people in the industrialized world eat today to what people ate then, it should come as no surprise why we now confront this modern epidemic of obesity, cardiovascular diseases, type II diabetes and cancer.

In the quest for optimal health, diet plays a central role. Many are ignorant about how much our food supply has changed. Few really care about what those pretty packets and cans contain beyond the good-tasting delights. Fewer still have an accurate understanding of how such foods affect health. Many assume that corn and corn flakes are essentially the same or that the "100% tomato juice" is the same as blending fresh organic tomatoes. There are literally tens of thousands of new foods that appear on the supermarket shelves with thousands more added each year.

I cannot fault the public for being oblivious to these changes since it is such an entrenched part of modern culture. But if you grew up in an environment where fish is sold freshly-caught, and where fruits arrive in your home freshly-picked, you would then understand why I highlight these concerns. This is not a minor matter. There is a bumper sticker that says, "If you think education is expensive, try ignorance." Ignorance of our food supply comes with a heavy price tag. The costs are to be measured in the form of ill-health and premature death from largely preventable diseases.

Processed foods in the Western diet are essentially a product of industrialization and the demographic changes that have accompanied urbanization (see Chapter 5). Food processing comprises any action that results in a change to the original plant or animal food product. Strictly speaking, slicing, washing, storing, refrigerating, and cooking are simple forms of processing. Simplistic prescriptions like "raw food is best" and "all processing is bad" are misleading statements. Most foods need to undergo some form of processing before consumption, however minimal that process may be.

Table 7-6. Traditional Food Processing Methods

Traditional Food Processing Methods
(these methods have been used for millennia)

1. Smoking (meats)
2. Drying (meats, grain)
3. Salting (meats)
4. Pickling (meats)

Traditional societies have, for millennia, relied on relatively simple ways of preparing and storing food. The grand vizier Joseph, of biblical fame, became renowned in ancient Egypt for preparing the granaries to store surplus grain to hedge against the predicted famine.[50] People around the world have practiced a number of methods and means of preserving and storing the fruits of their labor. The commonest of these are smoking, drying, salting, and pickling foods (Table 7-6).

Industrial Food Processing Methods

In food processing, the process is just as important as the final product. Processing affects the nutritional value of foods, and paying attention to these details can make a major difference in the health of individuals and populations.

Progress brings problems, and with increasing urbanization, demanding modern lifestyles and the entry of more women into the workplace, the stage was set for a consumer-driven demand for more convenience foods. The modern food-processing industry has no parallel in human history. Never before in mankind's history have we exerted so much control over food and food supply. This would have been impossible without the rise of the modern food industry.

Table 7-7. Early Industrial Food Processing Methods

Early Methods of Industrial Food Processing
(these methods have become popular since the
advent of electricity and the industrial age)

1. Heating and Chilling
2. Evaporating and Drying
3. Freezing
4. Fermenting
5. Preservation (with acid, salt, sugar)
6. Grinding and Mixing
7. Emulsification and Foaming

This highly technical industry has harnessed the best minds and techniques into what could be considered an industrial revolution in itself. Without passing any judgment on nutritional quality, the modern food industry should be lauded and given full marks for delivering Western populations from repeated threats of starvation barely a century ago. Today food insecurity (starvation) in the industrial world is almost unthinkable (see Chapter 3 "The Mid 1900s: Nutrition Forsakened").

The section will provide some basic insights into those processes that pose considerable health concerns, particularly with respect to chronic diseases. In the last one hundred years, Western societies have experienced a shift from inefficiency and insufficient food, to one of unparalleled agricultural and industrial surplus. This has largely been the result of improvements in basic industrial food processing methods that have evolved into highly efficient and automated processes (Table 7-7).

Spectrum of Food Processing Methods

Industrial food processing involve physical, chemical, and biological methods of food preparation, in addition to newer processes that now find increasing applications in food processing. These processes and their objectives are summarized below (Tables 7-8, 7-9, and 7-10).[51-53]

Table 7-8. Simplified Spectrum of Industrial Food Processing Methods
Physical Agents

Processing Agents	Method	Main Objective
Physical Agents	Heat (cooking, heating, pasteurization, UHT) and Canning	Preservation and change to more palatable form. Canning: *is the most vigorous form of heat treatment designed to kill bacteria and microorganisms.*
	Cold	Preservation

	Change of State
	  Evaporation, Distillation
	  Drying, Freezing
		Preservation

	Subdivision
	  Cutting, Chopping, Crushing
	  Milling, Grinding
		Change to more palatable form

	Separation
	  Sieving, Centrifugation
	  Filtration
		Change to more palatable form

	Mixing	Change to more palatable form
	Emulsifiers and Stabilizers;Gelling agents Anti-Foaming agents	Change to more palatable form Change to more palatable form
	Radiation	Preservation

Table 7-9. Simplified Spectrum of Industrial Food Processing Methods
Biological Agents

Processing Agents	Main objective	Medium employed
Biological Agents	Modification and transformation	Selected bacteria for production of yogurts, cheeses
	Fermentation	Alcoholic beverages, beer, cider wine, spirits and vinegar
	Fermentation and gas (carbon dioxide) production	Bakers yeast and bread production

Table 7-10. Simplified Spectrum of Industrial Food Processing Methods
Chemical Agents

Processing Agents	Main Objective	Medium employed
Chemical Agents	Preservatives	Acidity and alkalinity regulators, Salting, Brine, Curing salts Sugaring, Smoking
	Direct food additives (intentionally added to foods to perform a specific function)	Antioxidants (to prevent oxidation & rancidity): Natural: (*vitamin C and E*); Synthetic: *butylated hydroxyanisole (BHA) and butylated hydroxytoluene (BHT)*;
		Anti-spoilage agents, Flavors, Colorants (natural): *annatto, carmine, paprika, turmeric, beta-carotene, carrot oil, beet extract, fruit and vegetable juices,* Colorants (synthetic): *tartrazine, amaranth, erythrosine, methylsalicylate oil* Emulsifiers, Bleaching agents, Stabilizers, Sweeteners, Leavening agents, Vitamins Minerals
	Modification	Hardening of oils (partially hydrogenated) Resulting in trans-fatty acid production

The main goal in food processing is to convert raw food into more palatable forms before consumption and to prevent the spoilage of food. Techniques employed in the food processing industry generally involve a series of stages or a combination of methods during processing, but the details of these processes lie outside of the scope of this book.

Newer Food Processing Methods

Consumers are now more aware than ever before, that the type of processing affects the quality of food.
In response to this, the food industry has sought to discover new ways of minimizing the impact of processing on the nutritional value of food.

A number of novel approaches have been developed in response to consumer concerns over the safety, nutritional value, and the organoleptic quality of foods. For some time manufacturers and food scientists explored sundry methods that have sought to do just that. They include a number of physical processes using various forms of non-ionizing radiation, electrical, and other magnetic processes, as well as attempts to employ natural additives. To date however, none of these methods have gained widespread acceptance. For some, the reasons are economic, and for others, it is because of insufficient data on safety profile and related concerns.[54]

Processing and the Nutritional Value of Foods

The American diet is a costly health problem.
With 90 percent of the money spent on food being spent on industrially/commercially processed foods, it is important to take a closer look at how processing affects the nutritional value of foods.[54]

Let me be quite clear that this discussion is not intended to be alarmist, nor is it an anti-food processing campaign. Rather, it aims to inform people that industrial food processing often results in significant undesirable changes to the nutritional value of the original product. This concern was first introduced in Chapter 5 on the subject of the Western diet. In a modern society that is hard-pressed for time, convenience is an important commodity.

Details are important, but we live in a world where things are often judged by appearances. Go beyond the fancy wrappings and catchy words and delve deeply into the labels, and discover that canned juices are not the same as freshly-squeezed fruit juices. Corn-on-the-cob is a world away from corn flakes. Traditionalists argue that even the American sweet corn is significantly different from its ancestor growing across the border in rural Mexico. Most people just assume that there is very little difference, but informed people understand otherwise. So make sure you ask the right questions.

Processed fruit juices differ markedly from their freshly squeezed or blended counterparts. Late in 2002, I flew from Dallas to Boston, and chose the in-flight "100% tomato juice" over the orange juice made from concentrate. Interestingly enough, I drank heartily from the can, and then idly scanned the tomato juice label in more detail. The fine print read, "from concentrate with added ingredients." Knowing that processed tomato products contain more of the beneficial ingredient called lycopene, I felt I had made a good choice. Further scrutiny of these "added ingredients" revealed that this 11.5 fluid oz. (340 ml) can, contained 1,210 milligrams of sodium, or more than half the recommended daily sodium allowance! Suffice it to say that I left the remainder in the can. A month later, a diplomat invited me to the VIP lounge at the GW Bush Airport and offered the same apparently healthy 100 percent tomato juice. I opted for fresh fruit instead. Incidentally, this man had suffered at least one previous stroke and actually assumed that the tomato juice was a healthy choice—thanks to food processing and misleading labels.

It is important to clarify our definitions regarding foods and food sources. For example, when people say they drink a lot of fruit juices, what exactly are they referring to? These answers are significant in any discussion about promoting health. Industrial food processing and the food consumption patterns are major contributors to obesity and the chronic disease epidemic. Supermarkets and grocery stores now trade over 90 percent of the annual volume of all food and beverage consumed in the United States. Full-service and limited-service restaurants, which include fast food franchises, account for more than 80 percent of the annual volume of sales of all food and drink served in America.[55-57]

Fresh strawberries are good for you, although some worry over the presence of the potentially carcinogenic pesticides (e.g. methyl bromide) that may be used. Fresh strawberries contain plenty of protective antioxidant pigments called flavonoids , but strawberry-flavored drinks have nothing in common with strawberries except in name only. They are two completely different products, with different health implications.

The food industry has, nonetheless, made a tremendous contribution to food preservation and storage. In times of war, natural disasters, and famine populations would stand very little chance of survival without the ability to access adequate amounts of non-perishable food. This can save the lives of millions who languish in such deplorable environments. Improving food safety and minimizing losses has been one of the great triumphs of the modern food-processing industry (Table 7-11).

On any discussion about optimizing health and preventing chronic diseases, the debate must move beyond mere survival issues. Undernutrition is not the problem in industrialized societies. Rather, it is the over-consumption of (nutritionally speaking) inferior-quality and often highly processed foods (Table 7-12).

Table 7-11. Advantages of some food processing methods

A D V A N T A G E S	• **Food Preservation:** Avoids spoilage and minimizes losses • **Convenience** • **Improves safety**: by eliminating micro-organisms • **Extends shelf life** • **Increases digestibility:** of some foods • **Improves palatability:** of some foods • **Improves texture:** of some foods • **Improves availability of certain nutrients** • **Destroys toxins and anti-nutritional factors** (see in this chapter under—Raw or natural can be dangerous) • **Creates new types of foods** • **Availability of foods year round** • **Availability of exotic and cultural foods** • **Improves food security:** especially in times of natural and other disasters

Table 7-12. Disadvantages of some food processing methods

D I S A D V A N T A G E S	• **Hidden salt (sodium):** major source (70 percent), most salt in the diet is added to food long before it reaches the dinner table. It goes under many names other than salt or sodium chloride (see table below) • **Disturbs sodium/potassium ratio:** this important ratio is invariably altered or reversed by the common food processing methods. (see Chapter 5: Excess sodium; reduced potassium and magnesium) • **Significant losses of many nutrients:** especially vitamins destroyed during heating or storage, and the leaching of some minerals • **Hidden sugars:** these come in various forms (see table below) • **Hidden Fat:** (see Chapter 5) • **Trans-Fatty Acids (Partially Hydrogenated or Hydrogenated fats):** now recognized to be a major culprit that has worse effects on blood cholesterol profile than saturated or animal fat (See Chapter 5) • **Additives and Preservatives**

The remainder of this chapter will introduce some of the more important details of food processing that should not be overlooked. These details have important bearings on our health.

Hidden Salt (Sodium)

"Most dietary sodium *has been added* during processing and manufacturing. … Only small amounts of sodium occur naturally in foods, and most sodium *has been added* to food during commercial processing or preparation either at home or in a restaurant."

The 1995 U.S. Dietary Guidelines

Consumption of excess dietary sodium, especially at the expense of dietary potassium is a big contributor to hypertension. In the first edition (1980) through to the third edition (1990) of *Dietary Guidelines for Americans*, table salt as a source of sodium received only passing mention. There was no mention of excess sodium being a possible culprit in these guidelines. The major sources of dietary sodium are processed foods, condiments, sauces, pickled foods, salty snacks, and sandwich meats (Tables 7-13). The 1990 guidelines stated that sodium was found in "preservatives and flavor enhancers" added to foods (Table 7-14). The subsequent 1995 guidelines were more explicit. It declared that "most dietary sodium *has been added* during processing and manufacturing. … Only small amounts of sodium occur naturally in foods, and most sodium *has been added* to food during commercial processing or preparation either at home or in a restaurant." [58-60]

Table 7-13. Foods High in Sodium

Foods High In Sodium

- Processed meats, bacon, sausages, ham, pepperoni
- Canned fish, shellfish
- Canned soups, noodles—with or without meat
- Canned vegetables: beans, corn, peas, potatoes, tomatoes
- Breads, muffins, stuffing
- Dairy products: cheeses, butter, margarine, milks: whole low-fat, condense and evaporated, yogurts
- Snacks, chips, salted nuts, crisps
- Desserts, pies, puddings
- Condiments, spices, sauces, baking powder, baking soda
- Anti-gas medicines e.g. Alka-Seltzer

Estimates are that food processing methods are responsible for 77 percent of dietary sodium intake. Some 12 percent was naturally found in foods, 6 percent was added at the table, and 5 percent added in cooking. Tap water contributed an insignificant 0.1 percent.[62] So if you thought that going easy on the salt-shaker was the solution to your excessive sodium intake, you have overlooked the major culprit. The bulk of sodium has been added to food long before it ever reached your table (Table 7-13 and Table 7-14).[62]

Table 7-14. Hidden Sources of Salt and Sodium

"Hidden" Salt / Sodium	Food Sources
Baking soda (sodium bicarbonate)	Leavening breads, cakes
Baking powder	Leavening breads, cakes, muffins
Brine (concentrated salt water)	For pickles, sauerkraut, beef, snouts, tails
Disodium EDTA	Food preservative
Disodium inosinate	Food additive
MSG (monosodium glutamate)	Food additive
Sodium alginate	Food texturizer (ice cream and flavored milk)
Sodium ascorbate	Food additive
Sodium benzoate	Food preservative in condiments & dressings
Sodium caseinate	Food additive/texturizer in cakes and bakes
Sodium citrate	Food flavor and preservative
Sodium cyclamate	Diet drinks and desserts
Sodium hydroxide	Food texturizer for removing skin of fruits
Sodium nitrate & nitrite	Food preservative (prevents botulism)
Sodium propionate	Food preservative (anti-molds)
Sodium saccharin	Diet drinks and desserts
Sodium sulphite	Food preservative (dried fruits)
Table salt (sodium chloride)	Added salt

Hidden Sugars

When the term "hidden" is mentioned, it does not mean that the manufacturer deliberately hides the sugar content. It refers primarily to sources of sugar and excess calories that consumers tend to overlook, mainly because of ignorance. They are not all reflected on the food label as "sugar" and, therefore, go unnoticed by all but the most nutrition-savvy consumers. Sugars appear in processed foods under a myriad of names and forms (Table 7-15). Fructose (fruit sugar) is naturally found in many fruits and honey. Industrially prepared fructose, the most popular sweetener used in the soft drink industry, has nothing to do with fruit. It is manufactured from corn (high-fructose corn syrup) and can be a major culprit in elevating blood triglycerides levels.[63] The nutritional significance of excess caloric intake is discussed in Chapter 5.

Table 7-15. Some Food Sources of Hidden Sugars

"Hidden" Sugars	Food Sources
Acesulfame (Sunette or Sweet One)	Artificial sweetener (200x sweeter than sugar)
Aspartame (Nutrasweet and Equal)	Artificial sweetener (200x sweeter than sugar)
Corn Syrup	From cornstarch
Dextrose	From cornstarch (a.k.a. glucose)
Fructose (High Fructose Corn Syrup)	From cornstarch (a.k.a. fruit sugar)
Glucose	Form cornstarch
Honey	From bees (mainly glucose and fructose)
Maltose	Disaccharide sugar from starchy roots e.g. potato
Mannitol	Sugar alcohol from fruit or dextrose
Maple Sugar	From sap of maple tree
Maple Syrup	From sap of maple tree
Molasses	Extracted from sugarcane
Saccharin	Artificial sweetener (300 times sweeter than sugar)
Sorbitol	Sugar alcohol from fruit or dextrose
Sucrose	From sugarcane or beets
Xylitol	Sugar alcohol from fruit or dextrose
Sucralose (Splenda)	Artificial sweetener–becoming popular because of no aftertaste like other artificial sweeteners)

Impact of Processing On Vitamins

Many vitamins are destroyed by food processing, especially vitamin C and thiamin (vitamin B_1).
Fruits and certain vegetables are best consumed while fresh. Other foods are best when they are minimally processed. Eating a wide variety of recommended foods is the best guarantee for ensuring optimum intake of desirable nutrients.

A primary concern of food processing is its impact on the retention of vitamins. A list of the more common vitamins and their stability under different conditions is provided in Table 7-16.[64-70] Amongst the most labile of vitamins to physical and chemical influences are ascorbic acid (vitamin C) and thiamin (vitamin B_1). Manufacturers and food scientists use the retention of these vitamins to gauge the impact of different processing methods on nutrient losses. If there is good retention of vitamin C and thiamin, you can assumed that there is good retention of the other nutrients (Table 7-17 and Table 7-18).[71-73]

Table 7-16. Stability of Some Vitamins under Different Conditions

Vitamin	Air	Light	Heat	Cooking losses %
Retinol (Vitamin A)	U	U	U	0-40
Carotenes (Beta-Carotene)	U	U	U	0-30
Vitamin D	U	U	U	0-40
Vitamin E	U	U	U	0-55
Thiamin (Vitamin B1)	U	S	U	0-80
Riboflavin (Vitamin B2)	S	U	U	0-75
Niacin	S	S	S	0-75
Vitamin B6 (Pyridoxine)	S	U	U	0-40
Vitamin B12 (Cobalamin)	U	U	S	0-10
Vitamin C(Ascorbic Acid)	U	U	U	0-100

Losses depend on the duration of exposure to the conditions listed
(Modified from Harris & Loesecke 1960) [64]

S = Stable (no important destruction)   **U** = Unstable (significant destruction)

Remember the principle of "you win some, you lose some." It also applies to nutrition. Processing releases certain nutrients, but destroys others. Some natural chemicals found in plants, such as vitamins, minerals, and phytonutrients are made more available by some forms of cooking, while destroyed by others. Cooking tomatoes, for example, destroys much of the vitamin C, but there is a pigment called lycopene that is freed up when tomatoes are cooked. Lycopene, which gives tomatoes their blush, is poorly absorbed from raw tomatoes because it is too tightly bound to the proteins and fiber in the raw tomato. Consumption of tomatoes cooked in oil (best to use extra virgin olive oil) further enhances the absorption of lycopene. This is because lycopene is lipid-or oil-soluble.

A 1995 study by Harvard researchers indicated that men who consumed an average of ten servings of tomatoes and tomato-rich foods weekly, reduced their prostate cancer risk by almost 50 percent. Lycopene shows promise in lowering, not only the risk of prostate cancer, but also cancers of the lung, breast, and the gastrointestinal tract.[74]

Processing common staples like rice and wheat typically results in the loss of important nutrients. For example, excessive polishing of rice removes the outer covering (the bran and the germ) which is rich in thiamin (vitamin B_1). Parboiled or brown rice retains five times as much thiamin as polished white rice. The popular Asian practice of washing rice before cooking, and straining off excess water after cooking, serves only to reduce thiamin levels further. Milling wheat to produce white flour removes more than 50 percent of the minerals and vitamins.[55]

Table 7-17. Vitamin C Losses during Different Methods of Processing Green Peas

Sample	Vitamin C (mg) per 100 mg of green peas	Percentage retention of Vitamin C compared to raw sample
Raw	130	100%
Cooked (12 minutes):		
With minimum water	116	89%
With equal water	84	65%
Stored at ambient temperature in pod		
1 day then cooked (12 min.) with minimum water	90	69%
4 days then overcooked (18 min.) with minimum water	57	44%
Frozen and then cooked[d] In water (4 min.)	65	50%
Cooked[d] after frozen storage time of:		
3 months	61	47%
6 months	58	45%
9 months	63	48%
Canned and then cooked (5 min.)	50	38%
Cooked[d] after canned storage time of:		
3 months:	40	31%
6 months:	37	28%
9 months:	38	29%
[d] Cooked in minimum amount of water		

Effect of storing, cooking, freezing, frozen storage, canning on the Vitamin C content of garden peas
(on a dry weight basis)
Source: Campden Food Preservation Research Association (1987)

Raw or Natural Can Be Dangerous

Having been enlightened to the health hazards of industrial food processing, some people have taken it to ridiculous extremes.

There is need to dispel the notion that raw or natural always means "better." There are anti-nutrients naturally found in many foods that exert negative effects on nutrition (Table 7-19).[55] Many anti-nutrient factors act as natural toxins to protect plants from pests and predators. Anti-nutrient factors include anti-vitamins, plant estrogens, hallucinogens, and plant phenolic compounds.

The example of the soybean illustrates this point quite well. When laboratory animals are fed with raw soy foods, they exhibit reduced absorption of fats and retarded growth. This is due to protease inhibitors present in raw soybeans. Most of the protease inhibitors can be removed by heat treatment and processing. Raw soybeans also contain phyto-hemagglutinins that can cause clumping of red blood cells. This group of substances has been shown to cause deaths in mice. Raw soy foods also contain phytates that bind calcium, zinc, and iron, thereby reducing their availability to the body.[55,75-77]

Table 7-18. The Effect of Storage and Cooking on Vitamin C Content

Sample	Mg of Vitamin C per 100 mg of green peas	Percentage retention of Vitamin C compared to raw sample
Zero Time		
Raw	<57	<100%
Fried (Chipped) Cooked 190⁰ C/10 mins.)	<16	<28%
3 Months Storage		
Raw	<15	<27%
Boiled (equal water)	<7	<13%
Fried (chipped)	<20	<36%
6 Months Storage		
Raw	<13	<23%
Boiled	<22	<39%
Fried (chipped)	<6	<11%
Fried (frozen chipped) Cooked 190⁰ C/3 mins.)	<20	<36%
9 Months Storage		
Fried (frozen chipped—3 months)	<18	<32%
Fried (frozen chipped—6 months)	<14	<25%
ᵈ Cooked in minimum amount of water		
Effect of Storage, Cooking, Freezing, Frozen Storage, and Frying the Vitamin C content of old potatoes (on a dry weight basis) Source: Campden Food Preservation Research Association (1987)		

Cooking and processing soybeans and other foods effectively destroys many of these anti-nutrient factors. Failure to do so can result in negative side-effects listed in Table 7-19. What is quite interesting is that human societies, through the ages, have been able to identify and distinguish safe from harmful foods. In addition, they have devised effective methods of preparing potentially dangerous foods. This knowledge, handed down through several generations, was based on trial and experience. It is amazing how many cultures have combined certain foods and food groups, and extracted maximum benefits without the scientific justification that we possess today.

Table 7-19. Heat-labile Anti-nutritional Factors

Anti-nutritional Factor	Common Food Sources	Effects of Anti-nutritional factor
Proteinase inhibitors	Legumes, beans (many varieties), peas, peanuts, potatoes, sweet potatoes,	Interfere with protein digestion and growth
Trypsin inhibitor	Legumes, egg whites Potatoes	Inhibits the activity of the digestive enzyme trypsin
Hemagglutinins (phytohemagglutinins, Phytagglutinins, lectins)	Red Kidney beans Castor beans (ricin) Soybeans, peanuts, black beans, yellow wax beans	Induces clumping of red blood cells
Thiaminases	Fish, shellfish, Brussels sprouts, red cabbage	Destroys Thiamin (vitamin B1)
Avidin	Egg whites	Binds biotin (vitamin), making it unavailable
Lathyrogens	Chick peas	Disrupts collagen structure and disturbs development of bone and connective tissue
Goitrogens	Sweet potatoes, spinach Beans, cabbage, kale, cauliflower, Brussels sprouts, broccoli	Causes goiters by interfering with iodine absorption and utilization of iodine
Alpha-amylase Inhibitors	Cereal grains, peas, beans	Slows the digestion of starch

Source: Modern Nutrition in Health and Disease, Shils, Olson & Shike, 1994.

Enrichment and Fortification of Foods

The enrichment of foods cannot adequately replace the nutrients lost during industrial food processing. Nutrients in fortified products are often poorly absorbed.

The food industry often calls to our attention that they replace nutrients that are lost during processing. This process is called enrichment. Manufacturers, for example, add B vitamins to flour to replace those lost during processing. They sometimes claim that their processed product is actually a better source of a nutrient than the original product, by adding "enriched" or "fortified" to the food label. This conveys the message that such products are superior sources, akin to taking a vitamin supplement. "Fortified with vitamin C and calcium" frequently appear on the labels on beverages, cereals, and assorted foods. Food enrichment, despite the hype, does not restore every important nutrient that has been lost during processing. Furthermore, good nutrition goes far beyond supplementing with vitamins, minerals, or attaining recommended daily allowances.[78,79]

Nutrification or fortification programs add nutrients that are not normally present in the fortified product. These were historically designed as a part of public health programs to prevent deficiency diseases. Potassium iodide/iodate is added to table salt to prevent goiters, fluoride to drinking water, vitamin D to milk, vitamin A to butter, and vitamins like thiamin, niacin, and riboflavin (B_2) to processed cereal-grain products. Flour and wheat products are routinely fortified with iron in the United States. However, even though labels routinely flaunt that these products are fortified, consumers should be aware that their presence in the food, says nothing of the absorption or the bioavailability to our bodies. This is certainly true of iron, which is poorly absorbed.

Reducing Nutrient Losses While Cooking

Certain home-cooking practices can destroy more nutrients than even industrial food processes. Popular cooking methods, like grilling and barbecuing meats, can produce potent carcinogens.

Home cooking is not exempt from the problem of nutrient losses. A well-meaning cook can be more harmful to food than any industrial food chemist. Some methods of food preparation and storage in the home can lead to significant nutrient losses. Losses of nutrients during home cooking can easily exceed those of industrial-food processing. Make every effort to avoid the culinary habits listed in Table 7-20. Adding too much salt and overcooking vegetables are common ways of creating excessively-processed home-cooked food.

Table 7-20. Reducing Nutrient Losses while Cooking

When Cooking at Home Ways to minimize nutrient losses	• Do not overcook vegetables • Steaming and stir fry preferable to frying • Minimize trimming of fruits and vegetables • Excessive heat and leaching result in greater losses • Cook food in covered pans • Keeping food on a warmer (or low heat)results in continuing losses of heat-labile vitamins e.g. vitamin C • NOTE: Certain cooking methods e.g. Grilling, Barbecuing, Deep-Fat Frying (see below) can cause harmful changes in food preparation at home.

Amongst the cooking methods that result in a better nutrient retention profile is the traditional Oriental custom of low temperature stir-frying (see Chapter 6 "The Okinawa Formula). A special pot called a wok and a vigorous flame are the essential requirements. It is a great time saver and is excellent for preparing vegetables and meats. It can preserve and enhance the flavors of food and makes vegetables crunchy and tasty, in stark contrast to the taste of overcooked food and vegetables. Stir fry's are ideal for low-fat cooking.

Steaming is a good method for preparing seafood and vegetables. It has the advantage of being quick, fat-free, and with good nutrient retention. Pressure cookers and slow cookers are convenient, but they overcook foods and can result in significant nutrient losses. Therefore, they are generally not recommended for preparing vegetables.[80,81]

Health Concerns over Some Cooking Methods

Food Toxins Produced During Grilling and Barbecuing

Certain cooking methods can produce harmful toxins. Smoking, grilling, and charbroiling meat can generate cancer-causing heterocyclic amines (HCAs) and polycyclic aromatic hydrocarbons (PAHs) (see Chapter 5). The process is called pyrolysis, and PAHs are produced when fats pyrolyse. When fats melt from grilled or charbroiled meat and fall onto the coals below, pyrolysis occurs. The smoke that arises contains PAHs (from pyrolysed fats) which are absorbed into the meat, especially the exposed layers. Therefore, smoke arising from barbecues and grills can be doubly harmful.

PAHs also arise from wood-burning stoves and hydrocarbon fuels e.g. diesel, kerosene, and charcoal-lighter fluid. HCAs are formed when the meat itself is charred (burnt), causing the amino acids (e.g tryptophan in meat protein) to form potent carcinogens (e.g. carbolines and quinolines).[82,83] There are practical ways of minimizing the generation of these harmful agents when grilling or barbecuing. These measures include:

- Use lean meats, avoid fatty cuts.
- Partially cook or bake meat before grilling or charbroiling.
- Avoid burnt foods, and do not eat the blacked outer layer
- Wrap meat in foil, and keep grill lid open to disperse the smoke.
- Marinate in olive oil, lemon, and garlic.

Irradiated and Microwaved Foods

Irradiation of foods uses ionizing radiation to preserve foods. The very use of the word "radiation" evokes much fear in our era of "weapons of mass destruction." Alarmists are quick to incite fear that radiating foods amounts to "an industrially-sanctioned method of terrorizing our food, leading eventually to radioactive fallout that threatens the very future of man!" As paranoid as this idea is, in our day of fear and uncertainty, perception is often more important than reality.

Irradiation, cold pasteurization, and sterilization are food processing methods that use ionizing radiation e.g. electron-beams, x-rays, or gamma γ-rays, to kill microbes (e.g. E. coli) and prevent spoilage. Irradiation is a very effective method of sterilizing foods, delaying the ripening of fruits, and preventing the spread of parasites (e.g. Mediterranean fruit fly) from imported fruits.[84,85]

The concerns over the use of ionizing radiation to preserve foods are not totally unjustified. Consumer fears are based on two major concerns. The first is whether radiating food causing them to become radioactive, and the second is whether free radicals, (see Chapter 6), generated by the radiation of foods, pose a threat to human health. On the first issue of foods becoming radioactive, there is no evidence to support such claims. On the matter of free radicals production triggered by irradiating foods, these occur in proportion to the dose of radiation used as well as the type of food that is radiated, but free-radicals in foods are short-lived.

Microwaves are entirely different. They are radiowaves. They do not ionize, nor do they generate free radicals. Microwaves penetrate food (albeit unevenly, especially if food is thick—may not make it all the way to the middle) and excite food components all at once, delivering quick results and hence its popularity. Microwaves destroy fewer nutrients, but concerns exist over possible infiltration of chemicals from recycled paper products (e.g paper towels) or plastics into the food during cooking. Your more immediate threat from a microwave oven, however, is to avoid getting burns after microwaving hot liquids, and making sure that meat is properly cooked. As a rule, use only ceramics and glassware for cooking, as these do not absorb microwaves.

On Aluminum Pots and Alzheimer's disease

Aluminum toxicity generated alarm when it was discovered that aluminum deposits were observed in the brains of Alzheimer's victims at autopsy. Before all this, the real concern existed in patients receiving aluminum-containing dialysis fluids (for kidney failure) and chronic intravenous nutrition. The aluminum in these fluids accumulated within the blood, affecting the bones, the nervous system, and blood metabolism. This practice has since been discontinued.[86]

Aluminum is widely used in cooking utensils, food additives, and certain medicines (e.g. antacids). Increased public health concerns over Alzheimer's disease have led to increased scrutiny about the potential toxicity of aluminum. Preparing acidic foods and drinks in aluminum containers can leach aluminum and increase its content in foods. The same applies if such foods are canned or cooked in aluminum containers. Although conclusive proof is lacking, it is sensible to avoid such practices.

In 1989 the medical journal *Lancet* reported the findings of a British government investigation which showed that the risk of developing Alzheimer's was 50 percent higher in those areas of the British Isles where the drinking water was higher in aluminum.[87] There is no evidence to support speculations that aluminum foils and wrappings can increase aluminum content in foods.

Deep Fat Frying and the Reheating of Oils

Frying foods in deep fat can lead to the production of acrolein, an irritating gas that has carcinogenic (cancer-causing) potential. More recent concern, however, stemmed from the findings of a respectable study by scientists at Stockholm University in Sweden. They showed that acrylamide (a solid, colorless, crystalline substance) is generated when potatoes and cereal grains are fried. The United States Environmental Protection Agency (EPA) classifies acrylamide as a substance with significant carcinogenic potential.[88]

French-fries and crispy potato products contain relatively high levels of acrylamide, but boiling potatoes before frying seems to reduce its formation. Acrylamide levels in fried potato products are 10-100 times higher than that found in other protein-rich foods. Toasting bread produces a moderate increase in acrylamide formation. Frying carbohydrate-rich foods (e.g. beet root) also resulted in similar increases in acrylamide.

The researchers concluded that popular cooking methods (e.g. frying, microwave, and baking), with the exception of boiling, all lead to significant acrylamide formation in the potato. Therefore, if you are hooked on fried potatoes and worried about acrylamide, boiling your potatoes (before frying) may reduce your acrylamide consumption.

Trans-fats (see Chapter 5) are generated when oils are subjected to high temperatures, as in the deep-frying process. The high temperatures used to fry foods, a common practice in commercial food outlets, can generate these undesirable trans-fats even when healthy oils are used. The bulk of trans-fats in deep-fried foods, however, come from the widespread use of trans-fats e.g. vegetable shortenings that are used for frying in the first place. Trans-fats accumulate when oils are re-used. In the fast-food industry, vegetable shortenings are preferred because they are easier to use and can be re-used more often than liquid oil, and hence saves money. Using fresh oils during each frying session reduces the build-up of trans-fats and the subsequent intake of these unhealthy oils from foods. Low-temperature stir-frying inflicts far less damage to oils than high-temperature deep-fat frying.

Frying foods at high-temperatures is judged unhealthy, therefore, on at least three counts: It leads to an overall increase in fat/calorie intake and hence the risk of obesity; it can increase your intake of trans-fats (see Figure 5-7); and it can increase your intake of acrylamide formation along with its potential risks.

Concerns about Technology and Agricultural Practices

Food safety and food quality have become major issues in the industrial world. Consumers have expressed unease over the widespread use of fertilizers, herbicides, pesticides, antibiotics, and hormones in modern agricultural practice. The growing mistrust of federal institutions and the influence of the food industry lobby have given rise to a climate of suspicion. The official "everything is ok" version of the events no longer resonates well with the public, and there is no scarcity of those who go to the extreme to make merchandise of this growing rift. Uncertainty has resurrected renewed enthusiasm for organically-grown foods—foods that many consider as the best guarantee and protection against the profit-at-any-cost food industrial complex. However, balance, not sensationalism, should be the watchword.

Organic Foods; Alarm over Mad Cow Disease

Mad cow disease and food scares must be placed in perspective. It is good to know why the cows went mad, but let it not overshadow the bigger issues. Judging from the records, these are what kill 70 percent of Americans every year, not mad cow or any modern agricultural practices.

Growing up in Belize, Central America, was an enriching experience. A fixture in my childhood was the weekly trip to the farm to plant, as well as to harvest, whatever produce was in season. Most of the agricultural methods used were simple and traditional. Therefore, I find it interesting to see that such methods, hitherto belittled and considered backward, are now the new way forward. Their produce now fetch premium prices in the supermarkets of North America and Europe.

Modern agriculture has evolved into a giant industry that relies heavily on the use of fertilizers and pesticides. Intensive farming methods and single-crop farms have led to massive increases in productivity, agricultural surpluses, and falling food prices. All of this, however, has come at a cost. Intensive commercial farming has been guilty of contaminating waterways and soils with their environmentally-unfriendly practices, and their potential negative impacts on public health. Many who strongly oppose this alleged irresponsibility towards the environment, and many who have lost confidence and trust in politics and industry, are making their voices heard by opting for organic foods.[89] They cite the case of mad cow disease as the flagship example of how modern agri-industry threatens our health.

Bovine spongiform encephalopathy (BSE or "mad cow disease") and foot-and-mouth disease, that both rocked the British Isles in the 1990s, have their roots in intensive farming and feeding methods that are contrary to nature. Critics have mockingly referred to these outbreaks as cases of "mad human disease"—man unnecessarily tampering with the foods normally eaten by cows, and rearing pigs in overcrowded conditions. The practice of rendering the remains of dead animals as feed ("animal protein") to cattle took many people by surprise, but rendering has been an established practice in modern animal husbandry for decades. Feeding animal protein to ruminants, like cattle, was cheaper and led to increased meat and milk production, and therefore better profits. Worse still was the nauseating discovery by a hitherto ignorant public, that the "bone meal" fed to cattle was a euphemistic term for a pulverized mixture of dead animal remains—dead cattle, dead sheep, and beyond. This inadvertently led to the transmission of the scrapie agent from scrapie-infected bone meal into cows. Cows infected with the scrapie agent develop BSE or "mad cow disease"—a term that refers to the bizarre behavior seen in affected cows. BSE is an incurable and fatal infection of the brains of cattle. Both the scrapie agent and the BSE agent are strange proteins that are collectively referred to as prions (PrPSc). The diseases they cause are called prion diseases and are characterized by spongy-looking (spongiform) changes in the brains of their victims.[90]

The real alarm was not that cows could get sick from eating scrapie-infected meat, but on whether humans could get sick from consuming infected beef. What was even more worrying was that there was no scientific certainty on deciding which beef products were infected, and which were not. Even more nightmarish was that there were no known blanket methods (e.g. sterilization or cooking) to destroy the BSE agent. The challenge to the cattle industry was whether to destroy all cattle (not a viable economic option), or to seek ways of selecting and destroying the focus of outbreaks. They chose the latter.

There is a BSE-like disease in humans. It is called CJD (Creutzfeldt-Jacob disease—named after doctors who described it in the early 1920s) rather than simply HSE (human spongiform encephalopathy). The classic form of CJD is a rare, occurring sporadically at the rate of about 1 in a million people. It typically affects older adults between the ages of 55 to 75 years, culminating in bizarre behavior and death.

Scientists' worst fears were confirmed in 1996, when the CJD unit in Edinburgh, Scotland officially declared that New Variant CJD, now known just as variant CJD (vCJD), is a new disease pattern. British experts confirmed that that the most likely explanation for the variant CJD cases was due to the BSE agent. Variant CJD primarily affects young individuals with average age of onset at 27 years.[91] According to the UK Department of Health, monthly CJD statistics (June 2, 2003), the total number of British people with CJD since 1990 was 877, of whom 648 had the classic (sporadic) form, and 135 had the variant (vCJD) form. People with variant CJD are still being diagnosed in the United Kingdom, but the actual numbers of new cases are not by any means explosive. Monthly updates of CJD cases are available at the following UK government website: http://www.doh.gov.uk/cjd/cjd_stat.htm.

The nightmarish scenario created by BSE/CJD sent ripples through the global beef industry on both sides of the Atlantic.[90-91] Canada reported its first case of BSE in May 2003 and caused further anxiety in the North American beef industry. As of June 2003, no further cases of BSE have been confirmed in Canada. In an attempt to prevent BSE from entering the country, the United States placed severe restrictions on the importation of live cattle and related products from all BSE affected countries. Updates can be obtained from the Center for Disease Control and Prevention website: http://www.cdc.gov/ncidod/diseases/cjd/cjd.htm.

Organic Foods—Definitions

> The resurgent interest in organic foods is more about people expressing political views and environmental concerns than it is about health. The name "organic" is not synonymous with "better." There is bad as well as good organic food.

Organic foods are now a 10-billion dollar-a-year industry in America, and the market is growing by almost 20 percent annually. In times past, great confusion reigned over its definition. The U.S. Congress set new standards for the definition of organic foods, "USDA Organic," that came into effect October 21, 2002.[92,93]

"Certified Organic"

National Organic Rule
"USDA Organic"

Since October 2002, foods certified as "organic" must comply with the following United States Department of Agriculture (USDA) guidelines: "100% organic" and "organic" (at least 95% organic ingredients) *can only be used for* foods produced without pesticides, herbicides, insecticides, antibiotics, hormones, antibiotics, chemical fertilizers, genetic modification, or food irradiation. Producers who comply with these standards will qualify to use the "certified organic" label issued by the USDA.

http://www.ams.usda.gov/nop/Consumers/Seal.html

Prior to this ruling, there was much confusion about terms (e.g. "natural," or "made with nature's ingredients," etc). This led consumer advocates and the organic food industry to demand more clarity and transparency about the definitions. Their efforts were rewarded by the 1990 Organic Foods Production Act. This established national standards governing the production and marketing of organic foods. Official information can be accessed from their website—the National Organic Program: http://www.ams.usda.gov/nop/indexIE.htm.[94]

Organic foods come with a price tag attached; they cost more. This method of production is less intensive and less efficient (at least initially) than commercial farming methods, but it is now the fastest growing trend in U.S. agriculture. Does their presumed benefit justify the additional expense? Are organic foods more nutritious? Do they pose fewer health risks than the commercially grown varieties? The answers you get depend on your source of information. Respected sources, both with scientific community as well as among organic-food advocates, are generally agreed that organic foods do not impart significant additional health benefits.

New evidence, however, lends credence to the claim that organic foods may confer additional nutritional benefits. A study reported in the *Journal of Agricultural and Food Chemistry* (2003), by University of California at Davis researchers, compared the levels of total polyphenols and ascorbic acid (Vitamin C) content—known health-promoting nutrients—in blackberries, strawberries, and corn grown under three different conditions: organically, sustainably, and conventionally. The organically-grown berries and corn contained up to 58 percent more polyphenols and antioxidants than their commercially grown counterparts. Sustainably- or organically-grown blackberries contained almost 60 percent more, and strawberries contained 20 percent more polyphenols and ascorbic acid than commercially grown varieties.[95] The evidence provided by this study is compelling, but like any other scientific evidence, it will need to be backed up by further studies.

Organic foods taste better, in gastronomic terms. But like beauty, taste is often in the eyes of the beholder. My mother complains that "the new eggs are pale, without flavor, and seem artificial." Others consider organic eggs coming from free-ranging hens to be repugnant—the yolk is deeply orange and it has a stronger taste. Adherents of organic food are simply content with the psychological reassurance that their food is "natural" and free of pesticides or interference from the commercial food industry. The debates over organic foods will continue. A growing trans-Atlantic divide separates the U.S. and the European community's attitudes toward organic foods, particularly with reference to genetically-modified foods. A proper debate on this matter lies outside the scope of this book.

Mad cow has served to agitate emotions. Organic food devotees, for example, are still "hopping mad" over a last minute addition to the bill that allows dairy, meat, and poultry to be labeled "organic," even when fed with feed that is not 100 percent organic. If this enrages you, go organic, but remember that organic is not synonymous with "better." There is bad as well as good organic food. What is more important is to never lose sight of the big picture. The debates over food safety and food politics merit our attention, but they should not cloud our consciousness.

The biggest killers in our society have not stemmed from whether people choose organic foods or not. They have stemmed from over-consumption of foods that fatten us and deliver a barrage of unhealthy nutrients (see Chapter 5) at the expense of healthier varieties. It is good to know how cows go "mad," but more often than not, this adjective better describes some of our nutrition and lifestyle patterns. Let us clean up our own act—our nutrition and our lifestyle, while cleaning up the environment. Judging from the death statistics, this is what kills 70 percent of Americans every year, not mad cow or modern agricultural practices.

Genetically Modified (GM) Foods

Crossbreeding and selective breeding of plants and animals are as old as man. Today we are witnessing a new phenomenon.
Scientists now directly insert genes with desirable characteristics into plants e.g. drought and pest resistance, herbicide tolerance, additional nutrients, and improved yield. Critics argue that GM foods pose a potential threat to human health and sow the seeds of a future environmental nightmare.

Much of the grain that is consumed today is not the same as their ancestors. For example, the popular sweet corn varieties in the U.S. are very different from Central American maize. The rice varieties we consume today are much different from their wild rice ancestors. Breeding and crossbreeding of plants and animals, strictly speaking, is a form of genetic manipulation going back to mankind's very beginnings.

Plants and animals have been selectively bred to harness desirable qualities that help to survive drought, fend off pests, and improve yield. This has become increasingly popular in the United States. China and India, with almost half the world's population to feed, have embraced GM and its promises. Other countries are yet to be convinced. The Europeans and the Brazilians oppose their use, citing unknown potential hazards. Worldwide, 70 percent of all GM crops are grown in the United States. GM soybeans and GM corn accounted for more than 80 percent of all GM crops harvested in 2000, with lesser amounts of GM potatoes, tomatoes, cotton, and rapeseed (canola). More than 40 different types of crops are now being genetically modified.[96]

Genes, those crucial parts of the DNA molecule that determine the characteristics of living things, are now being transplanted across the species barrier. What caused public disquiet was that such GM foods, also called genetically modified organisms (GMOs), have been in the American, European, and global food supply for decades, but went largely unnoticed. The major reason for this is that in the United States, neither the FDA nor the USDA requires the labeling of GM foods. In Europe, they now require that such foods be clearly labeled. Some U.S. manufacturers, in response to consumer sentiments, have voluntarily begun labeling their products to be "free of GM ingredients." [97,98]

Why is there so much concern over GM foods? Advocates contend that it is simply an extension of traditional hybridization and cross breeding, but greatly accelerated in our era of scientific progress and genetic engineering. They point to the success of the U.S. corn and soybean industries as shining examples. The prospects of increased crop yield to feed the billions in China and India have made GM foods seem a dream-come-true for these countries. The golden rice breakthrough, in which the gene for beta-carotene (pre-cursor of vitamin A) was inserted into rice and its promise to eradicate the most common cause of blindness (vitamin A deficiency) in at-risk populations around the world, has been hailed as the humanitarian flagship for GM foods. [99,100]

Critics disagree and warn of potentially dangerous consequences akin to that of mad cow disease. They cite that GM foods go far beyond the normal same-species pollination/hybridization programs that have been in vogue for millenia. They consider GM foods to be gross tampering with nature, citing worrying trends such as that of taking genes from fish and inserting them into the genes of tomatoes. This has potential implications for the future of the tomato gene pool. Critics also attack food-industry motives which they dismiss as naked profiteering, and single out industry giants like Monsanto, whom they accused of promoting "suicide-seeds" that gave on one hand (high-yields), but robbed using the other (Monsanto's "terminator technology" caused crop seed to become sterile at harvest time). [100,101]

The future debates over GM foods are bound to be heated. Balanced reviews and resources on this subject can be accessed from the Tufts University School of Nutrition Science and Policy in Boston, Massachusetts (http://navigator.tufts.edu.) and the Social Issues Research Center in Oxford, England (http://www.sirc.org; public interest section).

Is The American Food Supply Too Clean?

The United States and the industrialized world place great emphasis on food safety and hygiene. Their stated intention is to protect and preserve the safety of the food supply. Is the American obsession with food safety justified? Are we guilty of solving one problem, while creating another?

There exists a larger world within easy reach of the North American shores where you have to be tough to survive. In that world, your best defense is not bottled-water or germ-free food. There, your best defense comes from within; it resides in having a robust constitution and well-rehearsed immune system. In this world, you have to be tough to survive. This is the world in which I was born.

I have been struck by how animals survive in nature. They live in a world where the fittest survive. I observed many creatures, both domestic and in the wild, which do not as a rule wash their food. They eat their food off the ground without getting sick compared to their privileged North American cousins or the imported breeds. Such breeds need to be treated daintily, so "humanely." Mongrel dogs survive by scavenging. They have no owners and they visit no vets. They survive in places where their privileged cousins cannot.

This poses a challenge that may bear great relevance to Americans. In one sense, North Americans are at a survival disadvantage in this era of germ warfare. I am not referring to biological WMDs (weapons of mass destruction). In my past capacities as the physician for the Peace Corps and U.S. embassy personnel overseas, I defined a proto-typical American as one who suffers from recurrent diarrheas after eating local food. American citizens traveling to many parts of the world often take extreme precautions to avoid contracting food and water-borne illnesses. People who can only survive within a hygienic bubble—where all food and drink must be germ-free—are at a survival disadvantage in the wider world. There is a microbiological jungle out there. Get used to it. You may not face it now, but through travel or otherwise, you may have to face it later.

Children in the tropics develop natural immunity to all manner of pathogens in their environment. A favorite pastime of children is to pick fruits off trees and consume them without (excessive) washing. Many may squirm at the very thought of such practices, but people who spend much time in the rugged outdoors know how important it is to be in harmony with the environment. It confers survival advantage. The North American romance with disinfectants and antibiotic-laden detergents may lead to an undesirable outcome. Microbiologists can tell you that you cannot kill all the "bugs" (bacteria). The more you try, the more "super-bugs" (resistant strains) you can create. Today, scientists express real fears about the emergence of resistant bacterial strains. Our repertoire of effective antibiotics is far less than people think.

There is medical evidence that the rising rates of certain immune system disorders (e.g. asthma) may be influenced by insufficient exposure to pathogens early in life. Excessive food hygiene is a likely culprit. Being sheltered continually from mischievous germs in our environment robs us of a natural form of lifelong immunization. Failure to do so can lead to an inexperienced, poorly-orchestrated immune response to unfamiliar germs later in life. As we know from the military, this can result in "friendly-fire," which, when translated into medical jargon, are called auto-immune diseases. While this is not a call for a change in food policy, it is a call to re-examine our attitudes towards excessive hygiene. We were never designed to live in a hygienic bubble, because at some point, bubbles usually burst.[101-103]

The Need for Balance

We need to look at the big picture, and become more agitated over the major killers that we see, rather than the snipers that we do not see. These were responsible for the deaths more than 1.5 million Americans last year. Another 100 million more are on the hit list. Obesity, cardiovascular diseases, cancer, and type II diabetes ambush someone on every street, in every town, and every city across this nation, and around the world. This is a national and a global priority.

Food scares, cover-ups, and continued uncertainty over food safety foment apprehension in many quarters, despite official attempts to re-assure consumers. The failure of governments and industry to be transparent in the past has provided fertile ground for the skepticism and distrust. But in the midst of these public health concerns, let us not lose sight of what kills more 1.5 million Americans each year. The answers to these do not rest with cover-ups by governments and industry; they lie much closer to home.

The modern food industry should be understood within the context of the demands of modern industrial society. Modernity cannot thrive in the midst of food insecurity. The potential of processed foods to cause chronic diseases must be weighed against the alternative. This includes death and disability from starvation and deficiency diseases—a scenario that was prevalent just a hundred years ago. Therefore in our quest to aspire for prevention and optimal health, we must be careful not to throw out the baby with the bath water.[104]

Food Labels

Many consider the new food labels as a great step forward to help consumers understand what is in their food. This is a positive step towards greater nutrition understanding, but this is only the beginning.

In 1990, U.S. lawmakers passed the Nutrition Labeling and Education Act (NLEA) that prescribed specific food labels on most foods with the exception of fresh meat, poultry, fish, and produce (fruits and vegetables). These must include the following: The common name(s) of the product, the name and address of the product's manufacturer, the net contents in terms of weight, measure, or count, and the ingredient list that names the ingredients in descending order of weight or predominance.[105-108] Nutrition labeling involves more than the mere stick-on label that appears on the food. It involves at least six separate nutrition components. They are the following:

- The food label itself (Figure 7-6) has three major components: the nutrients, the quantities and their units, and the serving sizes
- The ingredient label
- Health claims (Table 7-21)
- Adjectival descriptors e.g. "low sodium" (Table 7-22)
- Labeling for special dietary purposes
- Warning labels

Labeling legally includes any in-store placards and restaurant menus that provide nutrition information on the food in question. For the purposes of this discourse, the definition will be restricted to the printed (stick-on) food label and associated health (disease-specific) claims.[109-118]

Table 7-21. Health Claims Approved by Food and Drug Administration (2000)

Health Claims **Approved by Food and Drug Administration (2000)**
Health Claims (Specific food components: added or natural) Foods high in calcium: reduce risk of osteoporosis Foods with folate or folic acid: reduced risk of having a baby with neural tube defects Foods sweetened with sugar alcohols: reduced risk of dental caries Foods with whole oats or oat bran containing β-glucan: reduced risk of heart disease Foods with psyllium or fiber: reduced risk of heart disease Foods with soy protein: reduced risk of heart disease Foods with sterol or stanol esters: reduced risk of heart disease
Health Claims (Foods low in some components) Foods low in total fat and saturated fat: reduced cancer risk Foods low in saturated fat and cholesterol: reduced risk of coronary heart disease Foods low in sodium: reduced risk of hypertension
Health Claims (Natural content of specific components) Foods that are good sources of fiber: reduced risk of cancer Foods that are food sources of soluble fiber: reduced risk of coronary heart disease Foods that are good sources of vitamin C or β-carotene: reduced risk of cancer

The New Food Label

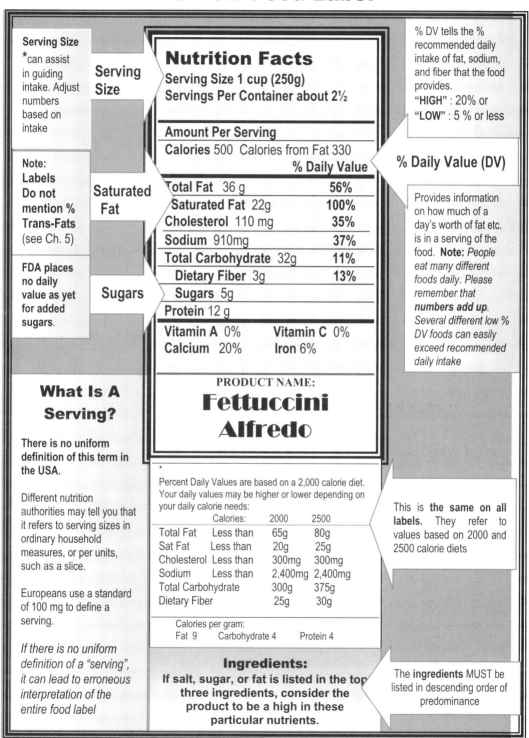

Figure 7-6. The New Food Label, annotated.

The New Food Label

What the food label fails to mention
may be more important than what it mentions.

The official line is that the new food label provides the consumer with an unprecedented insight into the content of foods. The intention is to enable consumers to choose healthier foods. The new food label is a useful tool not just for what it says, but also for what it does not say. Despite the insights it provides into identifying the major nutrients in food, there is much that is missing from these labels that have important health implications. Figure 7-6 illustrates an annotated example of food label.

Contrary to what you may have been told, the true meaning of the food label is not for the novice. There is more to understanding food labels than the print that appears. The waters are further muddied because of the use of verbal gymnastics that is permits clever marketing gimmicks that sometimes border on deception. I will illustrate this point with three personal examples.

Not even a postgraduate degree in nutrition spared me from being duped by slick food labeling. The first example of the "100% pure tomato juice" was mentioned earlier in this chapter under "Processing and the Nutritional Value of Foods." I was fooled a second time when I picked up a gallon of "Pure orange juice, 100% orange juice." In my tropical mind, such a label should mean what it says. My thoughts lusted after those wonderful home-squeezed orange juices. But alas, it left a cheap aftertaste as I knew that it was from concentrate. I felt violated, and my thoughts momentarily entertained that I should complain to the FDA. So I took a long second look at the label again, only to discover, barely visible and in very fine print, the words "from concentrate."

The third example was particularly upsetting. It is the classic example of what the food label fails to mention being more important than what it actually says. All olive oils are not the same (see Chapter 8, Table 8-6). Extra virgin olive oil is more expensive than olive pomace oil, but if you judge from the food label, the composition of both oils is identical. The percentage of monosaturated fat (the recommended healthy fats, see Figure 5-7) were identical on both labels. At the time, I had no idea about the manufacturing processes involved in the extraction of olive pomace oil, and that it was not edible, and therefore, could not be sold unless it was refined and improved with virgin olive oils. Based on the food label, I had begun advising my patients that olive pomace was a cheaper alternative with identical composition.

All olive oils are not the same. All monosaturated fats in olive oil varieties are also not the same. The label is absolutely silent on the percentage of unhealthy trans-monosaturated fat as it is not yet mandatory by law. These are the unhealthiest of all fats. This makes olive pomace oil not just nutritionally inferior, but potentially very damaging to your cardiovascular health (see Chapter 5 under Trans-Fatty Acids and Table 5-7). In this example, the food label failed miserably because of an important error of omission.

Dissecting Food Labels

Check the ingredients list:

Manufacturers are required by the FDA to place ingredients in descending order of quantities. The ingredients are generally listed in descending order of content. Avoid foods that list fat, sugar, or salt in the top three. This indicates a high content of such ingredients. People with cardiovascular diseases and diabetes need to exercise caution in such cases. Below are three examples of pitfalls while reading the ingredients list on a food label (refer to figure 7-6):

Flaw 1:
"Flexi-labeling" using the "and/or" or "may contain" clause is used especially with regard to fats or oils. Consumer groups oppose this practice because it prevents the consumer from knowing exactly which oil the product contains. The FDA countered that the uncertainty (over exactly which oil is used) could be deduced from checking the total and saturated fat content listings. Exactly which oil the manufacturer uses depends on which oil is cheaper. Manufacturers argue that they buy the cheaper oil in an effort to keep down the price of food.[119]

Flaw 2:
If the product lists that it contains meat, the natural tendency is to assume that it is made from whole meat. The term "meat" can include any or all parts of the animal ranging from muscle, to socially-objectionable organs, and mechanically recovered meat. The latter includes particles of flesh removed from the carcass by high pressure hosing. It strips the last shreds of meat and gristle from bones and the resulting paste can be seasoned and be legally labeled as "meat." This is what is used to produce potted meats.[120]

Flaw 3:
Check on "% Daily Value." Most people are unaware of the math involved in making calculations on the food label. Before you even begin to add, you need to first establish what it is that you are adding. What exactly do we mean by a "serving size"? In London where I studied nutrition, this was theoretically easy, because a serving meant 100 mg. This was impractical in my kitchen, as I never weighed food except in nutrition experiments. The definition of "serving size" in the U.S. varies according to which food is in front of you. Therefore there are many different

serving sizes. Worse still, my serving size will be different from your serving size. In this era of super-sizing, when stomach capacities have been re-sized, many conveniently underestimate their intake, and fool themselves in the process, wittingly or unwittingly.

If we have difficulty defining this yardstick—a serving size—(on which all other calculations that appear on the label are based), then we have in front of us a shifting road-map. It is then not surprising why so many get lost in reading labels. Therefore, despite its good intention, the U.S. food label is far from being a straightforward tool. If a thorough understanding of food labels were a necessary qualification for health living, few of us would graduate.

Deciphering "Labelese"

Deception or Misinformation about Whole Grains

Some nutritionists and dieticians salute the food label as though it was the best thing that happened to modern nutrition. Over the past few years, sober and expert voices, led by Walter Willet, M.D. Professor of Nutrition at the Harvard School of Public Health, have added some long-overdue sanity to the modern food debate. According to Dr. Willett, many Americans have heeded the message that cereals and "complex" carbohydrates are good for you. Slick marketing has, however, led many to make the wrong choices:[21]

> Most of the time … it takes a savvy shopper to separate the whole grain from the refined. You have to read food labels with the discriminating eye of a food critic, alert for subtle nuances that spell the difference between whole grain and refined grain. If the label says "made with wheat flour," it may be a whole grain product or it may be just an advertising gimmick—the silkiest, most refined white cake flour is made with wheat flour.

No Fat! Fat-Free! Low Fat! No Cholesterol!

There are about two dozen terms called "adjectival descriptors" that can appear on the food label. The headings above are examples of them.
They don't mean what many people assume.
They have specific meanings (Table 7-22).

The words "no cholesterol," "light and lean," and "lean cuisine" appearing on the food label give the impression that these are healthy alternatives. In the food label, the devil is truly in the details. Such buzzwords need to be consumed along with a healthy serving of skepticism. As discussed in Chapter 5, it is more important to look at the saturated fat content and the hydrogenated-fat ingredients rather than any claim of "no cholesterol." It can get even more confusing. Can the average consumer be expected to know that the terms—"fat-free, low fat, less fat, saturated fat free, lean, and light" have specific meanings? In fact, they do. These terms are called adjectival descriptors. They all have specific meanings and, therefore, reinforce my contention that the food label is far more than meets the eye (Table 7-22). My question is "do they expect us to memorize this table or take it along with us to the supermarket?" It is for you to decide.

Table 7-22. The Meanings of Adjectival Descriptors Appearing on Food Labels

Adjectival Descriptors	Requirements that must be met before using the claim in food labeling
Fat-Free	Less than 0.5 grams of fat per serving, with no added fat or oil
Low fat	3 grams or less of fat per serving
Less fat	25% or less fat than the comparison food
Saturated fat free	Less than 0.5 grams of saturated fat and 0.5 grams of trans-fatty acids per serving
Cholesterol-free	Less than 2 mg cholesterol per serving, and 2 grams or less saturated fat per serving
Low cholesterol	20 mg or less cholesterol per serving and 2 grams or less saturated fat per serving
Reduced calorie	At least 25% fewer calories per serving than the comparison food
Low calorie	40 calories or less per serving
Extra lean	Less than 5 grams of fat, 2 grams of saturated fat, and 95 mg of cholesterol per (100 gram) serving of meat, poultry or seafood
Lean	Less than 10 grams of fat, 4.5 g of saturated fat, and 95 mg of cholesterol per (100 gram) serving of meat, poultry or seafood
Light (fat)	50% or less of the fat than in the comparison food (ex: 50% less fat than our regular cheese)
Light (calories)	1/3 fewer calories than the comparison food
High-fiber	5 grams or more fiber per serving
Sugar-Free	Less than 0.5 grams of sugar per serving
Sodium-free or Salt-free	Less than 5 mg of sodium per serving
Low sodium	140 mg or less per serving
Very low sodium	35 mg or less per serving
Healthy	A food low in fat, saturated fat, cholesterol and sodium, and contains at least 10% of the Daily Values for vitamin A, vitamin C, iron, calcium, protein or fiber.
"High", "Rich in" or "Excellent Source"	20% or more of the Daily Value for a given nutrient per serving
"Less", "Fewer" or "Reduced"	At least 25% less of a given nutrient or calories than the comparison food
"Low", "Little", "Few", or "Low Source of"	An amount that would allow frequent consumption of the food without exceeding the Daily Value for the nutrient – but can only make the claim as it applies to all similar foods
"Good Source Of", "More", or "Added"	The food provides 10% more of the Daily Value for a given nutrient than the comparison food

FDA Specifications for Health Claims and Descriptive Terms

A health claim for a particular food is a declaration (on the food label) that describes the relationship of a nutrient or food ingredient to a disease or a health-related condition. For example, the adjectival descriptor reads, "Foods low in saturated fat and cholesterol reduce the risk of coronary heart disease" (Table 7-21). The health claims approved by the Food and Drug Administration (FDA) in 2000 should be based on the following criteria:[122]

> … totality of publicly available scientific evidence (including evidence from well-designed studies conducted in a manner which is consistent with generally recognized scientific procedures and principles), that there is significant agreement, among experts qualified by scientific training and experience to evaluate such claims, that the claim is supported by such evidence.

For a food to qualify for a health claim, it cannot contain more than a certain amount of any ingredient that is considered to place people at risk. These include total fat, saturated fat, cholesterol, and sodium (Table 7-22). In addition, such foods must contain at least 10 percent of the recommended daily intake of the following nutrients: vitamin A, vitamin C, iron, calcium, protein, and fiber.

Food Labels: A Personal View

> If a true understanding of food labels is necessary for minimizing our risks of chronic-diet related diseases, most of us would be at high risk.

The food label has a role, but quite frankly, with the multitude of potentially confusing terms, one cannot reasonably expect the average person to understand such detail. When shopping, my simple advice is to read fewer labels. This means shopping for produce, fresh foods, and other minimally-processed varieties that don't have labels attached. In so doing you waste less time, you lessen your risk of getting confused, and you simplify healthy eating.

> The balance of good health unquestionably weighs heavily in favor of choosing foods that do not require food labels.

A Question of Balance

The debates will continue about the pros and cons of processing and the need for labels. The role of the food industry in the food security of the Western world is undeniable. Progress has brought its share of problems. Additives, for example, have the potential to harm, but when weighed in its totality, the concerns voiced by alarmists are largely exaggerated.

In our drive towards improved nutrition and prevention of chronic diseases, the problem has to be one of balance. Highly-processed foods are not just unhealthy simply because they are processed, but because they substitute for healthier alternatives. This has played a major role in the global epidemic of chronic diseases that now confronts us. The challenge, therefore, is one of restoring a healthy balance and a clear perspective on healthy eating. This is the subject of the next chapter.[123]

Summary

The food choices that people make are perhaps the most vexing issues in nutrition, made worse by the bewildering array of choices that confront people living in modern urban societies. The reasons people choose the foods they do are complex. Personal, cultural, socioeconomic, and wider environmental issues all play important roles. Good choices should ideally commence during childhood, but social influences play significant roles throughout the life cycle.

Any serious discussion on health and prevention cannot ignore the central role of the industrial revolution on the quality of our food. This is where Americans spend ninety percent of their food dollar. Food processing has brought unprecedented food security, but it has swung the pendulum to the other extreme where we now face the problem of over-consumption and its pivotal role in the epidemic of obesity and nutrition-related diseases.

Food scares and concerns over the safety of our food abound, but these must be seen within the context of their overall contribution to death and disability. They merit our attention, but must never overshadow the glaring evidence it is over-consumption that plays a major role in the diseases that kill more than 1.5 million Americans each year.

Efforts like the introduction of the food label that were designed to enable the public to make healthier choices were well intended, but they fell fall far short of promoting healthy diets. The balance of good health clearly favors the consumption of fresh or minimally-processed foods.

******

PART V

Your Health
...Charting Your Future

The Way Forward Is Not Complicated.

Scientists have observed that ordinary people around the world
who follow certain traditional dietary patterns
exhibit excellent health and longevity.
The Prudent Cosmopolitan Diet is a simple plan that embraces the best
of these dietary patterns. This model answers the call to halt the modern
epidemic of obesity and the metabolic syndrome, cardiovascular
diseases, type II diabetes, and several forms of cancer.

But success calls for more than mere academic knowledge, it demands
sound insights and a clear strategy that can
translate knowledge into action.

Chapter 8

Nutrition Choices for Health and Disease

Chapter Outline

The Future is not "New" 315
Foods, Not Nutrients.. 316
The "Medicalization" of Nutrition... 319
The Scientific Evidence for the Role of Diet in Preventing Disease 323
    Keys Seven Countries Study 323
    Framingham Heart Study 325
    Lyon Diet Heart Study.. 325
    Italian GISSI Prevention Trial.. 326
    Asian Diet Studies... 326
    Dietary Approaches to Stop Hypertension (DASH) trial.................. 327
    The Nurses' Health Study 328
    Dietary Patterns and Type II Diabetes 328
    Lifestyle Heart Trial (Ornish) 328
Constructing a Prudent Cosmopolitan Diet 329
The Prudent Cosmopolitan Diet
    "The Best Diets All Under One Roof" 332
The Best of the Mediterranean Dietary Practices.................................... 332
All Olive Oils are not Created Equal 334
The Best of the Far East (Asian) Dietary Practices.................................. 336
Soy: A Great Oriental contribution... 338
Milk Consumption in the Far East.. 339
Orientals and Greens 339
Is Rice Fattening?... 340
Green Teas.. 340
Africa, Fiber and Whole Grains.. 341
Glycemic Index—Glycemic Load.. 342
Health Aspects of Some Fruits and Vegetables....................................... 344
Grapes, Tomatoes, Eggplant, Avocados, and Peppers 344

Citrus Fruits 345
A Wonderful Excuse for a Fruit Dessert 346
Spinach, Broccoli and Dark Leafy Greens e.g. Collard, Kale, Chard..... 346
Blueberries, Blackberries, Strawberries, Raspberries, Cranberries.......... 347
Garlic, Onion, Leeks, Chives, Allium Family 347
Soft Drinks, Reconstituted Juices, Water................................... 348
Summarizing the Prudent Cosmopolitan Diet............................. 348
Notes on Obesity: A Growing Epidemic 350
Obesity and Quality of Life Issues 351
Obesity and Medical Handicaps 352
Overweight, Obesity, Central Obesity, Visceral Obesity 352
Successfully Tackling Obesity: Perspectives and Principles 354
Needed: "Regime Change" 355
Practical Perspectives for Successfully Tackling Obesity................ 356
Say "No" to Counting Calories, Special Menus, etc. 357
Making Practical Choices When Shopping—Read Less Labels............... 358
Cooking at Home: Quick and Easy: The Way I Do It................... 359
When Eating Out Ask Questions, But Not Too Many 361
Understanding Global Cuisines 362
Conclusion and Summary 363

The role of science in nutrition is to establish why some dietary habits lead to higher rates of diseases, and others do not. Its role is not to discover some "new" diet. People the world over have a long history of healthy traditional eating patterns.

Looking at the whole diet is an important shift in approach because it mirrors how people eat. Previous studies using the single nutrient approach—looking individually at things like fat, sugar, and fiber—have provided results, but could miss the big picture.

Frank Hu, Assistant Professor [1] Harvard School of Public Health

One of the most consistent findings in dietary investigations is that people who consume a higher intake of fresh fruits and vegetables have lower rates of heart disease, diabetes, stroke, and cancer.[2-6]

...We identified and validated two major dietary patterns that we labeled "prudent" (characterized by higher consumption of vegetables, fruit, fish, poultry and whole grains) and "Western" (characterized by higher consumption of red meat, french fries, high fat dairy products, refined grains, and sweets and desserts)...Our findings suggest that a Western dietary pattern is associated with a substantially increased risk for type 2 diabetes in men.[7]

From Harvard School of Public Health, Brigham and Women's Hospital,
and Harvard Medical School, Boston, Massachusetts,
and National Institute of Public Health and the Environment, the Netherlands

§§§§§§§

The Future Is Not New

Today's media often trumpets sensational, but half-baked opinions about nutrition. Many people have been programmed to expect "new" diets and "new formulas" for optimal health. The evidence is clear—the new diets of tomorrow will not come in pills and packages. They will resemble the diets of yesterday.

Nutrition receives great coverage in today's media. It has moved from being a neglected subject to one that generates an intense level of debate, confusion, claims, and counterclaims. There is no shortage of self-styled nutrition experts proclaiming "new breakthroughs" on how to cure everything from obesity and cancer, to aging and Alzheimer's. As are the sellers, so are the buyers. There is likewise no shortage of people who subscribe to such claims that promise far more than they can deliver. There is a part of the human psyche that craves "new" things, especially quick fixes. This is a reflection of the pill-for-every-ill mentality described in Chapter 2.

Within the mainstream medical community, the responses have been varied. Doctors have successfully maneuvered themselves to center stage in the nutrition debates and now play host to an expectant audience. Today's headlines keep trumpeting many half-baked scientific discoveries on what is hot, and what is not. This has led many to perpetually anticipate a "new" diet for tomorrow. The balance of evidence is clear—the new diets of tomorrow resemble the diets of yesterday.

Healthy eating does not have to await new scientific discoveries for what's best to eat. People with such mind-sets place an unbalanced emphasis on isolated food components while disregarding the whole diet. Such people are prone to go overboard and subscribe to buzzwords depicting "new diets" and novel therapies. This chapter strongly discourages such approaches. There is a need to restore sanity and balance to the food debate.

Looking at the whole diet reflects how people normally eat. You cannot do limited experiments in laboratories and apply these to the real world. This is what much of television nutrition reporting is about. Cynically speaking, it often amounts to … Scientists "somewhere" did a new study (maybe in mice, or in a laboratory) to show "some" new finding that may lead to a spectacular breakthrough "sometime" in the future. When you get to the bottom of it, it equates to little more than news-grabbing headlines—full of speculation, but lacking in application.

If we have to wait for decades of research before discovering what to eat, most of us will not be around to digest the final conclusions. Healthy diets do not revolve around "new" discoveries. Healthy diets are here with us today. Our challenge is to draw upon the best of the healthiest diets that are now in vogue around the world, and apply these to our daily lifestyles.

Foods, Not Nutrients

The popular practice of championing a single vitamin, a nutrient, or a supplement can never be a substitute for healthy diets and lifestyles. Foods are complex mixtures of nutrients that act in concert (not unilaterally) on our metabolism.

People do not eat proteins, carbohydrate, fats, vitamins, and micronutrients. People eat food! Foods contain these nutrients—proteins, fats, carbohydrate, fiber, vitamins, minerals, and a host of other substances—*but foods are more than just nutrients.* They are related, but there is an important difference. Failure to appreciate this is like looking at Miami and calling it America.

Popular nutrition is guilty of very narrow definitions of nutrition. Pseudo-scientific claims about the benefits of single nutrients in isolation abound. For this reason, many people get swept away by "new herbs" and "special supplements" that promise to perform a wide range of miracles. Most of this is driven by naked profiteering. It is another reflection of the quick-fix mentality that dominates our "pill-for-every-ill" culture.

The bigger picture clearly illustrates that food components interact. They do not act in unilateral fashion. Failure to appreciate this has resulted in wrong conclusions. The case of tropical oils is one such example. Force-feeding rats with industrially-prepared tropical oils to clog arteries in laboratories is not a true reflection of centuries-old traditions of consuming home-made tropical oils. People have historically subsisted on coconut oil as their premier oil, but they have not exhibited high rates of heart attacks (see Chapter 5).[8]

Take the case of soybean (Table 8-1). This little bean attracts a lot of attention in nutrition circles today. It is packed with many ingredients. Popular science highlights its phytoestrogen component, particularly the isoflavones. The isoflavones or isoflavanoids are known for their weak estrogenic activity and so act in a manner comparable to the breast cancer drug, tamoxifen. The observation of high breast cancer rates in Western women and low rates in Oriental women who consume lots of soy, has led scientists to attribute the anti-cancer effect to isoflavones (the ingredient), rather than to whole-soy foods. The relationship, however, is not that simple.

Table 8-1. The Complex Little Soybean

The Soybean packs more than just isoflavones	Lower Incidence of disease associated with increased soy consumption
Protein (high grade) **Carbohydrate** **Fats** (unsaturated & omega 3) **Vitamins** (B vitamins, vitamin E, folic acid) **Minerals** (calcium, potassium, zinc, potassium, magnesium, iron **Fiber** **Glycosides** (2% of soybeans): phytoestrogens, soy saponins, isoflavonoids (genistein, diadzein, equol) **Phystosterols:** **Protease inhibitors** **Phytic acid**	Heart disease Lowers cholesterol Breast cancer Lung cancer Colon cancer Osteoporosis

Soybeans pack far more than one substance with anti-cancer properties. They also contain glycosides, phytosterols, protease inhibitors, and phytic acid, some of which exhibit anti-cancer as well as other beneficial health effects.[9-11] Soy foods, and not simply the isoflavone component, are linked to lower levels of chronic diseases. It is soy foods, not just isoflavones, that lower cholesterol. It is soy foods, not genistein, reduce menopausal symptoms. To attribute the benefits to a single constituent oversimplifies how foods exert their benefits. Trying to isolate a single ingredient from food and putting it inside a pill reflects a major misunderstanding of how food works.

Citrus fruits are another good example of fruits that provide many health benefits. Oranges pack far more than just vitamin C (Table 8-2). They contain two major types of anti-oxidants—vitamin C (ascorbic acid) and flavonoids, powerful oils called monoterpenes, the most potent of which is d-limonene. All three substances show promise in cardiovascular and cancer prevention, but consumption of citrus is more than just getting your vitamin C, flavonoids and terpenes. Citrus fruits pack a host of other vitamins, minerals, and other substances that impart important health benefits. These should be considered in any discussion of the relationship between citrus intake and disease prevention.[12-18]

Table 8-2. Citrus Fruits: Composition and Related Health Benefits

Citrus Fruits pack more than just vitamin C	**Lower Incidence of disease associated with increased Citrus and Fruit Consumption**
Protein (low grade) **Carbohydrate**	Hypertension
Fats and Terpenes (in the peel/rind and seeds) monterpenes: d-limonene	Immune response
Vitamins (vitamins C, B_1, B_2 etc.) **Minerals** (potassium, calcium)	Breast cancer
Fiber **Citric Acid**	Lung cancer
Flavonoids: hesperetin, hesperedin Flavones (tangeretin, nobiletin) Flavanones (naringenin)	Colon cancer

The discussions that follow will highlight foods and dietary patterns rather than their individual nutrients. The recurrent emphasis will be on the need for dietary patterns, rather than the reductionist models that try to isolate nutrients from their food sources.

The "Medicalization" Of Nutrition

The pill-for-every-ill mentality dominates the study of nutrition. Most research has focused on individual nutrients (e.g. fats, vitamin C, or calcium supplements, etc.) in place of whole diet studies. This can produce results that fail to accurately reflect normal everyday eating habits.

The resurgent interest in nutrition by the American public has awakened the attention of the medical community. This has led to a marked increase in nutrition research. Unfortunately, what predominates is a discussion on nutrients, rather than a discussion on food.

The "medicalization" of nutrition occurs when people simply trade pharmaceuticals for "nutraceuticals," to prevent and manage diseases. The nutrition debate has now been reduced to a question of nutrients versus drugs. What is often left out of the debate is the importance of the whole diet. This "nutraceutical approach" is good for business. It fuels a multi-billion dollar dietary supplement industry that caters to a population that has not departed from its quick-fix mindset, but has simply substituted supplements for drugs. We need to draw this distinction at the onset of this chapter. This is because it is crucial to dispel the mindset that majors on nutrients at the expense of nutrition.

People who consume higher intakes of fresh fruits and vegetables have lower rates of heart disease, diabetes, stroke, and cancer.[2-6] This is one of the most consistent findings in dietary investigations. Well-conducted studies on individual vitamins like vitamin C and vitamin E, on the other hand, have produced mixed results ranging from positive benefits in some trials, to no effects in others.[19-23] This is not to say that vitamin C or vitamin E is unimportant. In fact they are, but looking at these alone, while ignoring the entire diet, is an unbalanced understanding of nutrition.

Natural vitamin E as occurs in seeds, nuts, and grains is far more complex than the vitamin E that is sold in pharmacies (Table 8-3). Natural vitamin E consists of at least eight different naturally occurring substances with differing potencies. The most potent of these is d-alpha (α-) tocopherol (Table 8-4). There are also beta (β-), gamma (γ-), and delta (δ-) tocopherols. These are weaker forms of vitamin E. The most common and inexpensive types of vitamin E sold in stores are synthetic esters of alpha-tocopherol. These are significantly less potent than those listed in Table 8-4. These do not occur in nature.[24]

In the American diet, soybean and corn oil are the most heavily consumed oils. In both of these oils, 60 percent of the vitamin E is of the least potent variety—the gamma (γ-tocopherol) form. The best sources of vitamin E are nuts, seeds, and the oils found in wheat germ, sunflower, and safflower (Table 8-3). These pack more d-alpha or [d]-α-tocopherol, the most potent form of vitamin E.[25]

T 1. Table 8-3. Vitamin E (Tocopherol) Content of Some Nuts and Oils (mg/100g)

	Alpha (α-) tocopherol (most potent)	Beta (β-) tocopherol	Gamma (γ-) tocopherol	Delta (δ-) tocopherol (least potent)
Peanuts	9.7	--	6.60	--
Almonds	27.4	0.30	0.90	--
Sunflower seeds	49.5	2.73	--	--
Corn oil	11.2	5.00	60.20	1.8
Cottonseed oil	38.9	--	38.70	--
Peanut oil	13.0	--	21.60	2.1
Safflower oil	38.7	--	17.40	24.0
Soybean oil	10.1	--	59.30	26.4
Sunflower oil	48.7	--	5.10	0.8
Wheat germ oil	133.0	71.00	26.00	27.1

Modified from ource: Bauernfeind J: Tocopherols in foods: In Vitamin E: A Comprehensive Treatise.[24]

A vitamin pill or dietary supplement is a poor representation of its complexity in nature, as is illustrated with this example of vitamin E. Man-made vitamins and supplements are best considered supplements, but never substitutes for a healthy diet.

T 2. Table 8-4. Vitamin E—A Complex Group of Tocopherols

Different forms of Vitamin E	Vitamin E activity
[d]-α-tocopherol (MOST POTENT)(RRR-α-tocopherol)	1.49 IU/mg
[d]-α-tocopheryl acetate (RRR-α-tocopheryl acetate)	1.36 IU/mg
[dl]- α-tocopherol (all *rac*-α-tocopherol)	1.1 IU/mg
[dl]- α-tocopheryl acetate (all *rac*-α-tocopheryl acetate)	1.0 IU/mg
"[dl]- α-tocopheryl acetate" ("2-ambo-α-tocopheryl acetate)	1.0 IU/mg
[dl]-β-tocopherol	0.60 IU/mg
[d]-γ-tocopherol	0.15 – 0.45 IU/mg
[d]-δ-tocopherol (LEAST POTENT)	0.015 IU/mg

Modified from source: Farrell PA, Roberts RJ. Vitamin E. In Modern nutrition in health and disease, Lea & Febiger, 1994[24]

Therefore, a vitamin studied in isolation is not an accurate representation of its behavior in food. A "nutraceutical" or reductionist approach that studies vitamin E divorced from its food sources may be well intended, but misses the complexity of how vitamin E behaves within foods. This is the prime reason for introducing the concept of "foods, not nutrients" at the outset of this chapter.

The popular "nutraceutical" approaches to nutrition continually promote "superior forms" of vitamins, minerals, or nutrients that will vanquish tumora, lower cholesterol, or reduce heart disease. Even though individual nutrients may show beneficial effects beyond the prevention of deficiency diseases, singling them out from their food sources can lead to inaccurate conclusions about their effectiveness.[19] Furthermore, such views simply fail to reflect the way normal people eat food.

In 1994, I conducted a study that sought to address concerns arising out of an investigation by Professor Errol Morrison and colleagues in Jamaica. They had shown a diabetes-triggering effect of an annatto extract on anaesthetized dogs.[26] Malnourished dogs fed with an extract of annatto (the red carotenoid pigment from the red seeds of *Bixa orellana* plant) showed persistent elevation of their blood sugar (a diabetes-triggering effect) that lasted six to eight weeks. This effect was found to be the result of damage to the pancreas and liver of these dogs by the annatto exract. Well-fed dogs given the identical extract showed no such effects. Annatto (achiote), a popular food colorant in cheese, margarine, and processed foods, is a popular condiment throughout much of Latin America. My study, which looked 20 Hispanic adults in a Central American (Belize) population that heavily consumed annatto, failed to show any hint of annatto's role in triggering diabetes. Good scientific investigations, especially those looking at diet, may show results that do not reflect everyday realities.

The same principle applies when studying nutrients like the popular antioxidants. A wide body of research has consistently linked consumption of *foods rich in antioxidants* (vitamin C, vitamin E, beta-carotene, and flavonoids) with lowered rates of cancer and cardiovascular diseases.[2-6] Antioxidants are plentiful in fresh fruits, vegetables and nuts. However, studies that looked at *antioxidant in isolation* have provided mixed results.

The Cambridge Heart Antioxidant Study (CHAOS) analysed 2,000 patients with known heart disease who were given 800 mg supplements of natural vitamin E (alpha-tocopherol). An impressive 77 percent reduction in heart attack rates and an almost 50 percent reduction in cardiovascular complications were observed.[27] Another study called the Alpha-Tocopherol and Beta Carotene(ATBC) study showed a 38 percent reduction in recurrent heart attacks in people given vitamin E supplements.[28] The Heart Outcomes Prevention Evaluation(HOPE) followed up more than 9,000 patients who supplemented with vitamin E over a 5-year period. It, however, failed to show any benefits in reducing deaths from cardiovascular disease, heart attack, or stroke.[22]

This has led some experts to conclude that, "Unless new clinical trials in this area provide more positive information, there is no basis for recommending antioxidant vitamins to patients with chronic CAD [coronary artery disease]"[29] This statement refers to antioxidant supplements, and not to diets high in antioxidants. As has been reiterated several times throughout this book, it is *diets rich in antioxidants—plenty of fresh fruit, nuts, whole grains, and vegetables*—not antioxidant supplements, that have *consistently* demonstrated lower rates of cardiovascular disease, diabetes, and cancer. Again, comparing food ingredients versus their whole food sources can lead to different conclusions.

The debates about antioxidants are far from over. There is an excellent theoretical scientific basis on which to recommend them. As discussed in Chapter 6, they defend our bodies against free radicals attacks that play important roles in aging and disease. However, I see two extremes—the purists who believe that antioxidant supplements are useless in the face of inconclusive or conflicting studies on one hand, and those who contend that supplementation is the best guarantee for good health on the other. The truth is somewhere in between. Supplements can play a role, perhaps an important role, but never at the expense of good diets and lifestyles.

Foods, which contain thousands of nutrients that scientists are yet to comprehend, can never be replaced by dietary supplements. To relegate the entire antioxidant story to popping a few antioxidant supplements is again like looking at Miami and calling it America. At the same time, it is not wise to wait decades for conclusive medical research before taking some form of dietary supplements that show promise (e.g. vitamin C, E, flavonoids, alpha-lipoic acid, and a multivitamin). They are safe, and relatively inexpensive. Even those doctors, who do not advise patients to take dietary supplements, are themselves taking dietary supplements, but privately. Arrive at your own conclusions, but read on.

Dietary supplements are just that: … Supplements.
They can never be substitutes for healthy diets and lifestyles.
Much of the popular trends in nutrition
have simply traded pharmaceuticals for "nutraceuticals."
Both often promise more than they can deliver
—chiefly because they have ignored
the central role of nutrition and lifestyle,
and have opted instead, for quick fixes.

Scientific Evidence for Nutrition in Preventing Cardiovascular Diseases, Cancer, and Type II Diabetes

Good science helps us define the relationships between diet and disease. The dietary recommendations given in this book reflect sound and widely accepted scientific studies.

Just as the unbalanced Western diet led to an epidemic of obesity and chronic lifestyle diseases, so can prudent dietary practices reduce their prevalence. Nutrition plays a major role in preventing and managing both chronic diseases (cardiovascular diseases, type II diabetes, and cancer) and their risk factors (obesity, hypertension, and high blood cholesterol). This has been bolstered by good science that serves as the basis for the nutrition recommendations that follow.

People who eat more fresh fruits and vegetables have lower rates of heart disease, stroke, high blood pressure, and cancer. Both epidemiological and clinical trials have established that diets high in animal fats are major contributors to coronary heart disease. People who eat more fiber and whole grains have less heart disease, less type II diabetes, and lower rates of cancer compared to those who consume the highly-processed diets discussed in Chapter 5 and Chapter 7. High fiber diets and foods rich in vitamins and minerals have resulted in less heart disease, cancer, and diabetes.[19,30-33] A summary of the types of scientific studies used as the basis for good nutrition advice appear in Table 8-5.

Keys Seven Countries Study

No study of diet and its role in cardiovascular diseases would be complete without reference to the pioneer work of Ancel Keys, Ph.D. and colleagues from the University of Minnesota. "Monsieur Cholesterol," as he was dubbed by his University of Minnesota colleagues, conducted the first international survey of coronary heart disease among sixteen different populations in seven countries—Finland, Greece, Italy, Japan, the Netherlands, the United States, and Yugoslavia.[34-36]

The Keys Seven Countries Study, started in 1958, enrolled 12,467 men who were followed up every 5 to 10 years. Countries with the highest intake of saturated fats generally exhibited the highest rates of heart disease (East Finland), but with one major exception—the Greek population of Crete (Kriti), which indulged in one of the highest intake of fats (almost 40 percent of daily energy from fat—high intake of olive oil) exhibited the lowest rate of heart disease. Blood cholesterol and blood pressure levels accounted for most of the variation in heart disease rates across countries. Socioeconomic status, the degree of industrialization, lifestyle habits, obesity rates, physical activity levels, and cigarette smoking also made important contributions to the different rates of heart disease.

The Keys Seven Countries Study provided clear evidence that not all fats were bad. Virgin olive oils as consumed in the Mediterranean region, despite high intakes, proved heart-healthy.

Table 8-5. Understanding Nutrition and Disease Relationships

Types of Scientific Studies to Establish Relationships Between Diets, Diseases, and Prevention

Before sound advice could be given to people to embark on changes to prevent diseases, it is essential that nutrition claims be subject to scientific scrutiny. The most reliable conclusions are made when the different types of studies listed below are carried out—the relationship is strongest when there is harmony and consistency in the results.[19,30,31]

Epidemiological Studies:
designed to study the distribution and determinants of diseases.
3 Main Types:
Descriptive,
Observational
Randomized Controlled Trials

Descriptive Studies: describe basic disease patterns and as they occur in a particular place at a particular time. They include: *case reports, cross-sectional surveys, cross-cultural comparison and temporal trend studies.* (*e.g. Keys Seven Countries*).
Observational studies: (*case-control and cohort or prospective*) observe and do not interfere with the participants lifestyles, it analyses them as 'cases' or 'cohorts'(*e.g. Framingham Heart Study, Physicians' Health Study, Nurses' Health Study,* and *Adventist Health Study*).
Randomized Controlled Trials: or intervention studies—intervene and make changes in participants' lifestyles and measure the impact on their health. If well designed, they can provide a greater cause and effect relationship (*e.g. DCCT: Diabetic Complications and Control Trial*).

Basic Laboratory Research

Often involves test-tube and animal experiments.

Clinical Investigation or Metabolic Studies

Involves studying volunteers in hospital or clinic settings, and investigates the effects of diets etc.

Meta-analysis Studies

Provides an overview by combining the results of several comparable studies.

Cost Efficacy / Effectiveness Studies

Helps establish prevention guidelines, especially for these highly prevalent and expensive-to-treat chronic diseases.

A follow-up study of the same populations twenty-five years later, confirmed a direct relationship between cholesterol levels and coronary heart disease. Japan exhibited the lowest rates, despite their higher prevalence of smoking. The countries of

Northern Europe, with lower intakes of fruits and vegetables and higher rates of smoking, showed the highest rates of cardiovascular diseases. Ancel Keys was so impressed that he and his wife went on to publish several works about their findings, including a book, *Eat Well, Stay Well the Mediterranean Way.*

Framingham Heart Study

Started in 1948, the Framingham study, named after the town of Framingham, Massachusetts, was the study that "changed America's heart" (see Chapter 5). Its mission was to identify the causes of cardiovascular diseases. What we know today as the "risk factors" for cardiovascular diseases—cigarette smoking, high blood pressure, total cholesterol, obesity, and diabetes, were established by this important landmark study.[24] Framingham Heart Study has given birth to the Offspring Study (1971) that is observing the risk factors in the offspring of the original group, and the Omni Study (1995) that looks at risk factors in minority ethnic groups in Framingham.[24]

Lyon Diet Heart Study

The Lyon Diet Heart Study, headed by Dr. Michel de Lorgeril and colleagues, based in Lyon-Saint-Etienne area of southern France, examined the effect of a Mediterranean-style diet on 605 men and women who suffered a previous heart attack. Participants were to be followed up over a period of four years. Half the participants ate a Mediterranean-style diet—rich in fruits, vegetables, fish, cereals, beans, fiber, olive oil, and alpha-linolenic acids. The latter is a type of polyunsaturated omega-3 fat common in oily fish, flaxseed, canola, and walnut oils. The other half consumed an American Heart Association (AHA) diet that substituted linoleic acid (an omega-6 fat common in corn oil, safflower, soybean, and sunflower oils) for alpha-linolenic acid. Almost 30 percent of daily calories in the Mediterranean diet came from fat, with 8 percent from saturated fat. The AHA diet provided 34 percent of total daily calories from fat, with almost 12 percent coming from saturated fat. Dietary fiber intake was 3 grams higher in the Mediterranean-style diet.[39]

After only 30 months of follow up, those on the Mediterranean-style diet showed a 50 to 70 percent reduction in the recurrence of heart attacks, compared to the group on the AHA diet. Subsequent deaths (from all causes) were 70 percent lower in those who consumed the Mediterranean-style diet. There were fewer deaths from fatal and non-fatal heart attacks and fewer complications like unstable angina, stroke, and heart failure in those on the Mediterranean-style diet. The results were so convincing that researchers terminated the study after only two and a half years.

Alexander Leaf M.D., professor of cardiology at Harvard, hailed the study as a convincing directive to prevent heart attacks. Lamentably, the Lyon Diet Heart Study's results were largely ignored by mainstream cardiologists:[40]

Despite the striking findings in the first report of a 70% reduction in all-cause mortality due to a reduction in coronary heart disease (CHD) mortality and comparable large reductions in nonfatal sequelae, I have encountered few cardiologists here in the U.S. who are aware of the study and advise their patients accordingly. At a time when health professionals, the pharmaceutical industries, and the research funding and regulatory agencies are almost totally focused on lowering plasma cholesterol levels by drugs, it is heartening to see a well-conducted scientific study finding that relatively simple dietary changes achieved greater reductions in risk of all-cause and coronary heart disease mortality than any of the cholesterol-lowering studies to date.

This study is a bastion of support for the great contribution of Mediterranean-style diets, not just in preventing heart disease, but other diseases as well. It also indicates that a good diet can arrest the natural progression of heart disease and deliver great preventive benefits, including a reduction in complications and deaths from a host of other causes.

The Italian GISSI Prevention Trial

The GISSI-Prevenzione Study (Gruppo Italiano per lo Studio della Sopravvivenza nell'Infarto Miocardio, 1999) led by Dr. Roberto Marchioli and colleagues of Milan, Italy, investigated more than 11,000 Italian heart attack survivors, both men and women. This diet, high in vegetables, fish, omega-3 fatty acids, and monosaturated fats markedly lowered heart disease rates, and deaths from heart disease, compared to a Western-style diet.[41]

Participants who took a gram of fish oil supplements daily (containing the omega-3 fats—eicosapentanoic acid [EPA] and docosahexanoic acid [DHA])—reduced their risk of a second heart attack by 10 to 15 percent. They also reduced their risk of dying (from all causes, including stroke) during the four-year follow-up period by 20 percent. Vitamin E supplements were also given during the study, but did not show a strong protective benefit like that seen with the addition of the fish oil supplement.

Asian Diet Studies

Epidemiological studies of obesity, type II diabetes, breast, and prostate cancer have consistently shown lower rates of these diseases in Asian populations that follow their traditional diets. The same cannot be said of Asian populations, like the Japanese, who migrated and adopted the dietary habits of host populations in Hawaii and San Francisco. The latter exhibit substantially higher rates of heart disease compared to their compatriots living in Japan.[42]

This same trend is observed when Japanese, Korean, and Thai populations become increasingly westernized. Westernization of the Asian diet refers to the growing trend towards increased "protein and fat consumption at meals and the prevalence of American-style fast foods, such as hamburgers and fried chicken." Heart disease among Asians has risen sharply and is now the number one killer in Asia. The rates, however, are still far below those seen in North America and Europe.[43-44]

Asian women exhibit far lower breast cancer rates than women in the West. This five-fold difference in breast cancer rates is largely attributed to the traditional Asian diet.[45] Even though breast cancer rates are also low in other populations that do not consume soy products, populations with high soy consumption also exhibit lower rates of other cancers, including prostate, endometrial (uterus), stomach, colon, and lung cancers. This suggests a blanket effect of soy in preventing cancer. Increased soy consumption lowers blood cholesterol and cardiovascular disease risks as well (Table 8-1 and 8-9).[46-57]

The popularity of green tea is another feature of the Asian diet. Its consumption is linked to lower rates of cancer and reduced risk of type II diabetes. Both green and black teas have shown their ability to prevent every stage of carcinogenesis—the development of cancer. Green teas can reduce cancer rates by blocking the action of the cancer-causing nitrosamines. This action is chiefly mediated by protective polyphenol compounds known as catechins. These include epigallocatechin-3-gallate (EGCG), epigallocatechin (EGC), and epicatechin-3-gallate (ECG). Catechins comprise up to 40 percent of the solids extracted from tea leaves. They also possess potent antioxidant properties with wide ranging benefits including the prevention of cardiovascular diseases.[58-61]

Dietary Approaches to Stop Hypertension (DASH)

Dietary Approaches to Stop Hypertension (DASH, 1999) was a multi-center feeding study based at four clinical centers—Harvard, Duke, Johns Hopkins, and Louisiana State University. Three different dietary patterns were studied in 459 adults (49% women, 60% African American) and compared for their ability to lower blood pressure in the participants with untreated hypertension. The first group followed a control diet similar to the typical American diet, the second group followed a diet that had more fruits and vegetables, and the third group followed the DASH diet. The latter consisted of 4 servings of fruits, 4 servings of vegetables, and 2 or 3 servings of low-fat dairy foods daily.[62,63]

The entire group was monitored over an 8-week period, throughout which sodium intake, physical activity, and body weight remained constant. All participants on the DASH diet exhibited lower systolic and diastolic blood pressures, especially among African Americans. This blood pressure-lowering effect was seen as early as two weeks into the study.

The DASH study is significant for showing that there are practical effective, dietary patterns that can swiftly lower blood pressures in populations at high risk for high blood pressure, heart attack, and stroke.

Nurses' Health Study

Harvard Medical School researchers embarked on very large study that enrolled 121,700 female nurses between the ages of 30 and 55. The original design in 1976 was aimed at evaluating the long term effects of the increasingly popular oral contraceptive pill. Its popularity had sparked serious health concerns. It was linked to an increased risk of stroke, heart attacks, and blood clots.

It is the largest observational study, and one of the longest ongoing studies to follow up the health of its participants. It has yielded a wealth of information on lifestyle factors, diet, weight, smoking, and their relationship to health, disease, and life expectancy. An authoritative resource on this treasure of information is contained in *Healthy Women, Healthy Lives – A Guide to Preventing Disease from the Landmark Nurses' Health Study*, a book released by the Harvard Medical School research group. Among many other findings, the Nurse's Health Study revealed that diet and lifestyle can reduce the rates of heart disease by at least 80 percent in women.[64,65]

Dietary Patterns and Type II Diabetes

The first study to link the overall dietary patterns, rather than specific foods or nutrients, to the development of type II diabetes was published in 2002 as a collaborative effort between Harvard Medical School researchers and the National Institute of Public Health of the Netherlands. This large cohort of 40,000 male health professionals between ages 40 and 75, with no previous history of cardiovascular disease, diabetes, or cancer, was followed over a 12-years period.[66]

Those who followed a Western dietary pattern—with increased consumption of red meats, processed meats, french fries, high-fat dairy products, refined grains, sweets, and desserts—showed an increased risk of type II diabetes. Those who followed a prudent dietary pattern—increased consumption of vegetables, fruit, fish, poultry, and whole grains—developed less type II diabetes.

Lifestyle Heart Trial

Dean Ornish, M.D. and colleagues in California demonstrated that comprehensive lifestyle changes can improve the symptoms and angiographic evidence (special x-rays of blood flow to the heart) of heart disease.[67,68] People who adhered to a low-fat vegetarian diet, stopped smoking, and engaged in aerobic physical activity and relaxation therapies, showed impressive results after only 12 months on the program.

In those on the lifestyle heart program, the level of "bad" LDL-cholesterol dropped by almost 40 percent and the symptoms of angina pectoris (chest pains due to coronary artery disease) fell by more than 90 percent. Just as impressive was the angiographically-confirmed reversal of clogging of the coronary arteries. All this occurred within just one year of the program. The other group (the control group) that did not follow the program showed continued clogging of their arteries over time.

Dr. Ornish's program also convincingly demonstrated that continued benefit was possible with persistence on the program. Follow-up of the original group showed continued improvement five years later. Forty-eight of the original study participants were evaluated. They had all maintained their weight and their blood cholesterol levels remained 20 percent below their original baseline levels. Reversal of clogging within the coronary arteries continued for as long as they stuck with the program. This stood in marked contrast to those who continued in their old lifestyle habits, whose arteries continued to narrow over the same period.

In a congressional hearing in 1999, Dr. Ornish outlined the importance of his work for the American people. Importantly, he argued that it was never too late to embark on positive lifestyle changes:[69]

> One of the most meaningful findings in our research was that the older patients improved as much as the younger ones. When I began the research, I believed that the younger patients with milder disease would be more likely to show regression, but I was wrong. Instead, the primary determinant of change in their coronary artery disease was neither age nor disease severity but adherence to the recommended changes in diet and lifestyle. No matter how old they were, on average, the more people changed their diet and lifestyle, the more they improved. Indeed, the oldest patient in our study (now 83) showed more reversal than anyone. This is a very hopeful message for Medicare patients, since the risks of bypass surgery and angioplasty increase with age, but the benefits of comprehensive lifestyle changes may occur at any age.

Several other studies have demonstrated achievable benefits when people give nutrition and lifestyle a central place in their quest for optimal health, whatever their stage in life. The sum of these studies will serve as the scientific basis upon which to build a prudent diet. It draws upon the best of global dietary and culinary traditions with proven track records on health. These we will use to construct a logical plan for eating in a cosmopolitan urban environment.

Constructing a Prudent Cosmopolitan Diet

"The Best Diets All Under One Roof"

The Prudent Cosmopolitan Diet embraces the best of the healthiest diets in the world and places them all under one roof. This is a realistic prescription for eating in a modern cosmopolitan society. This simple model addresses the urgent need to halt the growing epidemic of obesity, cardiovascular diseases, type II diabetes, and some forms of cancer.

If you plan to improve your diet and your health, you will obviously not pursue those diets that exhibit high rates of cardiovascular diseases and cancer. Based on these criteria, we can dismiss those aspects of the North American and northern European diets that epitomize the unbalanced Western diet (Chapters 5 and 7). They are not good acts to follow. However, wherever you live, you should use as a nutrition foundation, the best available and affordable assortment of fresh fruits, vegetables, nuts, grains, fish, skinless-boneless poultry that you can muster. These good local choices should serve as your foundation for constructing a Prudent Cosmopolitan Diet (Figure 8-1).

Two important additions to this foundation are needed to construct our nutrition edifice to a higher level. These are the pillars that will bolster our nutrition plan. The first pillar is built from the best of Mediterranean-style diets and the second harnesses the best of Asian-style diets. It would also be naïve to assume that there is one Mediterranean or one Oriental diet. Indeed, there are hundreds of regional and dietary subcultures in China alone, but it is the best of those prevailing healthy choices in these diets, to which we should choose.

Thanks to globalization, access to Asian and Mediterranean foodstuffs is quite easy. Cuisines from around the world are now available where we live and work. As global cultures intermingle, the challenge is to exploit the best of this culinary mosaic and allow these to infiltrate your kitchen and your choices.

The borrowing of ideas and cuisines is as natural as cross-pollination. This is the history of mankind. Keep in mind, however, that the cuisines from many countries, in their drive to cater to Western tastes, have distorted many of their traditional cuisines. Westernized versions of these diets predominate in the fast food outlets common in Western cities. The merger of cultures has worked both ways. One unfortunate result is that many Latino, South Asian, and Oriental migrants to America exhibit higher rates of cardiovascular disease and diabetes than the local American population.[70-72]

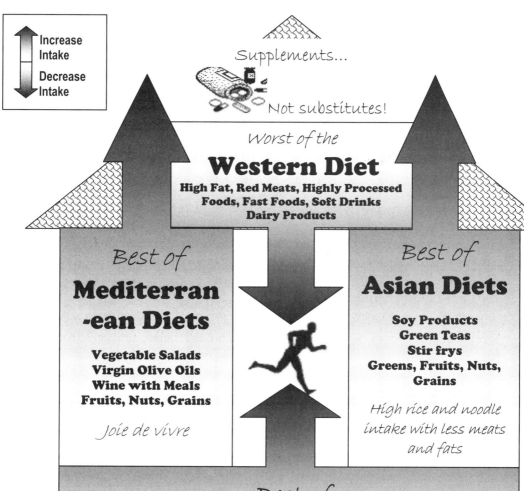

Increase Intake

Decrease Intake

Supplements...

Not substitutes!

Worst of the

Western Diet
**High Fat, Red Meats, Highly Processed
Foods, Fast Foods, Soft Drinks
Dairy Products**

Best of

Mediterran-ean Diets

**Vegetable Salads
Virgin Olive Oils
Wine with Meals
Fruits, Nuts, Grains**

Joie de vivre

Best of

Asian Diets

**Soy Products
Green Teas
Stir frys
Greens, Fruits, Nuts,
Grains**

*High rice and noodle
intake with less meats
and fats*

Best of

American, Regional or Local Diets
**Fruits, Vegetables, Whole Grains, Nuts, Fish-especially fatty
fish, Skinless-Boneless Poultry, & occasional Lean Meats**

Prudent Cosmopolitan Diet

"The Best Diets All Under One Roof"

Your Prudent Cosmopolitan Diet is a simple model of healthy eating that embraces the best of the healthiest diets in the world and places them all under one roof. It serves as a framework on which to build your personal strategy to prevent disease and optimize health.

See Chapter 8, Figure 8-3 and text "Constructing a Prudent Cosmopolitan Diet."

Figure 8-1. A dietary prescription for modern cosmopolitan societies

The Prudent Cosmopolitan Diet

The Prudent Cosmopolitan Diet
takes the best of the West
with the feasts of the East
and arranges a culinary marriage
that ends in harmony under a single roof.

The United States is the quintessential cosmopolitan society. The call is to exploit the best of the healthiest diets within the American mosaic. In much of Western Europe, and most urban cities worldwide, a similar cosmopolitan scenario exists. It is up to individuals within each community to open their doors and their minds to the best of these foods and cuisines. The Oldways Preservation and Exchange Trust, and the Nutrition Department at the Harvard School of Public Health in Boston, have been pioneers and advocates of using the best of traditional dietary practices from cultures around the globe.[73] Let us explore the contributions of these regions in more detail.

The Best of the Mediterranean Dietary Practices

This region is famous for its virgin olive oils, vegetable salads, pitta bread, feta cheese, and wines with meals.
The best of these diets is *the first important pillar* needed to construct the Prudent Cosmopolitan Diet. Mediterranean peoples hasten to add that their diet is as much about attitudes, as it is about food. The French call it the *joie de vivre*—the joy of living.

People in the Mediterranean region, whose per capita incomes are far below those of the United States and northwestern Europe, enjoy better health than their richer neighbors and relatives. The legacy of traditional Mediterranean cuisine has been in its contribution to greatly reduced rates of cardiovascular disease and cancer. There are noteworthy components of these diets that set them high on the pedestal of healthy eating patterns. A summary of the best of these ingredients is listed below and in Figure 8-2:[74-80]

- Extra virgin olive oils are the predominant oils used: These oils are high in monosaturated fats and free of the trans-fats or polyaromatic hydrocarbon (PAH) health alert warnings[81] that can result from the harsher extraction methods used to produce olive pomace oils. Virgin olive oils are produced cheaply in the Mediterranean, but become expensive by the time they reach foreign shores. Spain, Italy, Greece, and Turkey are the biggest producers of olive oils. Virgin olive oils lower artery-clogging LDL cholesterol and protect against heart disease. All olive oils are not the same (Table 8-6). How oil is processed can be as important as the source of the oil itself. Extra virgin olive oils of the "cold-pressed" variety have the best reputation for health. They are the only unrefined oils that are easily available on Western supermarket shelves. They appear green and hazy because of the presence of chlorophyll, plant sterols, vitamin E and other plant materials. Although there is no legal definition of what "cold-pressed" means, it generally refers to using less harsh extraction methods to extract the oil.

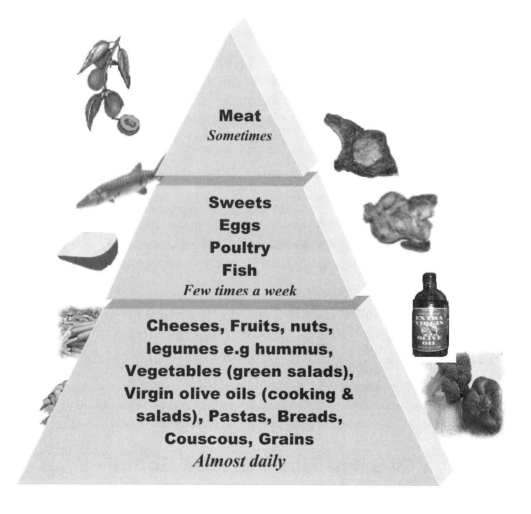

Figure 8-2. Mediterranean-style Diet Pyramid

- Lots of fruits, vegetables, legumes, nuts (pistachio, walnut, hazelnut, and almond), seeds (e.g. sesame and tahini), and grains (pasta, couscous, polenta, and bulgur wheat): These are excellent sources of fiber, vitamins, antioxidants, phytochemicals, and minerals that protect against cardiovascular diseases, obesity, diabetes, and cancer. What is impressive is the way Mediterranean peoples make vegetable salads. Compared to Western practices, a vegetable salad is not a side-show of coleslaw or potato salad soaked in high-fat dressings. Rather a salad comprises a separate dish of a medley of fresh vegetables, generously sprinkled with olive oil or olive oil-based dressings and lemon juice.

- Wine with meals: Although the predominantly Muslim inhabitants of North Africa and Turkey do not traditionally indulge in alcohol, the rest of the region is known for its practice of drinking wines with meals. Polyphenol substances such as resveratrol (an antioxidant) and ellagic acid in wines are known to protect against cardiovascular diseases and cancer. The benefit of wine drinking should be restricted to drinking within a social context, and not in excess. Taking alcoholic beverages on an empty stomach or drinking in excess is accompanied by its own share of gastrointestinal and social side effects (see Chapter 5, "Too Much Alcohol: Weighing Risks and Benefits." Non-fermented grape juices and fresh grapes also impart their share of health benefits.

- Mediterranean cuisine also includes increased consumption of fish and poultry, with fish consumption greatest in historically seafaring nations like Spain, Portugal and Italy. Consumption of red meat, eggs, and processed foods are lower compared to their Northern European and North American counterparts.

There is more to the Mediterranean diet than simply adding olive oil to your food. It includes a healthy dose of Mediterranean attitudes as well. Meals often last hours, and have meaning beyond mere nutrition in this region. Words like *bon appetit* and *joie de vivre* underscore the importance of enjoying food with family and friends on a daily basis, a commodity in short supply in Western urban societies. In today's fast-paced corporate culture, meals are akin to a stop at the gas pump—quickly filling up with much needed food, and then scurrying off to meet deadlines.

All Olive Oils Are Not Created Equal

Olive oils are the premier culinary oils, but marked variations in the composition of these oils can have significant health implications. Even good students of nutrition find the various categories of olive oil, which are regulated by law, quite confusing. Regulation of olive oils is a specialty in itself. A summary of the definitions of consumer olive oils appears in Table 8-6.[82]

Table 8-6. Grades of Consumer Olive Oil

Grades Of Olive Oils

Virgin Olive Oils (Cold pressed or first pressed)	Oils only obtained from the fruit of the olive tree by mechanical or other physical processes, under conditions, especially thermal ones, that do not cause alterations in the oil. These oils must not receive any treatment other than washing, decantation, centrifugation and filtering. This category does not include oils that have been obtained by using solvents, re-esterification processes, or mixtures with oils of different characteristics. **Extra Virgin Olive Oils:** Lowest free acidity (oleic acid) less than 1 gram per 100 grams. **Virgin Olive Oil:** Free acidity is not more than 2 grams per 100 grams. **Ordinary Virgin Olive Oil:** Free acidity is not more than 3.3 grams per 100 grams. **HIGHLY RECOMMENDED**
Lampante Virgin Oils	Sometimes, due to unfavorable climate conditions or deficiencies in the production process, virgin olive oils have a high degree of acidity or a defective flavor, color, or aroma. These oils, called **Lampante Virgin Oils,** must go through a refining process to correct these defects. This process reduces the degree of acidity and eliminates the defective color and aroma. Free acidity is more than 3.3 grams per 100 grams.
Refined Olive Oil	Refined Olive Oil is obtained from the refining process. A certain quantity of **Extra Virgin, Virgin** or **Ordinary Virgin Olive Oil** is then added to the oil to give it aroma and flavor. This is how the category called "Olive Oil" is obtained.
Olive Oil	**Olive oil** that consists of a mixture of refined olive oil and virgin olive oils, not including lampante, whose free acidity cannot be more than 1.5 grams per 100 grams.
Crude Olive Pomace Oil	Olive pomace or orujo is the solid residue or paste left behind after the extraction of higher grades of oil such as Virgin Olive Oil. This residue is treated with solvents to extract the oil as it contains **Crude Olive-Pomace Oil.** Olive oil obtained by refining virgin olive oils, whose free acidity, expressed as oleic acid, cannot be more than 0.5 grams per 100 grams and whose other characteristics are in accordance with those established for the category.
Olive Pomace Oil	As it is not edible, it has to undergo a refining process to obtain **Refined Olive-Pomace Oil.** This oil has no flavor, aroma or color and has to be improved with virgin olive oils. **Olive-Pomace Oil** (orujo or marc, *Spanish*) is the lowest quality and the cheapest of all olive oils sold to the consumer. **NOT RECOMMENDED**

Extra virgin olive oils are the most heart-friendly, but the most expensive variety. Far cheaper varieties like the olive pomace oil can contain significant amounts of trans-fatty acids due to the harsher extraction process (Table 8-6). Unfortunately, the trans-fatty acid content does not appear on food labels. Their listing is not yet required by law. Therefore, if you look at the food label, the composition of extra virgin olive oil and olive pomace oil would appear identical, but they are not the same. Oils with high trans-fats content are the most damaging of all oils (see Chapter 5, Table 5-7). In addition, there were concerns in 2001 that prompted health authorities to withdraw olive pomace oil from the Spanish and European market. This was due to the presence of excessive levels of polycyclic aromatic hydrocarbons (PAHs).[81]

Adopting the best of Mediterranean dietary practices is an important tool for optimizing health and preventing major chronic diseases (Table 8-7). The challenge for some people, is to adapt to the different tastes and flavors of the region, but most Westerners should have no difficulty doing so. Italian, Spanish, French, and Greek cuisines are now established features of the American culinary landscape. A Mediterranean-style diet should serve as a strong pillar in building your Prudent Cosmopolitan Diet (Figure 8-1).

Table 8-7. Summary of Health Benefits of the Mediterranean Diet

Summary of Health Benefits of the Mediterranean-style Diet

- Extends life expectancy
- Protects against cardiovascular diseases
- Protects against cancer
- Protects against type II diabetes
- Protects against obesity

The Best of the Far East (Asian) Dietary Practices

The Far East region, specifically Japan, China, the Koreas, Taiwan, and Indo-China are societies that have traditionally exhibited low rates of obesity, cancer, and coronary heart disease.
Despite recent shifts towards Westernization, the best cuisines of the region constitute *the second important pillar* in the construction of a Prudent Cosmopolitan Diet (Figure 8-1).

When most people think of "Chinese," one of the first things that comes to mind is food. Chinatowns in major Western cities highlight the important role foods play in varied culinary traditions and festivals of Asia. In the midst of this food-happy culture, it is quite striking that Asians as a group are far slimmer than their American counterparts. Asian societies are characterized historically by low rates of obesity, heart attack, and cancer, despite recent shifts in the opposite direction. The best of their cuisines serve as the second important pillar in the construction of your Prudent Cosmopolitan Diet (Figure 8-1).[46,73,83-95]

More than half the world's six billion people live in Asia, with almost 1.5 billion in mainland China alone. Various theories have been advanced as to the reasons for this, including the roles of Asian diets. What is clear, however, is that Western dietary patterns, with heavy emphasis on meat and diary products, would be impossible to sustain in Asia. An acre of farmland produces six times more energy if cereals are grown instead of grazing cows. The population pressures in this part of the world could only be sustained by dietary practices that emphasize plant-based food sources like legumes, rice, and wheat.

The Far East has evolved a rather peculiar blend of dietary practices, a legacy of thousands of years of tradition. These practices range from their use of chopsticks and metallic cleavers (used for more than just cutting), to the tradition of stir-frying foods in a large wok. Oriental concepts of health and disease, including the yin and yang philosophy, dazzle the average Western mind. The emphasis of Chinese medical tradition is to maintain good health compared to the Western emphasis on treating diseases. Western thoughts on disability and disease in old age tend to be seen in a different light than in much of Asia. Eastern traditions pay more homage to their elderly than in the West, and their attitudes towards old age do not merge with the retirement philosophies that are so prevalent in the West.

The Asian region, however, is far from being a homogeneous monolithic culture. In China alone, the world's most populous nation, the variety of cuisines is nothing short of legendary. Japanese cuisine features more raw foods than Chinese cuisine, and Thai food incorporates the use of coconut milk, curries, and the ever-present rice. These cultures are largely united by their love for rice, legumes and noodles. Northern Asians tend to consume more wheat than rice. Nevertheless, there are prevailing culinary practices that promote excellent health.

An important advice before adopting the best of Asian styled diets is that there is healthy as well as unhealthy Asian food. Asian restaurants across America and Western societies, whether they are Chinese, Japanese, Thai, or Vietnamese, generally cater to Western tastes. They serve larger portion sizes, especially meat, compared to what is served traditionally. The best of Asian diets exhibit healthy features listed below:[46]

- High premium on grains (rice and noodles)
- Far less meat: meat is not the centerpiece of the meal. Vegetables, rice, and noodles (from wheat, rice, and legumes) predominate
- Lots of vegetables incorporated into meals
- High intake of soy bean and whole soy foods
- Far less milk and dairy product consumption
- Unsweetened teas, especially green (non-oxidized) teas no milk or sugar
- Fish and seafood are very popular, especially in Japan
- Generous use of condiments, herbs, and spices, including garlic, onions, and ginger
- Less use of processed foods

- Sweet pastry not historically popular
- Stir-fry's: uses less oil and cooks quickly with less nutrient losses

Soy: A Great Oriental Contribution

Perhaps the most headline-grabbing Asian contribution to good health has been the observation that Asian women living in Asia exhibit far lower rates of breast cancer than women in the West. Although low breast cancer rates are also found in populations that do not consume soy products, soy foods are associated with lower rates of other cancers as well (e.g. prostate, stomach, colorectal, lung, and the endometrium) (see Table 8-1). Phytoestrogens, the soybean component that shows good anti-cancer potential) are not confined to soybean products. They are also plentiful in other legumes, flaxseed, eggplant, and sweet potatoes.[46]

The cholesterol-lowering effects of soy products have been confirmed by several studies. Soy protein intake (averaging 50 grams daily) can lower blood cholesterol levels by 10 to 13 percent. Soy consumption is linked to lower rates of prostate cancer and less hot flashes following menopause.[96-99] The United States is the world's largest producer of soybeans with half the world's production, but ost of the soybeans are for animal feed and oil production. Americans consume only about 3 grams of soy foods daily compared to about 20 to 80 grams in the average Asian diet (Table 8-8). Soy foods are a great addition to the diet, and is a highly recommended ingredient for your Prudent Cosmopolitan diet:[100]

> It is prudent for health-conscious persons to include soy protein as part of their dietary selections throughout the week. Soy protein is a complete protein, with clear advantages for those who would like to reduce their intake of animal-based foods or those with elevated serum cholesterol... Although it is not possible to suggest specific levels of soy product consumption, soy can be an important part of a balanced dietary approach to health.

As soy foods become more popular in the West, the emphasis should be increased consumption of whole soy foods (Table 8-8) rather than soy supplements. There is no shortage of soy supplements that laud the great benefits of individual soy ingredients. The evidence is in favor of consuming whole soy foods, and not simply isoflavones or protease inhibitors (Table 8-1):[102]

> There is also strong epidemiological evidence for the reduced incidence of several cancers in high soy-consuming populations. Because these populations ingest mostly foods derived from whole soybeans, and because the precise benefits of individual soy constituents have not yet been determined in humans, the authors suggest consumption of soy products that retain as much of the components of whole soy as practical.

The average Westerner may have some initial difficulties adjusting to the tastes, but there are now a wide variety of soy products—milks, burgers, sausages, meats, and ice-cream—that now cater to Western tastes, in addition to the varieties listed in Table 8-8). A better option is to visit a nearby Chinatown or learn from your Asian friends and colleagues. They can provide great insights into the traditional Asian way of preparing and consuming these foods. They may do so better than any cookbook can.

Table 8-8 Varieties of Soy Foods

Non-Fermented Soy Foods	Fermented Soy Foods
Green Soybeans (fresh)	Soy Sauce (high in salt)
Soybeans (dried)	Tempeh
Bean Sprouts	Fermented Tofu
Soy Milk (regular & flavored)	Fermented Soy Milk
Dried Bean Curd (tofu)	Miso
Soft Bean Curd (tofu)	Natto
Skimmed Bean Curd (skin of tofu)	
Soyflour, Okara, Yuba	
Soy and Isoflavone Dietary Supplements	

Milk Consumption in the Far East

A sharp distinction exists between traditional Oriental attitudes towards milk consumption compared to those in the West. In the traditional Oriental diet, there is a conspicuous absence of milk and dairy products from their traditional diets. Instead of the Western practice of milk-based beverages for breakfast, Asians traditionally drink unsweetened teas without any added milk. Rice and soy-based beverages predominate.

Lower rates of osteoporosis in the Orient dispel the popular Western belief that milk and dairy consumption are crucial to prevent osteoporosis. Contrary to what Westerners would expect, osteoporosis rates and hip fractures are actually markedly lower in those parts of the world where people consume very little meat and dairy products. The highest rates of osteoporosis are found in Western countries that have embraced higher intakes of milk, dairy products, and meat (see Chapter 5 "Milk and Dairy Products").[101,102]

Orientals and Greens

Among the world's cultures and cuisines, few do a better job of incorporating green leafy vegetables as a daily part of the diets, than do Asian cultures. Asians have a "culture of greens." Westerners, by comparison, eat very little green leafy vegetables, and when they do, they tend to overcook them or combine them with unhealthy salad dressings. These practices may improve palatability, but destroy vitamins like folate, and introduce excess calories and undesirable oils. The Western practice of using high-fat mayonnaise and dairy products on green salads is not recommended.

Dark greens can be easily prepared using a little sprinkling of extra virgin olive oil, garlic, a pinch of salt and light frying for a minute or two in a wok. This causes vegetables to remain crunchy and tasty, not overcooked and mushy. Alternatively, generous servings of greens can be chopped up and added to stir-fried fish or chicken. This will add the familiar flavor of your preferred protein sources, and increase the palatability of greens. For those who need to lose weight, adding plenty of greens to your regular meal is a healthy alternative that provides bulk and maintains satiety while simultaneously lowering total calorie intake.

Is Rice Fattening?

Questions have arisen about the wisdom of following the Asian dietary pattern of rice intake. All rice is not the same, and rice preparation methods differ immensely across the globe. Texas long grain rice is different in composition from Basmati rice from India. Starchy rice with high content of amylose (25 to 30 percent) is harder and fluffier to the taste and packs proportionately more calories; the rice grains remain largely separate after cooking. This variety is popular in South Asia (India, Pakistan and Bangladesh). The sticky rice popularly consumed in East Asia (China, Korea, Japan and Taiwan) is lower in starch (10 to 18 percent) content and less fattening. [103,104]

Asian methods of cooking rice traditionally use lots of water that is subsequently thrown off. Western methods usually cook rice with added oils, butter, and added seasonings. Many then consume this already fat-laden rice along with meat and high-fat gravies. Such methods of preparing rice can make a big difference in energy intake, especially if it is a daily practice and accompanied by sedentary lifestyles.

Therefore, the fattening potential of rice should be seen within the context of the methods of preparation, in addition to the prevailing lifestyle changes. Based on observations, it is reasonable to conclude that the types of rice consumed, and the preparation methods used in Asia, have not historically led to the fattening of China and the Far East.

Green Teas

Asian green tea and its role in reducing the risk of cancer and diabetes, has generated much interest in the scientific community (see "Asian Diet Studies" earlier in this Chapter). [58-61] Commercial teas fall into three major groups. Black or oxidized teas are the most popular in the West; oolong or partially oxidized teas, and green or non-oxidized teas are gaining in popularity. Asian green teas are packed with flavonoids and polyphenols—substances with powerful antioxidant properties. Green tea consumption has been linked to lower risk of cancers of the esophagus, stomach, and liver. The greatest anti-cancer activity has been shown with green teas, but there is experimental evidence to show that other types of teas can also benefit, though to lesser degrees. The message is this: Enjoy your tea, whether it is black or whether it is green. Refrain from adding sugar and milk, especially if you are a frequent tea drinker. A recent finding by Tuft's University researchers in Boston, gave credence to a possible role of green tea in lowering blood sugar in people with diabetes.[105] Studies are now underway to investigate previous findings of marked reductions in blood sugar (up to 20 percent) in diabetic hamsters that had the privilege of consuming green tea.

Table 8-9. Summary of Health Benefits of Asian Diets

**Summary of Health Benefits
of the Asian Diets and Lifestyle**

- Extends life expectancy
- Protects against cardiovascular diseases
- Protects against cancer (breast, prostate)
- Protects against obesity and type II diabetes
- Protects against osteoporosis
- Protects against post-menopausal symptoms

In summary, the best of Asian diets offer their important share of health benefits (Table 8-9). Even though aspects of Asian foods, cuisines, and preparation methods may initially appear quite foreign, the huge array of choices from this region provides plenty room for individuals to choose according to your tastes and preferences. Asian diets are the second important pillar you need to construct your Prudent Cosmopolitan Diet.

Africa, Fiber, and Whole Grains

Africa does not get much positive mention in nutrition circles, but this continent has provided the basis for some of the earliest research and recommendations about the importance of fiber in the diet—"Eat your roughage!" Dietary fiber, or roughage, is that indigestible part of plant foods that serves as packaging for nutrients. They are plentiful in many fruits and vegetables. By providing bulk to food, fiber provides bulk and satiety, and speeds up the transit time of food passing through the intestines. I was informed by a Sudanese colleague that many of his surgeon friends in Africa have never removed an appendix—one of the commonest operations in the Western world. The major reason for this is that appendicitis is rare among people who ate a lot of fiber.

Sub-Saharan Africans consume a staple of sorghum and millet cereals along with starchy roots and tubers. These are traditionally prepared and consumed as porridges of varying consistencies, along with local sauces. Pioneer research by Dr. Dennis

Burkitt and Dr. Hugh Trowell, both surgeons working in Africa in the 1940s, revealed that black Africans exhibited markedly lower rates of non-diarrheal gastrointestinal and cardiovascular diseases compared to European whites and the African diaspora:[106,107]

> In particular they rarely encountered the diseases known as the 'diseases of civilization', a group of 17 that included constipation, appendicitis, diverticular disease, hemorrhoids, colorectal cancer, coronary heart disease and gallstones. Trowell, observing that all the relatively common non-infectious diseases were rare in sub-Saharan blacks, speculated that the protective factor might be the soft and bulky nature of their stools, which were passed easily and frequently, which were the consequence of their high-fiber diet. Subsequently it has been shown that lack of dietary fiber is a major factor which could be involved in several gastrointestinal diseases. A highly refined diet results in hard, dry stools that pass sluggishly through the intestine and require a large increase in luminal pressure for their evacuation.

Dietary fiber falls into two main categories. Insoluble fiber is found in wheat bran, citrus, carrots, cabbage, and leafy vegetables and soluble fiber as found in oats, oat bran, beans, prunes, and fruits. Dietary fiber is called non-starch polysaccharide (NSP) in Europe, referring to the fact that fiber is a carbohydrate like starch, except that it is indigestible in humans. Herbivores or ruminants are equipped with a special rumen, staffed by bacteria that digest these NSP fibers in grass and hay. Chewing the cud is part of this complex digestive mechanism that extracts energy from these otherwise indigestible materials.

Glycemic Index—Glycemic Load

Far from merely providing bulk, fiber also serves as good packaging for nutrients and sugars, thereby preventing them from being released too rapidly from food. This leads to a slower and a more sustained entry of sugars into the bloodstream, compared to the rapid entry of sugars into the bloodstream following drinking a soft drink or eating sugary foods.

A gentler entry of sugar from the intestines into the blood leads to a more modest rise in insulin levels. This is why processing that eliminates fiber from grains can have such a negative impact on health. The differences in the glycemic index and the glycemic load of refined and unrefined grains are the result of processing. Removal of the outer bran of whole grains, as occurs during the milling process, leads to more rapid digestion and absorption of its contents into the bloodstream.[108,109]

Glycemic index describes the rate at which foods increase sugar (glucose) levels in the blood. University of Toronto researchers first used the glycemic index as a measure of how quickly different foods elevated blood glucose. High glycemic index foods were compared to white bread, which was assigned a high score of 100. High glycemic index foods lead to more rapid surges in blood sugar levels following consumption. They are generally represented by refined, high carbohydrate foods. Low glycemic index foods are those with a value below 60. They result in a more gradual and sustained rise in blood sugar levels. High-fiber and minimally processed foods represent this group.

The glycemic index of a food cannot accurately predict the extent to which food can elevate blood sugar. The reason is that fat and fiber content that of a particular food, affect the rate and the extent to which they raise blood sugar levels. The glycemic load (the glycemic index multiplied by the actual carbohydrate content) is the measure preferred by nutritionists. It is a better predictor of the glycemic effect of foods. Low glycemic index/low glycemic load foods are generally healthier choices.

Table 8-10. Glycemic Index and Glycemic Load of Common Foods

Lower Glycemic Index /Glycemic Load Foods	Higher Glycemic Index /Glycemic Load Foods
Whole unrefined grains (e.g. bran, and oatmeal)	White bread
Vegetables (non-starchy)	Table sugar
Lentils	Mashed potatoes
Nuts (e.g. peanuts)	French fries
Apples and pears	Candy
Dairy products	White rice
Many fruits are in the mid-range	Cornflakes
	Refined sugary cereals and grains
	Soft drinks and flavored drinks
	Reconstituted juices
	Pancakes

The consumption of whole grains plummeted in the Western diet with the rise of the food industry. Whole grain products were considered less sophisticated, too chewy, and took longer to prepare. They have made a comeback, but has generated some confusion (see Chapter 7 "Deciphering Labelese").

Whole grain confer good health benefits. In the Nurses' Health Study, women who ate more cereal fiber (whole wheat bread, cold breakfast cereals, oatmeal, and wild rice) lowered their LDL-cholesterol levels, and were one-third less likely to develop heart disease compared than those who ate less fiber.[64] Fewer deaths from heart disease has been a consistent observation in studies that compared dietary fiber intake and the risk of heart disease. Overweight women who ate more refined grains (white rice and white bread) were twice as likely to develop heart disease. An increased intake of dietary fiber protects against a variety of other diseases (Table 8-

7).[48-51,110,111] Increased fiber and whole grains in the diet is another important addition to your Prudent Cosmopolitan Diet.

Table 8-11. Whole Grains and their Health Benefits

Whole Grains	Summary of Health Benefits of Regular Whole Grain Consumption
Whole wheat products Wheat bran, wheat berries Barley Rye Brown / parboiled rice Wild rice Corn-on-the-cob Corn tortillas (traditional) Flaxseed Oat bran, oatmeal, whole oat kernel, steel-cut oats Bulgur wheat Couscous pasta Buckwheat Millet, quinoa, spelt	• Protect against cancer • Protect against heart disease • Protect against type II diabetes • Protect against gallstones • Lower cholesterol • Less bowel disorders including constipation, hemorrhoids, diverticular disease, and appendicitis

Health Aspects of Some Fruits and Vegetables

Grapes, Tomatoes, Eggplant, Avocados, and Peppers

Grapes are interesting, not just for their popularity as a fruit, but also for wines and raisins that are made from them. The health benefits of their polyphenolic ingredients like resveratrol include anti-cancer and anti-inflammatory effects that are mediated by an effect called cox-2-inhibtion.[112-117]

Tomatoes and most fruits contain plenty of potassium, minerals and vitamins including vitamin C (raw tomato). Tomatoes are also the major dietary sources of lycopene. Lycopene is a pigment with antioxidant properties more powerful than beta-carotene, and its consumption has been linked to reduced risks of prostate and digestive tract cancers. Lycopene is not readily available from fresh uncooked tomatoes, but is freed up after cooking. Therefore it is a good practice is to cook tomatoes in olive oil which increases the availability and absorption of lycopene. Although vitamin C is destroyed by cooking, your best option is to obtain this from other sources.[118]

Colored fruits contain powerful colored pigments known as carotenoids and flavonoids. Vitamin A and its pre-cursor beta-carotene, along with vitamin E, and vitamin K, are oil-soluble vitamins found in many plant sources. They all need fat in the diet for their absorption.[124] The eggplant (known variously as bygan, batinjeem, melongin) gets its description from its egg-like texture when cooked. Elongated tubular varieties are popular in the Far East. The pear-shaped purple variety is a close relative of the tomato. It is also a good source of plant estrogens (phytoestrogens) that may protect against breast and prostate cancer. Avocados, rich in the healthy monosaturated fats, are excellent in salads, and add smoothness and texture (See chapter 5). Guacamole, a seasoned avocado spread has become popular in the United States.

Peppers come in a wide array of sizes, shapes, textures, and colors. They impart flavor and excitement to food. They are rich sources of minerals and vitamins including vitamin C and the vitamin B group. Colored varieties are packed with carotenoids. Hot varieties such as bird peppers, habaneros, and jalapeños abound in Latin America, the Caribbean, sub-Saharan Africa and the Far East. Their hot flavor is due to the presence of capsaicin. They are potent appetizers.

Citrus Fruits

Citrus fruits (oranges, grapefruit, limes, tangerines, mangarines, etc.) are the most popular fruit juices. Citrus pulp provides extra fiber and satiety. Fresh citrus juices provide plenty of vitamin C, flavonoids, beta-carotene, and minerals including plenty of potassium. Citrus oils are the best source of a group of substances called terpenes (Table 8-2). One of them is called d-limonene, a monoterpene. Scientists have been impressed by its ability to cause regression (shrinkage) of all kinds of tumors, including breast, prostate, skin, and lung . D-limonene is also found in oils from caraway, cardamom, coriander, mint, and thyme.[12,13,18] To increase your intake of d-limonene, it is best to squeeze oranges using an old-fashioned mechanical presser. This expresses some of the citrus oils from the rind into your juice, giving it a characteristic taste. Some people love it, and some cannot tolerate it. Orange peels and rinds are popular in cooking and baking. These can serve as a source of d-limonene.

Citrus fruits are also among the best sources of powerful antioxidant substances called flavonoids, sometimes referred to as citrus bioflavonoids. Flavonoids show more potent anti-cancer and cardioprotective benefits than their more famous antioxidant relatives like vitamins C, E, and beta-carotene. Tangeretin and nobiletin, both flavonoids, have stimulated great interest for their anticancer effects. Tangeritin exerts its anticancer effects on human breast tissue in ways similar to the breast cancer drug tamoxifen, but there are concerns that tangeritin can interfere with the action of tamoxifen when both are used together. This effect clearly needs to be investigated further, but it does not mean stopping citrus if you are on tamoxifen.

The benefits of consuming citrus outweigh this potential negative effect.[125] You should consult with a knowledgeable physician, if this is an area of personal concern.

Grapefruit juice has generated serious concern over its ability to interfere with the metabolism of many drugs. Furanocoumarins present in grapefruit juice can interfere with alprazolam (Xanax), and atorvastatin (Lipitor). If you are on blood pressure medicines, cholesterol lowering medicines, or tranquilizers, it is best to avoid grapefruit until the matter is further clarified. The Nurse's Health Study also indicated that grapefruit juice consumption was linked to a marginal increase in kidney stones.[126,127] This is no reason to avoid grapefruit altogether, but if kidney stones are your problem, it is prudent to limit grapefruit intake.

A Wonderful Excuse for a Fruit Dessert

University of Maryland researchers published an interesting study in 1997 that showed pre-treatment with antioxidants—vitamins C (1000 mg) and vitamin E (800 I.U.)—abolished the negative effects of a high-fat meal (see Chapter 6, "Free Radicals and the Cardiovascular System: Blood Vessel and Cholesterol Effects").[128] Fresh fruits and vegetables are rich in antioxidants that can counteract free-radicals generated by high fat diets on blood vessels.

Fruit and nut desserts are therefore healthier alternatives with the potential ability to block the harmful effects of fatty meals. The popular custom of fat-laden desserts should be replaced by exuberant fruit salads. Chilled papaya, cantaloupes, and watermelons are easily prepared and make excellent post-meal desserts.

Spinach, Broccoli and Dark Leafy Greens e.g. Collard, Kale, Chard

Green salads deliver a host of vitamins, minerals, and antioxidants. Spinach and other dark leafy greens contain phytochemicals and vitamins like folate (folic acid), which can lower blood levels of homocysteine. Homocysteine is a known risk factor for cardiovascular disease and blood clots. Lutein and zeaxanthin, both components of green plants, show promise in preventing age-related macular degeneration (AMD), an age related condition that often leads to blindness.[129,130]

Greens serve as the best natural sources of dietary magnesium, a mineral that is important in maintaining blood pressure and cardiovascular health. Magnesium is found in every green plant. It is a central ingredient in chlorophyll, the pigment that gives plants their green color. Studies consistently show a drop in blood pressure in people who consume more magnesium. The chemical of form magnesium in the food or drink is important. Magnesium causes diarrhea if taken as magnesium sulfate (Epsom salts) or milk of magnesia because magnesium in these compounds is poorly absorbed and remains in high concentrations in the gut, leading to osmotic diarrhea. When magnesium is in the chelated form found in greens, it is well absorbed. It causes no diarrhea, and contributes to lowering of blood pressure. People with diabetes can benefit with better blood sugar control and reduced insulin requirements after supplementation with magnesium.[131]

Broccoli, especially its sprouts, is rich in indole-3-carbinol and sulphoraphane—phytochemicals with potent cancer-fighting activity. Increased consumption of broccoli is linked to a lowered risk of cancers of the breast, colon, and stomach. Fresh broccoli is a very rich source of vitamin C.[132]

Blueberries, Blackberries, Strawberries, Raspberries, Cranberries, Gooseberries

A USDA report (2000) on the health benefits of forty different fruits and vegetables showed that blueberries had the highest antioxidant activity. Blackberries, strawberries, raspberries, cranberries, and gooseberries followed closely behind. Anthocyanins, the pigment responsible for the intense blue color of these other berries, belongs to the diverse group of substances called flavonoids.[133-135]

These have shown promise in retarding the effects of aging in animal experiments, especially in motor functions and cognitive abilities. Cranberry juice is known for its antibacterial efficacy in fighting urinary tract infections.

Garlic, Onions, Leeks, Chives & Allium Family

Garlic, onions, and company evoke polarized global responses. In the minds of many Westerners, garlic or onion breath is socially undesirable. Garlic is loved in Eastern cultures. Mediterranean and Asian peoples consume garlic or onion in one form or another almost everyday.

Garlic (*Allium sativum*) is packed with organo-sulfur compounds called allyl sulfides (thiosulfinates, dithins, and ajoenes). These comprise about one percent of the dry weight of garlic. The most popular of these is called allicin. It is released when garlic is crushed and gives garlic its characteristic odor. Westerners have tried to eliminate the smell by manufacturing odorless garlic. Odorless garlic may be less effective than fresh unaltered garlic.

There is compelling evidence that garlic and its sulfur ingredients suppress the incidence of the breast, colon, esophageal, and lung cancers. Garlic suppresses the formation of (cancer-causing) nitrosamines from sodium nitrite preservatives in foods. A Chinese study concluded that consuming of 5 grams of garlic daily completely prevented the formation of these harmful nitrosamines. Evidence also supports garlic's ability to lower blood cholesterol, with one study showing cholesterol reduction by as much as 15 percent. Garlic also possesses anti-inflammatory and anti-infective properties. The organo-sulfur compounds in garlic can protect cellular DNA from attack and prevent the growth of abnormal cancer cells.[136, 137]

Soft Drinks, Reconstituted Juices, Water

Throughout much of the world, soft drinks and sodas are the most widely consumed beverage after water. An average can of soft drink delivers an extra 150 calories. Many have switched to fruit juices as healthier alternatives, but the overwhelming bulk of juices sold in shops and supermarkets are reconstituted from fruit concentrate, and are just as fattening.

It is best to consume freshly-squeezed juices (from fresh fruits). It is even better to consume whole fruits over juices, as this provides more bulk and fiber in addition to less calories overall. It is easy to overlook the additional calories that arise from drinking freshly squeezed juices. Juices from concentrate dominate the market and are less expensive. Fruit juices are converted to concentrate for logistical reasons; it makes it easier to store and transport. Vitamins and minerals are lost during processing, with losses dependent on the type of processing and storage methods employed. When juices are reconstituted from concentrate, water alone and in some cases, vitamins or minerals are added. Vitamin C losses can be significant with storage, heat, and pasteurization. Another health concern of consuming certain fruit juices is the addition of large quantities of sodium (see Chapter 7, "Processing and the Nutritional Value of Foods").

Soft drinks, juices, and fermented drinks are now such fixtures with meals that water, arguably the perfect beverage, has been largely forgotten. Water packs zero calories, but must compete with diet drinks for the low-calorie market. Tap water, despite its chlorinated taste, is not less healthy than bottled water. Enjoy water. Drink lots of it, and you will not have to worry about extra calories, or the potential side-effects of artificial sweeteners like saccharin and aspartame.

Summarizing a Prudent Cosmopolitan Diet

Lifestyles changes— smoking cessation, a Prudent Cosmopolitan Diet, and increased physical activity— are effective in the prevention and control of a wide range of nutrition and lifestyle related diseases: obesity, cardiovascular diseases, type II diabetes and several forms of cancer.

The Prudent Cosmopolitan Diet is a simple model of healthy eating that embraces the best of the healthiest diets in the world and places them all under one roof. This is a logical prescription for eating in a modern cosmopolitan society. (Figure 8-1 and Figure 8-3). It serves as a framework upon which to build your personal strategy to prevent disease and optimize health:

- The **foundation** is the *best of American or local foods* (Chapter 8). The upward direction of the arrow symbolizes the need to increase the intake of these foods.

- The **first pillar** is a *Mediterranean-style diet* (Chapter 8).The upward direction of the arrow ("chimney") recommends increased intake of these cuisines.

- The **second pillar** is an *Asian-style diet* (Chapter 5 and Chapter 8). The upward direction of this arrow ("chimney") recommends increased intake of these foods.

- The **ceiling** with the downward-pointing arrow ("chandelier") represents the advice to consume less of all foods that comprise *the Western diet* (Chapter 5 and Chapter 7).

- Hidden somewhere in the **attic** is a bottle of dietary supplements with the label marked "*Supplements ... not substitutes.*" These can play a role, but they are never substitutes for a healthy nutrition and lifestyle (Chapter 2, Chapter 6, and Chapter 8).

Good Choices in Nutrition and Lifestyle (Figure 8-3) summarizes the "big picture:" Your Prudent Cosmopolitan Diet, smoking cessation, and increased physical activity are the 3 key players to prevent and control a broad range of nutrition and lifestyle-related diseases: obesity, cardiovascular diseases, type II diabetes and several forms of cancer.

Just as smoking, unbalanced nutrition, and physical inactivity have gave rise to a spectrum of chronic diseases, so can the reverse of these behaviors be the major tools needed to halt them. Different diets are not needed to prevent high blood pressure as compared to heart disease. There really should not even be a special diabetic diet per se; neither should there be a special diet for obesity. If you follow a healthy diet, you can expect "multiple beneficial side-effects" These include a reduction in a wide range of risk factors and diseases listed in Figure 8-3.

The challenge is to lay hold of this nutrition plan and build upon it, according to your own tastes and preferences. Tailor it to suit your needs. Let it serve as the central core of a personal nutrition and lifestyle strategy for optimal health, which is the central purpose of this book.

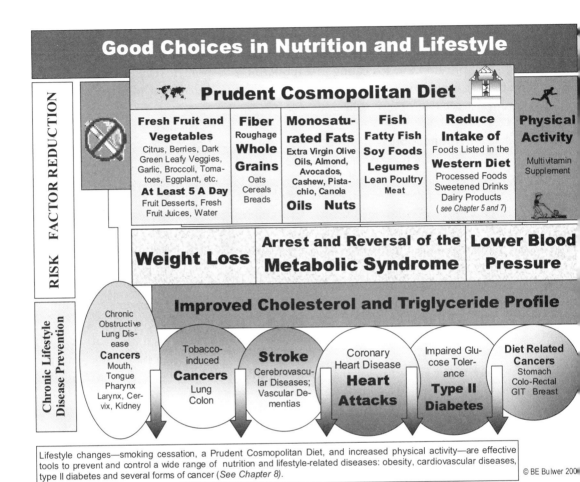

Figure 8-3. Summarizing the Big Picture: The Best Diets and Healthy Lifestyles for prevention and management of the major killers of modern mankind

Notes on Obesity—A Growing Epidemic

Excess body weight (overweight and obesity) lies at the hub of major health problems

The global epidemic of obesity has been fueled by profound changes in the way modern societies work, eat, and live. Consumption of high fat, energy dense foods coupled with marked reductions in physical activity are chiefly responsible.

Obesity needs to be singled out for special attention. It is the fastest growing cause of preventable death in America and is projected to soon overtake smoking as the number one cause of preventable death. An alarming report by experts of the International Obesity Task Force (IOTF) (www.iotf.org) showed that as many as 1.7 billion people around the world do suffer from some form of overweight and obesity. This figure is far higher than the previously reported figure of 300 million. Experts attribute this massive leap in the numbers as the result of stricter standards of measuring overweight and obesity. Evidence now points to a higher risk of chronic disease at levels of overweight previously thought to be medically insignificant. These are now known to be triggers for the metabolic syndrome and increased risk of premature death from many diseases (Table 8-12). Obesity lies at the core of several major chronic diseases. Obese people are more likely to die young and suffer more health problems than individuals of normal weight[138-140]

Table 8-12. Diseases linked to Overweight and Obesity

Diseases linked to Overweight and Obesity

- Metabolic (insulin resistance) syndrome
- Impaired glucose tolerance
- Type II diabetes
- Hypertension
- Dyslipidemia (abnormal cholesterol and triglycerides)
- Coronary heart disease
- Cancer, including breast and uterus
- Obstructive sleep apnea
- Gallstones
- Gout
- Osteoarthritis

Obesity and Quality of Life Issues

The costs of obesity should not just be measured in terms of medical complications, or medical care costs, but also in terms of the day-to-day quality of life and other handicaps. Harvard investigators using data from Nurse's Health Study noted that overweight and obesity exerted a negative impact on people's quality of life (Table 8-13).[64] Many of these are the predictable result of carrying excess weight. The musculoskeletal system bears the brunt of this strain. Although osteoarthritis and musculoskeletal problems are not covered in this book, they are among the commonest day-to-day complaints associated with excessive body weight.

Table 8-13. Overweight and Quality of Life

Lower Quality of Life among Overweight and Obese Individuals

1. More problems doing daily chores
2. Handicap proportional to the degree of obesity
3. More pain and disability
4. Less energetic compared to normal-weight individuals
5. Increased risk of musculo-skeletal injuries

Obesity and the Medical Handicaps

Medical caregivers may discriminate against obese patients in subtle and not so subtle ways. Nurses and paramedical personnel do not welcome the thought of lifting obese bedridden patients. There is increased risk of personal injury when lifting heavy patients. This can easily occur, especially if lifting aids are not readily available. Phlebotomy technicians often experience difficulty when withdrawing blood samples or setting up intravenous lines. Larger blood pressure cuffs are needed for more accurate measurements in obese patients. Inflating these cuffs can be hard work, especially if the customary two to three readings are taken. These can be unwelcome challenges, especially in a busy medical practice.

Certain physical signs of disease are easier to miss in obese patients, simply because of excess adipose tissue. Physical signs during examination of the abdomen and chest are more difficult to elicit and can be a tedious exercise. Obese patients are subject to frequent postponement of surgical procedures. Most surgeons advise significant weight loss in order to minimize intra-operative and post-operative risks. The risk of respiratory complications and deep vein thrombosis (blood clots) are increased following surgery in obese patients.[141,142]

Overweight, Obesity, Central Obesity, Visceral Obesity

The terms *"overweight" and "obesity"* to refer to measures of excess body weight in this section is deliberate. Such distinctions help to underscore that overweight, and not just its exaggerated form (obesity) has significant cardiovascular implications.[143]

What do we mean when we refer to someone as overweight or obese? Standardized *weight-for-height charts* have been used for decades by insurance companies. They use these charts to assess risk and establish life insurance premiums. Weight-for-height measures are easy to use, but must be interpreted with caution because of sex and ethnic differences. Using this simple standard, persons with more than 20 percent of ideal body weight for height are considered to be obese.[144]

The Quetelet's *body mass index* or BMI—the calculated weight in kilograms divided by the square of the height in meters [(weight(kg)/(height(m)^2)]—has gained widespread acceptance because it helps researchers to standardize and make easier comparisons across studies. Using this standard, individuals are placed in the categories that appear in Table 14.[145]

$$\text{BMI} = \frac{\textbf{Weight (kg)}}{\textbf{Height (m}^2)}$$	$$\text{BMI} = \frac{\textbf{Weight (pounds)}}{\textbf{Height (inches)}} \times 703$$

Table 8-14. **Degrees of Excess Body Weight and Body Mass Index (BMI)**

Classification of Excess Body Weight	Body Mass Index Kg/m^2
Normal	18.5 - <25
Overweight	≥25 - <30
Obesity (Class I)	≥30 - <35
Obesity (Class II)	≥35 - <40
Obesity (Class III)	≥40

Waist-Hip Ratio (WHR)

Waist circumference is the circumference of the waist (that region below the rib cage and above the buttock region at its *narrowest point*). Hip circumference is taken as the *largest circumference* around the buttock region. Calculate the ratio between the two (waist circumference divided by the hip circumference) The recommended waist hip ratio for women is below 0.95 and for men it is 0.85.[146]

Body fat distribution patterns influence the risk of developing disease. Two individuals can be of the same weight for height, or the same BMI, yet can exhibit different risks for developing cardiovascular disease. Overweight or obese individuals who exhibit a predominantly central (abdominal/visceral) pattern of obesity are at greater risk for the development of the metabolic syndrome, compared to similar individuals who carry a greater proportion of their body fat around their hip, and thighs. The former is sometimes called apple-shaped or upper-body/android obesity, and the latter as pear-shaped or gynecoid obesity.[147,148]

In recognition of the differential risks posed by the distribution of excess body fat, other measures such as the *waist-hip ratio* (WHR) or *abdominal circumference* have been adopted by many researchers in an attempt to categorize the differing degrees of risk.[146,149]

Other methods have been used to measure obesity in different settings. They include skinfold measurements, densitometry studies, bioelectrical impedance, deuterium dilution, and x-ray absorption methods. Skin fold measurements are widely used, but the other methods are confined primarily to studies done in research centers.

Each method of assessing excess body weight is subject to limitations that affect the validity and the precision of the measurements used. Such limitations can be minimized by using these methods in combination, thereby exploiting the strengths and advantages of each method.[150-154]

Successfully Tackling Obesity: Perspectives and Principles

Lifestyle Problems Need Lifestyle Solutions:

The reasons for the obesity epidemic are obvious: People's genes have not changed; their environments and their lifestyles have. People are consuming excess calories and expending too little energy. Lifestyle problems need lifestyle solutions, not genetic or pharmaceutical ones.

Many volumes have been written, and many programs created for tackling obesity in America and around the world. Armies of infomercials, products, and services fight for profits in the battle of the bulge. Some services are credible and convincing. Others are downright ridiculous and even dangerous.

Within the scientific community, researchers themselves are focusing on their own pet projects, going after genes and ignoring the glaring facts. The reasons for the obesity epidemic are obvious—People's genes have not changed; their environments and lifestyles have! Obesity may be affected by genes, but it has been clearly triggered by changes in lifestyles. People are consuming excess calories concomitant with too little energy expenditure (see Chapter 5 "Excess Calories"). Lifestyle problems demand lifestyle solutions, not genetic ones! This should be the major focus of our attention.

The emphasis throughout this entire book has been one of looking at the big picture and majoring on those big issues over which we have control (see Chapter 2 "The Root of the Matter"). This book gives scant attention is given to the role of genetics in obesity. This is for a very simple reason … Your genes are done deal. Our consumption excesses and sedentary lifestyles are the issues that deserve our attention. These are what we have control over.

Needed: "Regime Change"

Losing weight is not about dieting.
It is about eating (and living) differently.

The call to reduce calorie intake is not a call to dieting. This is what springs to mind when most people think about losing weight. Many have become discouraged and have simply tuned out. Reducing calorie intake, however, should not translate into a series of negative prescriptions. The quality of food is more significant than the mere quantity of food. Eating more does not automatically translate into getting fat. You can eat more and weigh less—sayings made popular by Dean Ornish, M.D. and Terri Shintani, M.D. in their books *Eat More Weigh Less* and *The Hawaii Diet*, respectively. This reflects a renewed emphasis on quality rather than mere quantity.[155,156] This is why many food lovers in the Orient, despite their indulgence in foods, remain much slimmer that their Western counterparts.(Chapter 5, Table 5-3). It is not about dieting. It is about eating differently. It is a "lifestyle regime change."

Psychologically, most people resent restrictive diets. In their book *Lifestyle Nutrition*, Professor Johanna Dwyer and James Rippe, M.D. sum up this phenomenon quite aptly:[157]

> Traditionally, nutrition intervention has focused on advice to *restrict* intake of certain foods or nutrients (e.g., reducing fat and saturated fat intake, limiting calorie intake, limiting sodium/salt). Yet the most often mentioned obstacle to achieving a healthful diet is not wanting to give up the foods we like. Basic psychological principles hold that when people are faced with a restriction, or loss of a choice, that choice becomes more attractive. In other words, focusing mainly on what *not* to eat, or on eating less of some types of foods, may evoke conscious or unconscious negativism in some people. As an alternative, emphasizing *additive* recommendations such as increasing intake of fruits and vegetables, or eating more fiber-rich foods…

These principles apply when addressing almost any habit. Appetites do not relish restrictions.

> The most successful way to get rid of bad habits
> is not so much about stopping them, as it is about
> replacing them with something better.

The more room you make for good choices, the less room remains for negative choices. It is that simple.

Practical Perspectives for Successfully Tackling Obesity

Textbooks have been written on obesity and its management. Central to all successful approaches are the roles of increased physical activity and dietary changes. The following perspectives are helpful to keep in mind, regardless of what program you choose to follow. The author does not subscribe to special weight-loss diets.

- *The most successful treatment for obesity is prevention.*
- Start *living differently*. If you want to see changes, some things have to change.
- Being overweight is not the problem; it is the consequence. Obesity did not happen overnight. It is insane to expect it to disappear the morning after.
- The sooner we start, the better. Obesity often starts in childhood. The problems of childhood are often tied to problems of parenting, peers, and politics. Women should not eat-for-two during pregnancy (see Chapter 5). Today's problems, if not tackled diligently, may become tomorrow's nightmare.
- Losing weight is not about dieting. If you go on a diet, you will one day come off that diet, and weight gain will recur.
- Do the right things: Eat differently, increase your daily physical activity, and then witness the "positive side-effects." It will reduce your weight, your diabetes risk, high blood pressure, blood lipid profile, and your risk of heart disease. But it will go beyond just preventing diseases. It will launch you on the road to optimal health, and produce results that last.

Throughout this book, the emphasis has been on knowledge and principles. Formulas for specific diseases have been deliberately shunned. This author is convinced that people need to focus more on healthy living and less on diseases. Develop the right attitude, eat right, exercise, stop smoking and expect good health to follow. Give it your best shot. You can't do better than that.

> If you take the prescription for a healthy lifestyle,
> weight loss will be one of its major side-effects.

Say "No" To Counting Calories, Special Menus, and Regimented Prescriptions

> Much of the dietary advice given for obesity and diabetes adds more
> burden to an already burdensome situation.
> Instead of regimented dietary prescriptions (e.g. reading food labels,
> counting calories, and dietary exchanges) that aggravate distress and
> cause poor compliance, the best way to proceed is to
> learn about healthy living. Keep it simple!

People are better off learning principles rather than regimented prescriptions. Life has enough problems of its own. To engage in regimented dietary prescriptions can easily dominate and frustrate the daily lifestyles for those affected. These look good on paper and in textbooks, and convey a semblance of science and credibility to your colleagues in academia, but they promote distress rather than improve compliance. Teach people nutrition principles, and they can then make good choices whether they live in urban America or in rural Botswana. Armed with sound nutrition principles, people will be able to make good choices at home as well as abroad. It is a liberating rather than a burdensome experience.

Nutrition principles promote understanding, and understanding can improve control, and improved control can lead to greater compliance. People with hypertension, high blood lipids, or coronary heart disease, and diabetes are already saddled with enough do's and don'ts. The last thing they need is further regimentation of their prescriptions. Some people benefit from being held by a short leash, but this should only be seen as a short term measure. If becoming diabetic means counting calories, reading every label, and memorizing food exchanges, these can instigate denial and poor patient compliance. It is not surprising, therefore, why many find the diagnosis of diabetes so depressing.[158]

On the matter of counting calories, Professor Willett of Harvard gives advice that should be heeded:[159]

> It isn't necessary to count fat grams or whip out a calculator to compare
> percentage of calories from fat. You have better things to do with your

time, the payoff is very small, and so far there is no solid evidence for adopting exact numerical goals for total fat intake. It does make sense to know what is in the foods you eat, or plan to eat, so you can make healthy choices. But I don't recommend keeping precise tallies all day long.

There will be those obsessive personalities who relish checking their blood sugars 4 to 6 times a day and counting every calorie, but for most people, this is the formula for major depression. The diagnosis of type II diabetes should be a wake-up call to embark on the journey towards optimal health, and not just better diabetes control.

Making Practical Choices When Shopping— Read Less Labels

Shopping for food at a supermarket has become much more difficult … it takes forever, and it is difficult navigating through the multitude of processed foods to find the few whole-food items that I need. In fact, there are so many products, so many labels to read, so many health factors to consider, that sometimes it's hard to grasp just how unhealthy a seemingly reasonable, time-saving choice may actually be.[159]

Miriam Nelson, Associate Professor
School of Nutrition Science and Policy, Tufts University, Boston

You need to know what you want. Otherwise, the dazzling and exceedingly tempting array of foods on supermarket shelves is bound to confound the aimless consumer. Going through today's supermarkets is an education itself— if just to marvel at the amazing variety of items that all scream to get your attention. The overwhelming bulk of the items on offer are of the highly-processed variety. Labels may be helpful, but for reasons described in the previous chapter, they can be very misleading. Fresh produce and minimally processed foods are the best alternatives if you are seriously interested in improving your nutrition. Therefore shopping for healthy living is not difficult (see Chapter 7 "Food Labels: A Personal View").

Most of the foods required for your Prudent Cosmopolitan Diet can be obtained from large supermarkets. However, I prefer open air markets or a visit to the green grocer for produce. A visit to a nearby Chinatown or Chinese food store can provide you with tasty greens not available in most supermarkets. There is also a wide variety of interesting soy products and original green teas.

Below are a few perspectives to adopt while shopping:

- Set your own agenda (make a shopping list), otherwise the supermarket will set it for you.

- If you are choosing foods with labels, make sure you know what you are looking for. The devil is often in the details. If you are a novice (most of us are), speak to a budding label expert, chances are they do not mind showing off a few skills to help you decide on an item or two.

- Know what you are paying for. The word "organic" does not mean better. (see Chapter 7)

Cooking At Home: Quick and Easy

The Way I Do It

> Many people spend too much time
> preparing and cooking food.
> Excellent and tasty meals can be
> prepared in less than fifteen minutes
> … quicker than it takes to collect a take-out meal.

Most people see cooking as a chore. Much of this has to do with the demands of urban living and the perception that cooking is inconvenient, takes up too much time, plus you have to wash the dishes! Having led a very demanding life during medical school and beyond, and for a variety of reasons, I specialized in quick cooking methods.

Cooking has been learning experience, one that continues to this day. Living, traveling, and studying in Latin America, the Caribbean, Europe, the Middle East, and Asia have given me a great first-hand education in global cultures and cuisines. Through the years and across the continents, it has been my pleasure to receive commendation for my experimental style of cooking—using no cookbooks, no weights, nor measures. Learning came through trial and error, and a willingness to experiment (along with a long list of human guinea pigs).

As a busy doctor, speed continues to be of the essence, and therefore quick, tasty, nutritious meals are what I can speak about. I give much credit to my global friends who taught me many of their secrets. Sample one of my recipes; it actually won an award. It took me less than ten minutes to prepare. Do not ask me about baking or any meal that takes more than an hour to prepare. But be forewarned, every real chef knows that the final taste of a meal depends on a personal touch, which no recipe can accurately convey.

Dr. B's Cosmopolitan Jerk-Chicken Stir-fry

Eliminate All Hassles over Foods and Recipes

If preparing and eating food means frequent weighing, measuring, constantly looking at the clock etc., then cooking is bound to be quite a chore. As this is the popular way of writing cookbooks, it is not surprising why so many hate to cook.

Ingredients:
Chicken breast—skinless, boneless *(2 pieces)*
Snow peas *(handful or as desired)*
Fresh onions *(handful—more or less, if you choose)*
Fresh sweet pepper *(one or two if you choose)*
Garlic *(crushed, finely chopped according to preference)*
Ginger *(grated or finely chopped in blender)*
Extra virgin olive oil *(preferably cold pressed)*
Optional: Jamaican jerk seasoning (hot & spicy or mild) or Marie Sharp's pepper (from Belize)—*for pepper addicts*). Fresh hot peppers are best and add excellent flavor. If you cannot tolerate hot food, try using whole uncut pepper for its wonderful aromatic flavor.

Instructions:
Use knife or cleaver to quickly cut chicken breast into small pieces (dice or shred—bigger or smaller portions if you choose *(15seconds)*. Add a little table salt or squeezed lemons for an interesting twist.
Heat wok (Chinese) using medium heat *(30 seconds)*
Add extra virgin olive oil just enough to cover the bottom of the wok, add garlic, ginger and jerk seasoning or whole peppers. Do not burn. *(10 seconds)*
Place chicken in the wok and stir *(about 3 to 4 minutes)*
Add snow peas *(during final minute)*
Add onions—rings or angular cuts *(during final minute)*
Add chopped sweet peppers—I recommend at least two *(final 30 to 40 seconds)*
Serve (as is or with whole grain bread or preferred grain)

Dining:
Eat with a merry heart
Drinks: water or freshly squeezed juices
For dessert: fruit plate made with tropical papayas (paw paws) are excellent digestion aids (contain papain, an ingredient in meat tenderizers); watermelon, cantaloupes or add a few nuts of choice.
Salads: green salad with tomatoes, peppers, cucumber, spring onions (escallion), or parsley.
Optional: sprinkle extra virgin olive oil, guacamole or fresh avocado chops, French or Italian dressing on salad or lemon juice.

Useful Kitchen Equipment:
- Stove with vigorous flame or heat: gives better results with quick stir-fry's.
- Oriental-style wok and accessories: They are excellent for meats and vegetables
- Vegetable steamers: they cause less leaching of nutrients compared to boiling.
- Juicer: they extract fresh juices from fruits and vegetables. Carrot juice is wonderful and it takes just seconds to fill a cup. If you prefer chilled juices, store fruits at the bottom of the fridge before juicing.
- Blender/food processor: these are excellent for drinks, fruits, and vegetables.
- Multiblade extruder presser *(e.g. LePresse):* for rapid cutting or pressing of fruits and vegetables and avoids tedious preparation work (good for a big family).
- Mechanical citrus juice presser: these seem a strange addition to a hi-tech kitchen. This form of squeezing releases some of the potent cancer-fighting ingredient (d-limonene) in the citrus oil and provides extra fiber (pulp). In addition, it gives you a chance to exercise those arm muscles. Some people find the taste of rind too harsh, in this case, peel oranges before squeezing.

Some principles:
- Quick Meal: The entire procedure should take no more than 10 to 15 minutes. This is ideal for a busy individual.
- No need to overcook, otherwise chicken gets tough, vegetables lose their crunch, and you do not destroy too much vitamins. Avoid overheating wok which can cause oil to overheat; this can result in unhealthy changes in the oil
- Use whatever vegetables you prefer.
- Health tip: use fish, skinless-boneless poultry or lean meat, but it is not the center of attraction
- Becoming a good cook comes with time and experimentation.
- Stop being regimented about diets and learn the principles of healthy eating.

When Eating Out Ask Questions,
But Not Too Many

Excessive preoccupation with healthy living
can be an unhealthy thing
Eating out is not the time to be too fussy,
unless this is your daily lifestyle. Enjoy the outing.
Enjoy the company. Enjoy the food.

Remember this … Whenever you eat out, you lose control of what is in the food, even after you have sought reassurance about what's supposed to be in the food. In my experience, the truth may not be forthcoming from restaurant staff, simply because they themselves may not know. This is not a call for ordering the least healthy cuisine, but eating out has excellent benefits beyond mere nutrition. Family and social relationships are all essential ingredients for optimal health and happiness (see Chapter 1, "Healthy Living is not a Killjoy").

If eating out is an occasional event, the nature of the ingredients is much less of a concern, than if you eat daily in such establishments. My frank advice is to forget about the ingredients, enjoy the food, enjoy the company and don't be a spoiler. If eating out is a daily part of your lifestyle, the popular buffet-style restaurants give you greater control over choices. Pertinent questions include:

- The type oils used: If this is really important, ask to see it. I once asked for olive oil to sprinkle on my vegetable salad, only to be offered olive pomace oil instead (see discussions earlier in this chapter). I graciously declined. Choose extra virgin olive oils (plain) or olive oil based sauces and dips for salads.
- How the food is prepared: Fried foods deliver far more calories. Deep-fat frying causes negative changes (see Chapter 7).
- Avoid fish, poultry, or meat prepared in batter. Avoid fatty cuts.
- It is hard to escape salt, but ask for low salt options if high blood pressure is your concern.
- Choose fresh fruit dessert when available.
- Choose water as your preferred beverage, especially if you want to reduce your calories (it does not mean that you are a cheapie). Opt for freshly squeezed juices in place of reconstituted (made from concentrate) varieties.
- You do not have to eat all the food. It is okay to ask for a "doggie bag."
- As for fast foods, these epitomize the unbalanced Western diet and the health implications of such choices are discussed in Chapter 5 and 7.

Nevertheless, please do not be a nuisance or embroil yourself in nutrition or medical hubris. This is uncalled for at the dinner table. If you still feel very strongly, graciously decline certain foods without preaching a sermon. Stirring up a melee at the dinner table can be bad for your blood pressure or give you a heart attack. It is also a great way to ensure that you never get invited to dinner again, or at best, only reluctantly.

Understanding Global Cuisines

You will never truly understand global cuisines from a cookbook or a restaurant. Get to know the "people of the cuisines," either through travel, or through personal interaction. Many cookbooks and restaurants provide Westernized versions of global cuisines that cater largely to Western tastes and portion sizes.

Global cuisines serve as important pillars within the Prudent Cosmopolitan Diet (Figure 8-3). There are a large number of cookbooks on international dishes. This is the preferred choice for many. Some people receive their introduction through restaurants and other ethnic outlets, while others learn through foreign travel.

Americans need to remember that many restaurants have tailored their menus to suit American tastes and expectations. Ethnic restaurants "Amerisize" their portions and include significantly more meat. Any native from these cultures can tell you the difference between restaurant foods versus home-cooked meals.

The major cuisines espoused in this book can be found in most cities of the world, thanks to globalization. It would be an injustice to discuss them in a passing paragraph. Get to know people and their cultures. Many will be happy to share insights into their cuisines. Through the years, I have nurtured a heartfelt appreciation for the wonderful salad of global cuisines. Getting to know people and their culinary contributions to healthy eating have proven both an eye-opening, as well as a mouth-watering experience.

Conclusion and Summary

Good nutrition plays a central role in preventing disease and optimizing health. Low rates of chronic diseases have been consistently linked to healthy diets. As scientific evidence emerges on the details of nutrition, it has encouraged a popular tendency towards a reductionist or "nutraceutical" approach to nutrition. This has led to an unbalanced emphasis on individual nutrients at the expense of the broader diet.

Scientific studies have confirmed the key role of nutrition in the prevention and management of several chronic diseases. Certain global dietary patterns, specifically the traditional Mediterranean-style diet and the Asian/Oriental-style diet, have been historically linked to lower rates of obesity, cardiovascular diseases, type II diabetes, and cancer. These, along with other traditional diets, are the best way forward in our quest for preventing diseases and optimizing health.

In a modern cosmopolitan setting, a logical way to proceed has been summed up in the Prudent Cosmopolitan Diet. It is a simple model of healthy eating that embraces the best of the healthiest diets in the world and places them all under one roof. It serves as a framework on which to build a personal strategy to prevent disease and optimize health. Dietary supplements can play a role, but they should be seen within the context of the whole diet. They are supplements, but never substitutes for good nutrition.

Obesity deserves special mention. It is soon to overtake smoking as the number one cause of preventable death. Obesity plays a central role in the genesis of the metabolic syndrome, cardiovascular diseases, and type II diabetes. Successful strategies for tackling the obesity epidemic should focus on primary prevention. Treatment strategies are best approached within the wider context of pursuing a healthy lifestyle, rather than the singular aim of losing weight.

******

Chapter 9

Lifestyle Physical Activity
...Get Moving

Chapter Outline

Victims of Our Success 367
Physical Activity Levels in America 368
Definitions 369
Increased Physical Activity: It's Role in Prevention 370
Benefits of Increased Physical Activity 370
The Evidence for Physical Activity on Health and Longevity 371
The Institutionalization of Physical Activity 372
Can Sexual Activity Qualify as Exercise? 373
It All Adds Up 374
Targeting the Children 376
Exercise Modalities and Health Benefits: A Summary 376
Why Wait Until…? 377
Potential Hazards of Exercise: Be Sensible 378
When to Check with Your Doctor 379
"On-the-Job Training" 380
The Television and Computer Age: Creative Solutions Needed 381
Overcoming Psychological Barriers 381
Barriers to Exercise: Foreign Considerations 382
A Good Habit is as Hard to Break as a Bad One 382
Exercise and Physical Activity—Personal Reflections 383
It is All about Choices 384
Summary 384

Current low rates of regular activity in Americans may be partially due to the misperception of many that vigorous, continuous exercise is necessary to reap health benefits. Many people, for example, fail to appreciate walking as "exercise" or to recognize the substantial benefits of short bouts (at least 10 minutes) of moderate-level activity. [1]

Physical Activity and Cardiovascular Health
National Institutes of Health Consensus Development Conference Statement,
December 18-20, 1995

Moderate exercise is just as essential to a healthy life as good nutrition, seat belts, and avoiding cigarettes. [2]

Surgeon General of the United States and the
Centers for Disease Control and Prevention
Report on Physical Activity, 1996

§§§§§§§

Victims of Our Success

> In one sense, we have made tremendous strides, but at the cost of marked reductions in physical activity levels.

Progress brings problems. Nowhere is this more pertinent than the impact of modernity on physical activity levels. The emergence of market economies that promote improved efficiency and productivity has led to increasing mechanization and automation of previously labor-intensive agriculture and industry. Urban migration and the love affair with the automobile accelerated the march towards physical inactivity. The lives we live today are far removed from those of our ancestors less than a century ago.

In one sense we have gained. We now enjoy more comfortable and less physically demanding lifestyles. We have more time for leisure, relaxation, and the finer things in life. The arrival of the television, the computer, and the Internet has mellowed things further. As we became more efficient and more indulgent, we faced new challenges brought on by modernity. This trend is not confined to industrialized nations. As developing countries follow in the footsteps of industrialized nations, the consequences of sedentary lifestyle are being globally felt. The emergence of mega cities, massive population shifts, and increased fast-food consumption have given birth to unprecedented levels of sedentary lifestyles and obesity.

Not only has modernity ensnared today's societies with its new charms, but it has also extended its tentacles to our domesticated friends. Even dogs and cats have not been spared revolution in their lifestyles. The most privileged among them now enjoy effortless access to highly processed foods. They sit idly in couches rather than foraging outdoors. Cats and dogs have become increasingly obese, developing diabetes, and dying from cardiovascular diseases just like their owners.[3]

All this has come at a heavy price. Sedentary lifestyles and unhealthy eating now claim at least 300,000 deaths in America and 76 billion dollars in direct medical care costs. The other side of the physical inactivity coin, vis-à-vis obesity, inflicts more than 115 billion dollars in damages. [4,5]

Physical Activity Levels in America

Physically inactive lifestyles are the norm for more than 60 percent of American adults. The figure is not much different for American youth. Up to half of all youngsters in high school level are ominously inactive. Data on physical activity levels in America are presented in Table 9-1 and 9-2. [6-8]

Table 9-1. Physical Inactivity / Sedentary Lifestyle Levels in U.S. Adults

Quick Facts on Physical Activity Levels in the United States

1. 25% of Americans age 18 and older (about 50 million) report no leisure-time physical activity.
2. 22% of American adults report sustained daily physical activity lasting 30 minutes or more 5 times a week.
3. 15% of U.S. adults engage in regular vigorous physical activity 3 times a week for at least 20 minutes.
4. 60% or more of U.S. adults did not achieve the recommended amount of physical activity.
5. Physical inactivity is more prevalent among these groups: women, African-Americans, Hispanic-Americans, older adults, and the less affluent.
6. The relative risk of coronary heart disease associated with physical inactivity ranges from 1.5 to 2.4. This increase in risk is comparable to that observed for high cholesterol, high blood pressure or cigarette smoking.
7. Up to 50% increased risk of developing high blood pressure in physically inactive individuals.
8. At least 250,000 deaths a year in the United States are attributed to a lack of regular physical activity.

The Centers for Disease Control and Prevention (CDC) recommends at least 30 minutes of moderate exercises like walking five times a week, or 20 minutes of vigorous exercise such as running, three times a week. Such recommendations remain largely ignored. Americans failed to make any meaningful changes in their physical activity levels over the last 10 to 15 years (Table 9-2).[9]

Table 9-2. Physical Activity Levels of U.S. Adults[8,9]

Physical Activity Levels of U.S. Adults		
Physical Activity	**1990** Percentages (%)	**1998** Percentages (%)
Recommended Amounts	24.3	25.4
Insufficient Amounts	45.0	45.9
No Physical Activity	30.7	28.7

According to the Centers for Disease Control and Prevention, exercise habits did not change much between 1990 and 1998

Definitions

Most people equate physical activity with exercise. Many believe physical activity means intense athletic or sporting pursuits. This misconception has caused many to ignore the call.

Physical activity includes any daily activity that requires movement. Walking, climbing stairs, and manual labour all involve physical activity and therefore qualify under the label.[10] More structured physical activities that require increased energy expenditure and muscular activity are called exercises. These include simple activities like walking and jogging or more organized pursuits in gymnasiums, fitness centers, and sporting arenas.

These distinctions are needed because people often get the wrong message. Many perceive exercise to be the privilege of athletes and individuals dedicated to sports and fitness. Paying more attention to lifestyle physical activity can send the important message that no one needs to feel left out. You do not need to don exercise paraphernalia or purchase special gadgets to become more active. Linda Pescatello, assistant professor School of Allied Health and director of the Center for Health Promotion at the University of Connecticut, summarized these perceptions and the consequences as follows:[11]

> The traditional exercise prescription of the 1970s and 1980s strove to improve physical fitness by promoting participation in vigorous types of endurance exercise. The general belief was that if a person did not exercise within a given heart-rate range or exercise intensity, the benefits of the program would be minimal. In hindsight, it is not surprising that these

recommendations did not inspire approximately 85% of American adults to become physically fit. Common barriers to achieving this task include lack of time, the program being "not fun" or "too hard," and musculoskeletal injury. Consequently, 60% of the American public remains sedentary.[9]

Lifestyle physical activity, as defined in the *American Journal of Preventive Medicine*, is "the daily accumulation of at least 30 minutes of self-selected activities, which includes all leisure, occupational, or household activities that are at least moderate in their intensity and could be planned or unplanned activities that are part of everyday life."[11] This encourages non-athletic individuals to make the most out of their daily physical activity chores. Lifestyle physical activity can result in improved cardiovascular and metabolic health, particularly in middle-aged, overweight men and women.[12-21]

Increased Physical Activity: It's Role in Prevention

Good nutrition is paramount in the pursuit of optimal health, but good nutrition without physical activity misses an important ingredient for optimal health. Our bodies were designed to be active. Physical activity expends excess energy and prevents accumulation of excess fat within body tissues. Physical activity can compensate for excess food intake that is so prevalent in America and the industrialized world. Many professional athletes, despite their ravenous appetites, gain weight only after they retire from active sports or during the lay-off season. Food excess certainly matters, but it matters even more when physical activity levels are low. Increased physical activity can offset many of the excesses of the Western diet, and prevent a large number of premature deaths.[22]

Physical activity is an exceptionally common modifiable risk factor for coronary heart disease (CHD). In a study of all CHD deaths occurring in the United States in 1986, more than 205,000 were attributable to physical inactivity, second only to the 253,000 attributable to hypercholesterolemia (high blood cholesterol).

Benefits of Increased Physical Activity

How does physical activity help in the prevention of chronic lifestyle diseases? Epidemiologic studies have shown that physically active people suffer less cardiovascular and chronic diseases than their more sedentary counterparts. Physically active lifestyles reduce cardiovascular diseases by 35 to 55 percent.[22] Increased physical activity and exercise impart great benefit to both mind and body. A summary of these benefits appear in Table 9-3.[12-21,23]

Table 9-3. The Benefits of Physical Activity and Exercise

The Benefits of Physical Activity and Exercise[12-21,23]

Cardiovascular benefits
Lowers resting heart rate
Lowers heart rates in response to exercise
Increases blood supply to the heart
Decreases oxygen demand by the heart
Improves heart contractions
Increases electrical stability to the heart
Elevates HDL or good cholesterol
Decreases LDL cholesterol
Lowers blood pressure
Lowers risk of a heart attack and stroke
Musculo-skeletal benefits
Increases muscle strength
Increases bone strength
Increases over all body tone
Prevents bone loss (osteoporosis)
Mental-psychological benefits
Increases energy
Improves mood
Relieves stress and reduces symptoms of depression
Improves self- image and psychological well-being
Enhances psychological well-being
May reduce the risk of developing depression
Other Disease risks
Lowers risk of type 2 diabetes by ~ 50 percent
Lowers risk for cancer (endometrial, colo-rectal, breast)
Effects on Body Weight
Maintains weight
Helps in weight control and is a key part of any weight loss effort

The Evidence for Physical Activity on Health and Longevity

Several landmark studies have provided clear evidence of improved health with increased physical activity. Increased physical activity and exercise are known to reduce the risk of sudden death, coronary artery disease, type II diabetes, and stroke.[24-36] People whose jobs require more physical activity experience lower rates of coronary heart disease compared to their sedentary co-workers. You do not have to be an athlete to experience the benefits of increased physical activity. Engaging in half an hour of brisk walking daily provides almost the same prevention benefits as running 30 to 40 miles per week (Table 9- 4).

Table 9-4. Studies on Physical Activity and Health

Studies on Physical Activity and Health

London Double Decker Buses: Drivers vs. Conductors*(Morris 1953) [30]

American Letter Carriers vs. Mail Clerks* (Kahn 1963) [31]

San Francisco cargo handlers vs. warehousemen* (Paffenbarger 1975) [32]

College Students and Alumni in various activities*(Paffenbarger 1978) [33]

The British Civil Servants Study♦[34]

The U.S. College Alumni Study♥[35]

The Institute of Aerobics Research ♠[36]

Studies that show benefit in both men and women, who engage in simple physical activities such as brisk walking, ranging from lowered rates of heart disease, type II diabetes, and stroke. [24-29]

* The first four studies listed above showed that *people whose jobs required more physical activity generally experienced lower rates of coronary heart disease* compared to their more sedentary co-workers.

♦British civil servants who engaged in *vigorous physical exercises and sports exhibited far less coronary heart disease rates and deaths from heart disease* that their less active work mates.

♥A study of Harvard alumni (1916 to 1950) commenced in the1960s noted that *the most physically active participants exhibited 50% less coronary heart disease compared to the least active of their colleagues.* Light to moderately-vigorous recreational and sports activity led to a 20 to 40% lower risk of heart disease compared to their inactive or non-sporting colleagues: *The benefits of vigorous physical activity and sports in youth fade unless activities are continued in later years;* being athletic in college is *no* guarantee of good health in later life.

♠ This study provides evidence that *you do not have to be an athlete to experience the benefits of increased physical activity. Engaging in half an hour of brisk walking daily, provides almost the same prevention benefits as running 30 to 40 miles per week.* This follow-up study of 15,000 healthy men and women over an 8-year period showed that deaths from all causes (including deaths from heart disease and cancer) were lower in active individuals compared to the physically inactive.

The Institutionalization of Physical Activity

Current low rates of regular activity in Americans may be partially due to the misperception that vigorous, continuous exercise is necessary to reap health benefits.

National Institutes of Health (NIH) Consensus Development Conference Statement
on Physical Activity and Cardiovascular Health[37]

Given the clear benefits of increased physical activity and exercise, and given the enormous popularity of sports worldwide, why do so many choose to remain spectators? It is not surprising why the majority of Americans equate physical activity with organized exercises. The popular perception remains that you are not really "physically active" until you play regular sports or join a gym.

These notions are fueled by many social and economic pressures to institutionalize physical activity. Cable television and the magazines heavily promote such ideas. These must be dispelled if most people are to move beyond being mere spectators. This mentality further fuels the socioeconomic divide and undermines public health efforts to reach the majority who seem content with their status as spectators. The socio-economically disadvantaged, because of limited access to sporting facilities and fitness clubs, have less incentive to increase their physical activity. However, this can be offset when people understand that there are many alternatives for becoming more active, outside the confines of a stadium or a gym.

People need to appreciate that increased physical activity can take place where they live, at work, and on the way to and from work. The National Institutes of Health (NIH) Consensus Development Conference Statement on Physical Activity and Cardiovascular Health acknowledged that the "current low rates of regular activity in Americans may be partially due to the misperception of many that vigorous, continuous exercise is necessary to reap health benefits."[37] The challenge, therefore, is to expend as much energy during the normal activities of daily living.

Can Sexual Activity Qualify As Exercise?

Physical health promotes sexual health, and vice versa.

There is a prevailing mindset that sees physical activity and exercise solely in terms of unpleasant activities. Human sexual expression, an innately pleasurable experience, can involve considerable energy output. The question is this—can sexual activity make a meaningful contribution to good health? The answer is yes, but with some clarification. Sexual activity includes mental and emotional expenditure in addition to physical energy output. These effects are additive and they increase with increased frequency and duration of the activity.

In his book, *Secrets of the Superyoung*, Dr. David Weeks presented data on the youth-enhancing effects of sexual activity.[38] Sexually active people were noted to look up to ten years younger (see Chapter 6, "Skin Aging and Sex"). Individuals with physical and other disease impediments may find such advice too demanding, but "sexercise" (especially since many Americans seem confused over the definition) is more than sexual intercourse. Sexual expression involves every step on the road to the summit.

An imaginative mind can discover it to be a good outlet for burning extra calories while at the same time building intimacy. A detail description of such methods and means lie outside the scope of this book.

Sexual activity delivers other benefits—physical and otherwise. Susan McCrensky Heitler, clinical psychologist and author of *The Power of Two: Secrets to a Strong and Loving Marriage* summarizes this point quite well:[39]

> As a physical boon, sex appears to be an all-time winner: For men, sexual arousal increases testosterone and flushes out the prostate gland. For women, regular lovemaking increases levels of estrogen, which protects the heart, keeps vaginal tissues more supple, sustains the brain at its cognitive best, and even helps ameliorate premenstrual syndrome. The endorphins released with sex, as well as the accelerated blood flow throughout the body, can reduce pain from any number of bodily ills, arthritis ... to headache to whiplash. And, like other forms of exercise, sexual encounters burn calories, enhance the immune system, and suffuse the physical body with feelings of relaxation and well-being.

Physical exercise, in turn, can improve sexual performance. Vigorous activities, the equivalent of walking two miles or burning an extra 200 calories a day, can significantly reduce the incidence of erectile dysfunction or impotence in middle-aged men. Both the cardiovascular benefits and improved muscle tone that result from exercise can improve sexual performance. According to a University of Texas report, this is yet another excuse to exercise regularly. Physical health promotes sexual health. The better your health, the better is the potential for a vigorous calorie-burning sexual relationship.[40]

It All Adds Up

Every bit counts. You do not have to be a super-athlete. Studies on physical activity and health have shown that even mild increases in physical activity, such as walking just an average of 30 minutes a day, reduced the risk of premature death to the same degree as running 30 miles a week (Table 9-4). The benefits extend beyond premature death. Deaths from all causes, including deaths from cancer and heart disease, are lower in people who engage in physical activities that fall way short of vigorous exercises.[36,37]

Previous recommendations stressed the need for sustained physical exertion to obtain the desired benefits, but experts now reject this. There is a big difference between being athletically fit and being a physically active person. The advice is to become physically active, not to become an athlete. The more rigorous the physical activity, the greater is the potential for injury, as the world of sports can clearly attest.

Most people will never become athletes, and most people will never join a fitness center. Therefore it is comforting to know that you don't have to climb all ten stairways at once. You can still benefit if you climb them one stairway at a time throughout the course of the day. This is what is to be encouraged, and not the host of popular misconceptions that surround advice on physical activity and exercise (Table 9-5).

Table 9-5. Misconceptions about Physical Activity and Exercise

Popular Misconceptions* about Exercise

1. *It's best to engage in sports, join a gym, or an advertised program.* The emphasis should be to increase your physical activity. Exercise is simply a structured way of increasing one's physical activity. This works best for some people.

2. *"No pain, no gain"* This myth stems from a "machismo" mentality. Proponents often indulge in grueling and non-pleasurable approaches to exercise and fitness by pushing their bodies to the limit. The risk of injury and sudden cardiac death increase in direct proportion to the intensity of exercise, especially if one is unaccustomed to exercise. Walking (briskly) can provide many health benefits with minimum risk of injury or sudden cardiac death. Those loud grunts and groans at the gym can be quite a nuisance.

3. *You must become athletically fit before you can reap the benefits of exercise.* It is good to be an athlete, but great benefits to protect against chronic disease occur with modest increases in physical activity, way short of physical fitness.

4. *You must exercise continuously to gain benefits.* The evidence is that it all adds up.

5. *Being athletic in your early years exerts a protective effect against disease later in life.* "Used to be" does not protect against heart disease later in life.

6. *Exercise is the best way of losing weight.* Exercise can provide great health benefits with or without weight loss. Paying attention to nutrition choices can be even more important. Paying attention to both is best.

7. *If you are a highly conditioned athlete, you cannot have a heart problem.* Sudden death amongst physically conditioned athletes is by no means rare. Usually it is due to an underlying genetic, structural, or physiological heart abnormality.

8. *Sexual activity has no health or cardiovascular benefits.* A mutually satisfying committed sexual union has the capacity to provide great emotional, psychological, as well as physical and medical benefits.

*Misconceptions appear in *Italicized* print

Targeting the Children

Today's youth face challenges to physical activity like no other generation in history. Television, video games, and the Internet have robbed many children of much time that was previously spent on outdoor activities. School exercises that were the norm in previous generations are being progressively phased out in many schools across the country. Such unfortunate trends, coupled with easy access to high-calorie junk food, have led to unprecedented levels of obesity in youth (see Chapter 7, "Targeting the Children" and "The Media and Food Choices"). These are vexing issues for public health authorities.[45,46]

Children spend the bulk of their weekday hours at school. It is paramount, therefore, to cultivate physical activity and exercise patterns early in this captive population.[47-48] Only 50 percent of American youth between age 10 to 20 years get the extra activity they need. Enrollment in physical education classes has declined from 42 percent in 1991 to 25 percent in 1995. Less than 20 percent of high school students get more than 20 minutes of daily physical activity during physical education classes.[49]

Exercise Modalities and Health Benefits: A Summary

Despite the well-deserved emphasis on increased physical activity, as opposed to structured exercises in this chapter, the latter helps millions to become more active. Exercises can be classified in terms of their impact on the cardiovascular and musculoskeletal systems. Aerobic exercises, strengthening exercises, and flexibility exercises are a simple popular method of classifying them.

Aerobic exercises provide an excellent workout for the lungs and the cardiovascular system (Table 9-6). These forms of exercises are so named for their impact on calorie consumption using the oxygen or the aerobic pathway for burning calories. These forms of exercise have the greatest potential to increase heart rate and improve respiratory function.[50-55]

Strengthening or resistance exercises have not received much attention from health advocates in the past, but the loss of strength is an important part of the aging process. Although aerobic exercises are better for cardiovascular health, the importance of restored muscle mass and renewed strength should not be overlooked. Regain of lost strength is mentally and physically rejuvenating. These benefits are also available to the elderly population, even among those who suffer from poor health (see Chapter 6, "Strengthen those Muscles and Keep Active").[56-58]

Physical activity experts like Miriam Nelson Ph.D., from Tufts University in Massachusetts, encourages women to "start off strong." In her book *Strong Women*

Stay Slim, she considers resistance exercises as ideal for improving strength, balance, flexibility, and avoiding injury.[59] An overriding concern among many women is the unjustified fear of becoming too muscular. This is simply not the case for the overwhelming bulk of women who exercise. Weight training exercises reduce the risk of osteoporosis, a common problem for post-menopausal women.[55]

Table 9-6. Types of Exercises and their Health Benefits

Types of Exercise	Health Benefits
Aerobic Exercises Walking Jogging Swimming Dancing Cycling (outdoors) Stationary cycling Treadmill walking Sports: baseball, tennis, basketball, football	Cardiovascular workout increase heart performance, lowers blood pressure Diabetes prevention—physical activity alone can reduce risk of type 2 diabetes by ~ 50 percent Improved strength, preserves muscle during weight loss procedures
Strengthening Exercises Weight training, Bodybuilding Resistance training Various forms of home gym equipment e.g. Total Gym®, Bowflex®	Metabolism booster, strength training can increase your metabolism by ~ 15%. In practical terms, this translates into an extra 300 to 400 extra calories burnt per day Improved balance by strengthening muscles and joints and improves flexibility Rejuvenating, literally reverses and slows down the aging clock—you literally look and feel better
Flexibility Exercises Warm up exercises Various forms of yoga Winsor Pilates® type exercises	Protects against osteoporosis

Why Wait Until ...?

The time most people neglect their health is the very time their bodies need the most attention.

The demands of work, family, or academic pursuits cause many to neglect their health during their most productive years. It is so easy to get bogged down with the responsibilities of career and family. The time most people neglect their health is the very time their bodies need it most. Those times of greatest physical and mental stresses are the times our bodies need the best nutrition, adequate physical activity and excellent sleep. Ironically for many, this is precisely the time they get none of the above.

It sometimes takes a tragedy before people pay attention to their health. Do not wait for negative events to occur before you start paying attention to your health. Unfortunately, this is what it takes for most people to pay attention—negative triggers (Table 9-7).

Table 9-7. Trigger Factors for Healthier Lifestyle and Physical Activity

Some Trigger Factors for Healthier Lifestyle and Physical Activity
1. Development of new illness (e.g. heart attack, diabetes, or erectile dysfunction) or failing health
2. Unfavorable blood test or laboratory report
3. Failed medical checkup
4. Awareness of the ravages of illness in a loved one, relative, or friend
5. Sudden death of someone you know
6. Encouragement from family or friend
7. Doctors orders

Potential Hazards of Exercise: Be Sensible

In a multitude of counsellors, there is safety (Sayings of the Wise 24:6) [60]

You know you need to get active, so what's next? Should you just put on your jogging shoes or start pumping weights? If you have a significant medical illness or if you are totally out of shape, you are best advised to get a professional opinion before proceeding. The older you are, the more careful you need to be. People unaccustomed to exercise need professional advice before embarking on activities that require major physical exertion. Critics of exercise highlight the number of people, including highly conditioned athletes, who die from vigorous physical exertion. Even though such numbers are small, caution is certainly in order.

The watch words are, "Be sensible." Tune in to your own body and go at your own pace. Your body has a good way of telling you what it can tolerate and what it cannot. Do not push yourself past your limit, and there is no need to try and impress onlookers. Excessive exertion is more likely to precipitate heart attacks or primary cardiac arrest in previously unfit sedentary individuals. Sudden cardiac death has followed precipitous bouts of exertion. For these and other reasons, a graded exercise program is the sensible way to proceed.

Individualized instructions are especially important before commencing strength training exercises that involve lifting weights. Serious harm can result if advice and supervision are not sought. This is especially true for beginners who have no experience with weight lifting. At-risk groups need medical clearance before embarking on these programs (Table 9-8 and Table 9-9).[61-63]

Table 9-8. Conditions that can increase the Potential Hazards of Exercise

Conditions that can increase the hazards of exercise
1. Any illness or prescription medications
2. Obesity
3. Adverse climatic conditions: hot weather, high humidity, high altitude (increased risk of hyperthermia, heat exhaustion, heat stroke)
4. Recent meals (increased risk of nausea, vomiting, reduced performance)
5. Physical exhaustion
6. Insufficient sleep
7. Alcohol or illegal drugs

When to Check With Your Doctor

A visit to the doctor is the sensible step when risk factors are present, or uncertainty exists (Table 9-9). A family history of cardiovascular diseases or sudden or unexplained death is especially important. As the practice of medicine is now highly specialized, it is best to consult with a doctor who has a special interest or training in cardiovascular diseases and exercise.

Having a disease does not disqualify you from being physically active. Very few conditions exist that absolutely forbid exercises, and the few exceptions are more likely to be found at the intensive care units in hospitals. Even immediate post-operative patients are encouraged to get moving once the anesthesia wears off. Patients with hip-replacement surgery are mobilized the following day. People with arthritis and obesity are better off being active than sedentary. Non-weight bearing exercises such as swimming or cycling are better options for some patients.

People on diabetes medications must know that dangerous episodes of hypoglycemia (low blood sugar) can occur both during and following exercises. People with diabetes, especially if controlled on insulin or other oral hypoglycemic drugs, should have a glucometer to detect and prevent these life-threatening episodes. These can occur without warning or also occur several hours following exercises. People on cardiovascular drugs or pacemakers need to be in touch with their cardiologists. Advice must be tailored to the individual. One size does not fit all.[64-68]

Table 9-9. Conditions to Check before Starting Exercises

Check With Your Doctor Before starting exercises if any of the following applies

1. Overweight or obesity
2. Heart disease (especially if family history of heart attacks under age 55 years), pacemakers, defibrillators etc.
3. Family history of heart disease
4. High blood pressure
5. Type II diabetes mellitus, special caution if on diabetes medicines, especially insulin
6. 35 years or older
7. Arthritis or joint problems
8. Prescription medicines
9. Smoker

"On-the-Job Training"

For those whose activities are markedly reduced by modern technology, a major challenge is to creatively weave increased physical activity into their daily lives.

We live in a different time, and there is no turning back. The tools of efficiency and productivity are not going to disappear. The challenge for today's generation is to match modernity with activity. We need creative ways of incorporating as much physical activity as possible in our daily lives. We must cast aside the notions that physical activity or exercise only takes place after work. Ten hours of exercises weekly is only 10 hours out of a weekly total of 168. There are simple ways of becoming more physically active (Table 9-10). It all adds up.

Many companies know the benefits of a physically active staff. Simple safe ways of strengthening the arms and thighs can be done in a busy office. Desk push-ups, arm curls, chair squats, chair dips, and calf raises need just a little imagination and no special equipment. On-site facilities and gym-membership incentives have helped in this effort. In many ways, such provisions prove only to be a win-win situation for both employers and employees. It can lead to increased job satisfaction, increased productivity, and better health. [64-68]

Table 9-10. Lifestyle Physical Activity Strategies

Lifestyle Physical Activity Strategies
1. Walk or cycle to work, school, or on errands
2. Use stairs instead of elevators and escalators, and do some extras, e.g. on tip-toes or with an extra "spring" in the step
3. Leisure time sports, walks, and family activity
4. While at work, fidget
5. Office Exercises: desk push-ups, arm curls, chair squats, chair dips, calf raises
6. Lift weights and strengthen muscles while at work or at home

The Television and Computer Age:
Creative Solutions Needed

These gadgets of modernity—television and the personal computer—can dominate so much of our daily routine. Because of this, they need special attention. The simple advice to watch less television or spend less time on the computer will not win many converts, but it is hard to see how we can both embrace modernity and technology without pursuing innovative yet simple strategies.

Using a treadmill or a stationary bike while watching television is a simple strategy to counteract the couch-potato lifestyle. Computer users can do simple leg, shoulder, and neck exercises while stroking keys and remaining glued to the computer screen. There are Internet programs that can walk users through a series of exercises breaks. Some are designed to reduce the risk of repetitive strain injury (RSI) and eye strain. These are certainly a better break than playing computer games.

Busy people will need to meet the challenges of harmonizing modernity with increased physical activity. It will be up to each individual to decide what works best and tailor these activities accordingly. The financial and other pressing demands of modernity need not ruin your health while you make a living.[69,70]

Overcoming Psychological Barriers...Why Many
Do Not Get Enough Physical Activity and Exercise

The way to hell is paved with good intentions.

It is time to stop making excuses. People can do those things that they really want to do. Life is never always smooth sailing. Constraints are bound to arise. The demands of time and competing priorities will forever confront us. Work, family, and social responsibilities will continually make demands on the activities of daily living. The list can go on.[71-74]

But one thing is evident: People make time for those things that they consider important. So if your health is really important to you, you will make time for it. It is that simple.

> People make time for those things
> that they want to make time for.

Barriers to Exercise: Foreign Considerations

Living overseas and travelling to countries have made me keenly aware of a number of socio-demographic attitudes that militate against the call to increase physical activity. In many cultures, certain lifestyles and physical activity patterns carry potent symbolisms. Being overweight in many countries is a symbol of prosperity, contentment, and material success. Walking or cycling may equate to being lower class. Driving an SUV (sports utility vehicle) makes a powerful statement of upward social mobility. This is the reality in much of the globe and within many communities in the industrialized world. The call to increase physical activity and lose weight in these settings often falls on deaf ears. Even educated and accomplished individuals in these societies may not be swayed. Social connotations and attitudes can be simply too overwhelming.

Fortunately, the medium of television that propagates unhealthy lifestyles is the same medium that promotes new trends for better health. But herein lies another problem. Many people in the developing world define exercise by the trends that they see on U.S. television. Fitness trends, Taibo, Bowflex, Total Gym, and whatever new trend is on offer are seen around the world. As many in the developing world cannot afford or access such equipment, many have opted to remain spectators.

A Good Habit Is As Hard To Break As a Bad One

> A thought becomes an act,
> ... an act becomes a habit,
> ... and a habit becomes a lifestyle.

Human beings are creatures of habit, and a good habit is as hard to break as a bad one, especially if immediate benefits are forthcoming. What is it that makes some people love to exercise while others do not? Why is it that some people make time and effort to exercise while others don't?

During the middle stages of writing this book, our facility played host to Sarah Neumann, an intern from Arizona. Sarah was hooked on exercise and physical fitness. It did not take long before she accused me of being a real slacker. I had refused her daily invitations to the gym that lay just a hundred yards across the street in a five-star hotel. Two tennis courts occupied the foreground of our facility, a soccer field was to the right, and two swimming pools were literally a stone's throw away. If those were not incentives enough, the beautiful Caribbean Sea and a lovely seafront cornice were within easy view. Worse still, I had a Total Gym tucked under my bed! Her statements were completely justified. You can surely take a horse to water, but you certainly cannot make him drink. In my mind, I had to finish the book. I used to be a fairly conditioned athlete, but I had become a complete slacker.

Nagging sometimes pays off. Some people are highly motivated, but most people are not. Most people need an initial push to get them underway. Once people get into the rhythm of regular exercises, many become impressed by the benefits. The increased sense of wellbeing and improved physical performance are enough incentives for many to continue. I can now understand why some people get hooked on exercising, even to the point of becoming obsessed or narcissistic. The benefits that accompany renewed vigor and a handsome body are the highs on which many exercise junkies ride. Better a good habit than a bad one, but as explained in Chapter 1, even a virtue can become a vice.[64-68]

Exercise and Physical Activity
—Personal Reflections

> The time to make time is the very time
> that you say that you don't have the time.

My father was a radical and fiercely independent man who was never afraid to speak his mind. He left home at the age of twelve to earn a living. This was the customary age in 1930s Belize when a boy left home to learn a trade. This certainly left its mark on him. His reality was to survive and provide food and education for a string of children—a dozen in toto, most of whom pursued academic excellence abroad. In his mind gymnasiums and sports were luxuries, gimmicks, and antics. Exercise for a struggling man meant the weekly trip to the family farm to till, to plant, and to harvest. Weekdays meant manual work in the carpenter shop. For my father these paid great dividends, not only in providing sustenance, but also in learning principles for successful living and the value of hard work and perseverance.

Once upon a time I was a slacker; the never-ending treadmill of medical studies robbed me of much needed physical exploits. My renewed interest in exercise is now in its third year. It has been truly rewarding, and I have not looked back since. I no longer make excuses. I have learned that the very time we need to make time is the very time we say that we don't have the time.

It Is All About Choices

Many say they have no time to exercise, yet somehow find three or more hours *daily* to watch television.

Enough has been said about the need for more physical activity and exercise.[75] Get moving. These are action words. Remaining sedentary and physically inactive is a choice. The opposite is also true.

Summary

Physical inactivity is a major risk factor for many chronic diseases. Increasing urbanization and modernity has bred sedentary lifestyles. This has helped to fuel the present global epidemic of obesity, cardiovascular diseases, type II diabetes, and cancer. The benefits of being physically active are many. Physical, mental, and psychological benefits are achievable even without the need for athleticism. Increasing physical activity and exercise can lead to improved management and prevention of several chronic diseases. Structured exercises can provide much needed discipline for many who confront the pressures of modern living. As good as structured exercises may be, they are not for everyone. Populations and individuals need to be encouraged to find practical ways of weaving increased physical activity into their daily lifestyles.

Many have reaped the rewards of physically active lifestyles. For those who are yet to get moving. It is worth the reminder that physical activity is not something you say— it is something you do.

******

Chapter 10

Making Choices That Last
...From Knowledge to Action

Chapter Outline

Refuse to Be Confused 387
A Simple Perspective: Complicate it Not 388
Needed … Nutrition Education 389
People Can Change 389
On Attitudes, Perspectives, and Behavior 390
What is it that you Want, What are you aiming for? 392
Making Choices That Last Means Going Beyond Circumstances 392
Good Changes Do Not Occur Overnight 394
Going for the Long Haul 395
People Who Succeed Are Willing To Take Responsibility 395
Beyond Nutrition and Lifestyle 396
Summary and Conclusion 396

Successes have come about where people have acknowledged that the unnecessary premature deaths that occur in their community are largely preventable and have empowered themselves and their civic representatives to create health-supporting environments. Beyond the rhetoric, this epidemic can be halted—the demand for action must come from those affected. The solution is in our hands.

Joint WHO/FAO Expert Report[1]
on Diet, Nutrition and the Prevention of Chronic Disease
Executive Summary, March 2, 2003.

Better is the end of a thing than the beginning…
[It is not how you start … it is how you finish]
The Teacher (Ecclesiastes)[2]

Knowledge is important...but what you do with knowledge is far more important.
Why is it that so many people know…yet still so many fail to do?

§§§§§§§§

Refuse To Be Confused

Then we will no longer be infants, tossed back and forth by the waves, and blown here and there by every wind of doctrine ... (Letter to residents of Efes 4:14)

The body of nutrition knowledge itself seems unstable, ideas change quickly, and recommendations tend to contradict one another, so that physicians tend to distrust even the nutrition data they receive. For example, within a short time, margarine was good for you and not good for you. Fish oil was important and not important (aside from its expense and non-palatability). Protein sparing fasting as a treatment for obesity was put on the map by one of the most respected authorities in the field from Harvard, and shown within a year to be potentially lethal. The Joslin Clinic pushed low calorie diets that a human being could hardly follow. The National Institutes of Health suggested low fat and low cholesterol diets in ways that were difficult for both professionals and lay people to understand.

Commentary by David Singer, M.D.
Harvard Medical School

Your Doctor Can't Make You Healthy is a trustworthy account of important perspectives needed to equip you for better health. The first ten chapters discussed facts wrapped up with insights that provide a comprehensive grounding on lifestyle and health. Readers should now be well-equipped to separate the wheat from the chaff. It is my hope that you have grasped, in just a few pages, the essence of what it took me half my life to learn.

The challenge that lies ahead, however, will not be so much a matter of "knowing," but a matter of "doing." This is the focus of this chapter. The maxim, "some people make things happen, some people watch things happen, and some people wonder what happened," is expounded in this chapter.

This is the shortest chapter in this book, but it can easily be the most important. For here is where the rubber meets the road. After reading all these books and learning all this knowledge, it would be tragic if the information fails to make a difference. My wish is that you could insert a few coins into the health machine, pick up your can, and drink 12 oz. of healthy lifestyles. But it does not work that way, and furthermore, no part of this book is about hype and quickies.

As I have grown older, I have become far more impressed with what people do than with what they know, or say that they know. There is a principle which says that "knowledge without application is abortion" (in the true sense of the word). My primary concern is that we achieve results, and results that will last. The principles outlined herein are not my invention, but they are principles that work. They have been tested through the ages and have relevance for more than just challenges for good health. They also bear wider relevance to life. This what has worked for me, and this is what I share.

A Simple Perspective: Complicate It Not

Just as bad choices can lead to a host of health problems, so can better choices prevent, halt, and sometimes reverse many of these same problems. It is that simple.

Our bodies function best when they are treated the way that they were designed to be treated. In the same manner that cars were assembled to use certain fuels and foundations built to support certain structures, so were our bodies meant to receive special care. We were designed to inhale clean air, not smoke; to eat good food, not junk; and to be active, not sedentary.

We are witnessing the fallout resulting from a failure to appreciate the fundamental connection between design and purpose. If we have successfully re-formulated almost everything in our food supply, and if we have pursued the path of unbridled excesses, how can we reasonably expect to reap anything other than the seeds we have sown? With 60 percent of Americans overweight and 50 million affected by the metabolic syndrome (the forerunner of cardiovascular diseases, diabetes, and premature death) are we not reaping the harvest from the seeds of unhealthy choices?[3]

As are the problems, so are the solutions. The same way we dug ourselves into this predicament is the same manner through which we must extricate ourselves. Just as bad choices led to a host of health problems, so can better choices prevent, halt, and sometimes reverse many of these same problems. It is that simple.

A healthy lifestyle can help you not only lose weight, but it can simultaneously lower your blood pressure, your cholesterol, and your triglycerides. These in turn can lower your risk for having a heart attack, type II diabetes, and cancer. When good nutrition is accompanied by increased physical activity and avoidance of smoking, these escort you a long way on the road to optimal health. These have been summarized in the charts at the beginning of this book. This is the big picture. Do not get distracted by majoring on the minors.

Needed: Nutrition Education

Nutrition education is not an overnight affair. Making good choices in today's world is an unprecedented challenge. We no longer live in those days when you had little choice but to marry the girl or the guy next door. That was in a time when people simply settled for whatever was on offer. Today we are bombarded by so many options, in so many ways, using so many means which makes it easier to understand why people seem so bewildered by the confusion. No generation of earthlings in the history of mankind has had to endure such an unrelenting barrage of choices.

Therefore, navigating through this maze requires knowledge. But this demands more than academic knowledge. This knowledge must be able to see clearly through the haze, strong enough to survive the storms, and exit thereafter with its focus still intact. This is the knowledge that will lead to choices that will last. It is encouraging to see more people making just such choices.[4]

Whatever the motivation, efforts to prevent lifestyle-related diseases mandate the need for a clear understanding of diet-disease and diet-health relationships. These issues have been settled in the previous chapters. The task now is to embark on making the necessary changes, but lasting changes must first begin in the mind. This is an individual decision, but it is a crucial prerequisite for change.

People Can Change

Change starts by making choices.
Choices then become habits, and habits, lifestyles.

Human beings, despite inclinations towards excesses, are endowed with the power to choose. The real challenges are the following: Do people really want to change? And if they do, what will it take for them to translate what they know and what the want into what they really do? This is an age-old struggle of humankind.

A study appearing in the journal *Appetite* examined certain characteristics that influenced people's choice of healthier foods.[5] They noted that vegetarians or people who took dietary supplements were more likely to pursue healthy choices. Being married, having a college-level education, and a higher socioeconomic status were reasonable predictors of positive lifestyle choices. These individuals are more likely to translate what they know into what they practice.

There is a less encouraging story. According to Maslow's pyramid of needs, people who are "broke, busted, and disgusted," may be struggling just to survive (see Chapter 7). In this scenario, having a satisfied stomach becomes a priority. It is easy at this level of the pyramid to be heavily preoccupied with securing food and drink. This is where many find refuge and great contentment. People in distress care little about future health concerns. They are served a far less exciting menu—survival, finding a job, or keeping the family safe and well fed. In such settings recommendations to increase fruit and vegetable intake are more likely to fall on deaf ears.[6,7]

Nevertheless, even in such settings, people can be empowered to embrace good choices. Despite socioeconomic and other hurdles, people can change. This was the finding of the "Atherosclerosis Risk in Communities Study" (ARICS). Poor people would like to be healthy too. Urban American populations, especially minority groups, made significant changes to their food choices when provided with the same opportunity. Unfortunately, these communities are far more likely to be saturated with fast-food outlets and corner-shops instead of green grocers and supermarkets.[8]

On Attitudes, Perspectives, and Behavior

Why is it that so many people know…
yet still so many fail to do?

Attitudes affect choices (Figure 7-1). Attitudes often have roots that extend deep into culture, upbringing, and value systems. Knowing the issues that affect choices is one thing. Implementing them is an entirely different matter. Why is it that so many people know, yet still so many fail to do? Changing attitudes towards healthy lifestyles are crucial for making choices that last.[5]

Tackling attitudes is never easy. It is a highly personal affair that individuals must sort out for themselves. This book is a presentation of knowledge wrapped up in my attitudes. It is a reflection of a mindset that has been cultivated by a combination of my upbringing, training, and experience. Doctors are often guilty of practicing medicine in an unreal world. I was one of them until a reality-check occurred after I came face to face with real people, without medical insurance or social safety nets, who often exhausted their hard earned money on medical bills.

I found it tragic that patients would return for visits month after month and year after year with the same problems, or rather frequently, with complications. These things troubled me. My conscience refused to allow me to keep going through the motions. We had to seek solutions. I developed a reputation for telling patients that "I am too old and too busy to waste your money and my time, if we are not going anywhere." Every doctor knows that there are things that we can fix, and there are things that we cannot fix. What we are talking about here are not magical cures, but the simple changes outlined in this book. These are things that can work.

The longer I observe human behavior, the more it becomes clear why some people succeed, while others do not. But to achieve results, we need to engage in self-examination, not out of narcissism or lack of anything else to do, but because we strive towards a goal. As the saying goes—if you fail to plan, you plan to fail. People who succeed are not interested in taking diversions that lead to nowhere. They remain focused. Speed bumps, potholes, and bridges are also part of the journey, but keep your hands on the wheel and your eyes focused on your destination.

It is all well and good for people to quote studies and statistics, but these will not be very relevant when it comes to looking at yourself in the mirror. For there you will see your face—in the prison of your own mind, trying to sort out your own issues, your decisions, and those things that make you tick. Having struggled with my own issues and working with friends and patients who aspire to live healthy, I will outline strategies that should prove useful. These are strategies and perspectives that have worked in my life, and I have seen them work in the lives of others (Table 10-1).

Table 10-1. Perspectives for Making Choices that Last

Helpful Perspectives for Making Choices that Last
• What is it that you want? What are you aiming for?
• Making choices that last means going beyond the circumstances
• Good changes do not occur overnight
• Going for the long haul
• People who succeed are willing to take responsibility
• Beyond nutrition and lifestyle

What Is It That You Want, What Are You Aiming For?

Set your own agenda ...
Lest someone else will set it for you.

It has been my custom to ask patients what they wish, or expect, from their consultation. Some patients are quite focused. They want their quick fixes, and then hastily exit. Others tarry longer, preferring a deeper and more meaningful encounter. Many patients have become accustomed to short consultations where only their immediate problems are addressed. Most settle for what is on offer because their options are few. Others, because of previous experience and negative perceptions of the medical profession, show up only after something is dreadfully wrong.

If prevention is your aim, you need to know that it should start at whatever your age, whether you are 15 or 50, and at whatever your stage, whether you are sick or enjoying good health. But the decision is yours. You must choose if you will simply settle for what is on offer, or whether you will do your best to look after your own health. The benefits have been outlined throughout this book.

If your aim is to settle for the mere treatment of disease, then that is largely what you will get. But there is another way, clearly outlined in this book, which goes beyond the customary servings of medical care. You can settle just to treat your disease, or you can decide to aim for optimal health. This is where it all starts. You will have to decide what it is that you want before you can move to the next stage.

Making Choices That Last means Going Beyond the Circumstances

The road to self care and optimal health is fraught with
negative challenges that militate against success.
These can either be seen as
stumbling blocks or as stepping stones.
What you see depends on *how* you perceive.

There is a culture of blame that is prevalent in today's world. Name the problem, and you will see the many faces of the games that are played. Slavery, wars, terrorism, poverty ... just name it. Who must we blame? The world is far from a perfect place, but there are those who still believe that the way to go is to trade an eye for an eye. Logic would dictate that if this principle is followed to the letter, it will leave us so blinded that we will be unable to see the way forward. So here lies another challenge. Adverse circumstances in life are bound to come, but what am I / you doing to be a part of the solution and not a part of the problem? Those who never-endingly harp on blaming others, typically do very little to strive for solutions.

People love a David and Goliath story.[11] Part of the human psyche loves to support the underdog. We love to hear stories of people succeeding against great odds. This is the intrigue of the Nelson Mandela story, the man who went from prisoner to president, reminiscent of Joseph in Pharaoh's Egypt, who escaped the pit and prison before becoming prime minister.[12] If these people had focused solely on their prevailing negative circumstances, such stories would have never been told. We all know of many such stories that are closer to home.

I have great admiration for the young lady with the charming smile who became the first woman to win five track-and-field Olympic medals in a single Olympics (Sydney, 2000). This is what Marion Jones is famous for, and rightly so. Few people know (or care) what I admire her most for. Marion triumphed despite serious fractures to her limbs—the very tools she needed to make her mark in athletic history. Fewer still may know that this young lady, who made America proud, has her roots that hail from the country of my birth. You can never truly appreciate a product without delving into the processes that produced that product. In life, most people never see beyond the gloss and the headlines. We adore the product, but pay scant regard for the process.

Attitudes

Life is 10 percent of what happens to you, and 90 percent of how you react to it.

Insights for Living, Chuck Swindoll[13]

This is why I like biographies. They often reflect the accounts of ordinary human beings who triumphed in the midst of difficult circumstances, and provide touching insights into some of the most remarkable stories of our time. People who have lost limbs, or deaf, or blind, have gone on to climb mountains, composed the finest music, or sing the most evocative songs.

Adversity is the mark of a man (and a woman). The challenge is to make the most of your circumstances. Turn your mess into a message. Give it your best shot. Do what you are supposed to do, and aspire always to be a part of the solution and not a part of the problem.

This is what the behavior therapists know as self-efficacy.[14] It describes as an individual's confidence in his or her ability to make decisions and persevere in the midst of life's hurdles and challenges. Psychologists describe this attitude in their social cognitive theory (SCT) of human behavior. One of its tenets is that people learn by personal experience as well as the experiences of others. If she or he can succeed, so can I. Setting goals and exercising the required discipline and perseverance, are crucial ingredients for success.[15-19]

What does all this have to do with nutrition and choices? These principles can prove successful when applied to the hurdles that stand in the way of healthy nutrition and lifestyles. The hurdles of socioeconomics, demographics, and others that are listed in Chapter 7, will pale in comparison to the barriers others face. In many parts of our world today, people are struggling just to eat enough to survive; in our indulgent societies many are eating themselves to death.

Where there is life there will be obstacles, but these we must move beyond. The task is not insurmountable. It is not a call to go to the moon. It is a down-to-earth challenge to encourage you to make simple choices for your health. And just in case you don't really care much about yourself, at least consider doing it for those who care about you.

Good Changes Do Not Occur Overnight

A journey of a thousand miles begins with a single step…
Chinese proverb

Chronic diseases never occur overnight. This is one instance in medicine when you don't have to hesitate to use the word "never". People never gain 50 pounds overnight, and serious harm can befall those who insist on pursuing such schemes. Therefore, let us stop all the madness about quick fixes and overnight solutions (see Chapter 2, Chapter 8). Show me instant success, and I can show you a disaster in the making. Fad diets have led not only to loss of fat but also to the loss also of vital proteins in essential organs, including the heart. These have even resulted in heart rhythm disturbances and death.[20-21]

Life involves a continual process of learning and unlearning. My journey towards good nutrition was not an overnight affair. I am still learning. During my early university years, nutrition choices were held hostage by a meager student budget. Eating for health purposes was never a deciding factor. Convenience and costs had the final say. As I moved from being a student to a doctor, so did my options. Foods have since taken on new meanings, and these I have sprinkled throughout this book. My journeys around the world have been a great source of practical insights that complemented my academic knowledge. The choices I now make are the result of this ongoing re-education process, but the changes in my behavior and lifestyle took time.

Going For the Long Haul

> Better is the end of a thing than the beginning…
> [it is not how you start…it is how you finish]
> The Teacher (Ecclesisastes)[2]

To persevere on this path, we need to off-load a major hindrance to long-term success. We live in an "instant" culture where patience seems no longer a virtue and where convenience has all but replaced commitment. People's attention spans are getting shorter, and few dare watch television without the ever-present finger on the remote control. We have become experts at changing horses in midstream. If you translate this attitude into your lifestyle, and then see healthy living as a complete drag, the odds are unlikely that you will ever persevere.

Healthy living is to be enjoyed every step of the way. It must never be a killjoy or a sadistic exercise (Chapter1). The lifelong journey towards optimal health should be like switching gears while biking, but never losing sight of the wonderful scenery, or forgetting to stop and smell the roses.

People Who Succeed Are Willing To Take Responsibility, They Take Charge

> Like a city whose walls are broken down
> is the man/woman who lacks self-control [discipline].
> Sayings of the Wise (Proverbs) [23]

On this journey, success requires a deep understanding of personal responsibility. People who succeed are not in the habit of making excuses. Neither do they wait for their environment to change before committing themselves. The pressures of modern living are here to stay. The media houses will advertise what they are paid to advertise. The supermarkets will sell whatever they decide to sell. No one is going to tie your hands or place blinders over your eyes while you stroll along the supermarket aisles. That is a choice you must make for yourselves. It is up to you (and your wallet) to decide.

A disciplined lifestyle is not a call to extremism. I do not subscribe to the cliché that says you are what you eat. People are more than what they eat. But the foods people eat can reflect broader insights into their lives. Show me someone who buys everything in sight and eats everything in sight, and I will show you someone who is completely out of control. We are responsible for our choices. The blame game is for losers.

Beyond Nutrition and Lifestyle

Good choices in nutrition and lifestyle are best pursued by paying attention to the whole person—physical, psychological, social, financial, and spiritual.

Being a physically healthy person is good, but becoming mentally, physically, and spiritually healthy is far better. The physical realm is the mode in which many problems manifest themselves. We are naturally drawn to what is seen and pay scant attention to what is unseen. This explains why the thief stole the monitor and tried to sell it as the computer. He had no clue where the real processes occurred.

It is easy to focus only on a person's weight, their diabetes, or their heart disease. We often fail to recognize that there are deeper issues going on in people's lives, beyond those things that we see. A sermon on diet and exercise may be the last thing this person needs. People are better off getting a grip on their life before they can be expected to get a grip on their health. Therefore, in our efforts to promote healthy lifestyles, we must not confuse the monitor with the computer, but remember that we need both.

I invite you to embark on the journey towards good health. Don't wait until you lose it before you start to appreciate it. It is my sincere hope that the arguments and the perspectives outlined in these pages will go the distance in your journey towards optimal health. At least give it a good try, you have nothing to lose and everything to gain.

Summary and Conclusion

A lot has been said. It is time to embark on the journey. We are no longer spectators; we are participants. The call for good health is a call to a better lifestyle. To all who dare to embark on this journey, I encourage you to follow the perspectives outlined in this book. This is the final chapter, but it is not the end. Keep on learning. There is good reward for making good choices.

******

PART VI

Book Resources

References

Book Resources

General Index

References

The scheme used is Vancouver style superscript system Journal names are abbreviated according to the style used in Index Medicus used by the following: the U.S. National Library of Medicine: http://www.nlm.nih.gov/tsd/serials/lsiou.html, or as appears in the "Journal Database" of PubMed: http://www.ncbi.nlm.nih.gov/entrez/query.fcgi?db=PubMed. Where online references are cited, every effort was made to source established websites.

Introduction

1. Victoria Declaration on Heart Health: A call for action. Declaration of the Advisory Board. International Heart Health Conference. Victoria, Canada 1992:p 15. Retrieved May 2002 from http://www.med.mun.ca/chhdbc/pdf/victr_e.pdf.
2. U.S. Surgeon General. The Surgeon General's report on nutrition and health. U.S. Department of Health and Human Services, 1998.
3. National Center for Health Statistics. Births and deaths—United States, 1996. Monthly Vital Statistics Report 1997;46(Suppl 2).
4. The World Health Report 2002—Reducing risks, promoting healthy life. Geneva, World Health Organization, 2002.
5. Hoffman C, Rice D, Sung H-Y. Persons with chronic conditions: their prevalence and costs. JAMA 1997;276:1473-9.
6. Ginzberg E. Ten encounters with the U.S. health sector, 1930-1999. JAMA 1999; 282: 1665-8.
7. Anderson R, Kochanek K, Murphy S. Advance report of final monthly statistics. Monthly vital statistics report. Hyattsville (MD): National Center for Health Statistics; 1995.
8. Cohen JW, Krauss NA. Spending and service use among people with the fifteen most costly medical conditions, 1997. Health Aff (Millwood) 2003, 22(2):129-38. Last retrieved April 2003 from www.healthaffairs.org/1100_table_contents.php.
9. U.S. Department of Health and Human Services, Healthy People 2010 Objectives: Draft for public comment. Office of Public Health and Science 1998.
10. Mokdad A, Serdula M, Dietz W, Bowman B, Marks J, Koplan J. The spread of the obesity epidemic in the United States from 1991 to 1998. JAMA 1999;282:1519-22.
11. Mokdad A, Ford ES, Bowman B, Nelson DE, Engelgau MM, Vinicor F, et al. Diabetes trends in the U.S. from 1990 to 1998. Diabetes Care 2000;23:1278-83.
12. International Diabetes Federation. Triennial report and directory from 1991 to 1994; 1994.
13. American Diabetes Association. Direct and indirect costs of diabetes in the United States in 1992. Alexandria, (VA): American Diabetes Association;1993.
14. Rubin RJ, Altman WM, Mendelson DN. Healthcare expenditures for people with diabetes mellitus in 1992. JCEM 1994;78:809A-F.
15. American Diabetes Association. Economic consequences of diabetes mellitus in the U.S. in 1997. Diabetes Care 2000;21:296-309.
16. Centers for Disease Control Diabetes in Managed Care Work Group. Diabetes mellitus in managed care: complications and resource utilization. Am J Manag Care 2001;7(5):501-8.

17. Diabetes Control and Complications Trial Research Group. Lifetime benefits and costs of intensive therapy as practiced in the Diabetes Control and Complications Trial. JAMA 1996;276:1409-15.

18. King H, Aubert R, Herman W. Global Burden of Diabetes 1995-2025: Prevalence, numerical estimates, and projections. Diabetes Care 1998;21(Suppl 9):1414-31.

19. Dalen JE. Health Care in America: The good, the bad, the ugly. JAMA 2000;160:17.

20. Gruman JC. Letters. Newsweek Magazine, February 7, 2001.

21. Kamm R. Letters. Time Magazine, February 5, 2001.

22. Eskin F. Public health medicine: the constant dilemma. J Public Health Med 2002;24(1):6-10.

23. Williams RD 2nd. Restructuring Medicare: a synthesis of the NASI Medicare projects. Medicare Brief 2003;(9):1-8.

24. Relman AS, Angell M. America's other drug problem: how the drug industry distorts medicine and politics. New Repub 2002;227(25):27-41.

25. Kuttner R. The American health care system: Health insurance coverage. N Engl J Med 1999;340:163-8.

26. Hoffman C, Rice, Sung H-Y. Persons with chronic conditions: their prevalence and costs. JAMA 1997;276:1473-1479.

27. Patrick WK, Cadman EC. Changing emphases in public health and medical education in health care reform. Asia Pac J Public Health 2002;14(1):35-9.

28. Ssemakula JK. The impact of 9/11 on HIV/AIDS care in Africa and the Global Fund to Fight AIDS, Tuberculosis, and Malaria. J Assoc Nurses AIDS Care 2002;13(5):45-56.

29. Harris Interactive Health Care News v2 i9. Cyberchondriacs Continue to Grow in America 2002 Retrieved June 2002 from http://www.harrisinteractive.com/news/newsletters/healthnews/HI_HealthCareNews2002 Vol2_Iss09.pdf.

30. Bendich A, Deckelbaum RJ. Preventive nutrition throughout the life cycle. In: Bendich A, Deckelbaum R, eds. Primary and secondary preventive nutrition. Totowa (NJ): Humana Press Inc. 2001; pp 427-441.

31. Willett WC. Potential benefits of preventive nutrition strategies: lessons for the United States. In: Bendich A, Deckelbaum R, eds. Primary and secondary preventive nutrition. Totowa (NJ): Humana Press Inc. 2001; pp 450.

32. Block G, Patterson BH, Subar AF. Fruit, vegetables, and cancer prevention: a review of the epidemiological evidence. Nutr Cancer 1992;18:1-29.

33. Reaven GM. Banting Lecture 1988. Role of insulin resistance in human disease. Diabetes 1988;37:1595-1607.

34. Reaven GM. Insulin resistance: a chicken that has come to roost. Ann NY Acad Sci 2001;892:45-57.

35. Field AE, Coakley EH, Must A. Impact of overweight on the risk of developing common chronic diseases during a 10-year Period. Arch Intern Med 2001;161:1581-6.

36. Reaven, Lithell, Landsberg. Hypertension and associated metabolic abnormalities—the role of insulin resistance syndrome and the sympathoadrenal system. N Engl J Med 1996;334:374-81.

37. Joint WHO/FAO Expert Report on Diet, Nutrition and the Prevention of Chronic Disease. Executive Summary 2003. Department of Noncommunicable Disease Prevention and Health Promotion. Retrieved March 2003 from http://www.who.int/hpr/nutrition/expertconsultationge.htm.

38. Willet WC. Nutritional Epidemiology, 2nd Edition. Oxford University Press. New York;1998.

39. Willet WC. Overview of nutritional epidemiology. In: Nutritional Epidemiology, 2nd Edition. New York: Oxford University Press; 1998; pp 11-12.

40. Underwood A, Springen K, Davis A. Cancer and Diet. Newsweek 1998:48-54.

Chapter 1

1. Anderson GF. Americans worry about chronic illness, look to Congress for help – Press Conference (2000). Retrieved August 1, 2001 from Reuters: http://www.medscape.com/reuters/prof/2001/02/02.27/20010226plcy001.html.
2. Bagshaw JL. Time Magazine, Letters. 2001.
3. Smith DR. Porches, politics, and public health. Am J Public Health. 1994;84:725-6.
4. Lown B. The lost art of healing: practicing compassion in medicine. New York: Ballantine Books, 1999. pp xiv,xv,xvii.
5. Health Law Reporter. 2001;10:389. Retrieved August 1, 2001 from http://subscript.bna.com/SAMPLES/hlr.nsf/.
6. Ginzberg E. Ten encounters with the U.S. health sector, 1930-1999. JAMA. 1999; 282:1665-8.
7. U.S. Department of Justice, Office of Justice Programs, Bureau of Justice Statistics. Prison Statistics: summary findings 2002. http://www.ojp.usdoj.gov/bjs/prisons.htm.
8. Kuttner R. The American health care system: Health insurance coverage. N Engl J Med 1999;340:163-8.
9. Hoffman C, Rice, Sung H-Y. Persons with chronic conditions: their prevalence and costs. JAMA 1997;276:1473-1479.
10. Wolf A, Colditz G. Social and economic effects of body weight in the United States. Am J Clin Nutr 1996;63:466S-469S.
11. Lown B. The lost art of healing: practicing compassion in medicine. New York: Ballantine Books, 1999. pp xiv,xv,xvii.
12. Berg C, Jonsson I, Conner M, Lissner L. Perceptions and reasons for choice of fat- and fibre-containing foods by Swedish schoolchildren. Appetite 2003 ;40(1):61-7.
13. Kearney JM, McElhone S. Perceived barriers in trying to eat healthier--results of a pan-EU consumer attitudinal survey. Br J Nutr 1999;81 Suppl 2:S133-7.
14. Scalera G. Effects of conditioned food aversions on nutritional behavior in humans. Nutr Neurosci 2002;5(3):159-88.
15. van Dam RM, Rimm EB, Willett WC, Stampfer MJ, Hu FB. Dietary patterns and risk for type 2 diabetes mellitus in U.S. men. Ann Int Med 2002;136(3):201-209.
16. Jospipura KJ, et al. Fruit and Vegetable Intake in Relation to Risk of Ischemic Stroke. JAMA 282 1999:1233-9.
17. Ness AR, Poles JW. Fruits and vegetables and cardiovascular diseases. A review. Int J Epidemiol 1997;26:1-13.
18. Cohen JH, Kristal AR, Stanford JL. Fruit and vegetable intakes and prostate cancer risk. J Natl Cancer Inst 1977;58:825-32.
19. Temple NJ. Fruits, vegetables and cancer prevention trials. J Natl Cancer Inst 1999;91(13):1164.
20. Garcia-Closas R, Gonzalez CA, Agudo A, Riboli E. Intake of specific carotenoids an flavonoids and the risk of gastric cancer in Spain. Cancer Causes Control 1999;10(1):71-5.
21. Trichopoulou A, Katsouyanni K, Gnardellis C. The traditional Greek diet. Eur J Clin Nutr. 1993;47 Suppl 1:S76-81. Review.
22. Murcott A. The cultural significance of food and eating. Proc Nutr Soc. 1982;41(2):203-10.
23. Popkin BM. Nutrition in transition: the changing global nutrition challenge.Asia Pac J Clin Nutr. 2001;10 Suppl:S13-8.
24. Fraser D, Abu-Saad K, Abu-Shareb H. The relative importance of traditional and "modern" foods for Israeli Negev Bedouins. A population in transition. Nutr Metab Cardiovasc Dis. 2001;11(4 Suppl):66-9.
25. Caballero B, Rubinstein S. Environmental factors affecting nutritional status in urban areas of developing countries. Arch Latinoam Nutr. 1997;47(2 Suppl 1):3-8. Review.
26. de Oliveira SP. Changes in food consumption in Brazil.Arch Latinoam Nutr. 1997;47(2 Suppl 1):22-4. Review.

27. Musaiger AO. Changes in food consumption patterns in Bahrain. Nutr Health. 1990;6(4):183-8.
28. Papadaki A, Scott JA. The impact on eating habits of temporary translocation from a Mediterranean to a Northern European environment. Eur J Clin Nutr. 2002;56(5):455-61.
29. Jarvis WT. Food faddism, cultism, and quackery. Annu Rev Nutr. 1983;3:35-52. Review. No abstract available.
30. Frankle RT, Heussenstamm FK. Food zealotry and youth: new dilemmas for professionals. Am J Public Health. 1974 ;64(1):11-8. No abstract available.
31. Bratman S, Knight D. Health Food Junkies: Orthorexia Nervosa: Overcoming the obsession with healthful eating. JAMA 2001;285:2255-6.
32. Pratt EL. Historical perspectives: food, feeding, and fancies. J Am Coll Nutr. 1984;3(2):115-21.
33. Freedman MR, King J, Kennedy E. Popular diets: a scientific review. Obes Res 2001;9 Suppl 1:1S-40S.
34. Dietary Guidelines for Americans. USDA Home and Garden bulletin No. 232. 3rd ed. Washington, DC. Government Printing Office (1990-272-930), 1990.
35. Lown B. The lost art of healing: practicing compassion in medicine. New York: Ballantine Books, 1999. pp xiv.
36. Hersey H. New Answers To Old Questions: The free radical story. West Palm Beach, FL. HMHT Corporation.1989. pp Introduction August, 1989.
37. Stewart M. Towards a global definition of patient centered care. Br Med J 2001;322:444-5.
38. Alspach G. Patient satisfaction with healthcare services: time to listen up. Crit Care Nurse 1997;17(3):10-1.
39. W.H.O. Division of Noncommunicable Diseases and Health Care Technology. W.H.O. Guidelines for the Development of a National Programme for Diabetes Mellitus. Division of Noncommunicable Diseases and Health Care Technology. W.H.O. 1991:5.
40. Dalen JE. Health Care in America: The Good, The Bad, and The Ugly [Electronic version]. Arch Intern Med. 2000;160:2573-6.
41. Aston G. Surplus now, but red ink looming in Medicare forecast. American Medical News 2001;1(1).
42. Editor's choice. Restoring the soul of medicine. Br Med J 2001;322:444-5.

Chapter 2

1. Nebergall PJ. Obesity and Diabetes: No quick fix. Retrieved March 2001 from http://www.nfb.org/.
2. Epstein AM, Drazen JM, Steinbrook R. Editorial, Health Policy 2001, A new series. N Engl J Med 2001;344:10.
3. Burkitt D. Canadian Medical Association Journal 2000. Burkitt D. Related disease – related cause? Lancet 1969;2:1229-31.
4. Schaffer Library of Drug Policy. Historical research on drug policy—general historical reviews. Retrieved March 2001 from http://www.druglibrary.org/schaffer/History/HISTORY.HTM
5. Deuteronomy 28:1-28. Holy Bible, New International Version 1978, Committee on Bible Translation.
6. Blumenthal, D. Controlling Health Care Expenditures. Health Policy 2001.[Electronic version] N Engl J Med 2001;344:9.
7. Prescription Drug Expenditures in 2001. Another year of escalating costs. Revised May 6, 2002. A report by the National Institute of Health Care Management Research and Educational Foundation. http://www.nihcm.org/spending2001.pdf.
8. Editorial 2001. Br Med J 2001;322:804.
9. Rosenbaum M. Marketing to schools. The Guardian 1993.

10. Lee Bowman.Scripps Howard News Service. 2000. Retrieved August, 2001 from http://www.reporternews.com/2000/ads/health2/drug.html.

11. Wilkes MS, Bell RA, Kravitz RL. Direct-to-consumer prescription drug advertising: trends, impact, and implications. Health Aff (Millwood) 2000;19(2):110-28. http://www.healthaffairs.org/Library/v19n2/s10.pdf - 254.1KB

12. Bradley LR, Zito JM. Direct-to-consumer prescription drug advertising. Medical care 1992;35(1):86-92.

13. Judd J. Truth in advertising? FDA says many prescription drug ads are deceptive. ABC WorldNews Tonight, 2001 3; Retrieved January 2001 from http://abcnews.go.com/sections/wnt/.

14. Bowman L. Pill-pushing ads fuel prescription drug industry. Scripps Howard news service 2000. Retrieved December 2000 from http://www.reporternews.com/2000/ads/health2/.

15. Yamey G, Drug-free Practitioners. West J Med 2001;174:163.

16. Lexchin J. What information do physicians receive from pharmaceutical representatives? Can Fam Phys 1997;43:941-945.

17. Lexchin J. Interactions between physicians and the pharmaceutical industry: what does the literature say? CMAJ. 1993; 149:1401-7.

18. Wazana, A. Physicians and the Pharmaceutical Industry: Is a gift ever just a gift? JAMA. 2000; 283, No 3.

19. Chren MM, Landefeld S, Murray TH. Doctors, drug companies, and gifts. JAMA 1989;262:3448-51.

20. Griffith D. Reasons for not seeing drug reps. BMJ. 1999; 319: 69-70.

21. Lexchin J. Doctors and detailers: Therapeutic education or pharmaceutical promotion? Int J Health Services. 1989;19:663-679.

22. Shaughnessy AF, and Slawson, DC. Pharmaceutical representatives (editorial). BMJ. 1996;312:1494.

23. Shaughnessy AF, Slawson DC, Bennett JH. Separating the wheat from the chaff: identifying fallacies in pharmaceutical promotion. J of Gen Int Med. 1994; 10:563-8.

24. Waud DR. Pharmaceutical promotions--a free lunch? N Engl J Med. 1992;327:351-3.

25. Wolfe, SM. Why do American drug companies spend more than $12 billion a year pushing drugs? Is it education or promotion? J of Gen Int Med. 1996.11; 637-9.

26. Chren MM, Landefeld CS. Physicians' behavior and their interaction with drug companies. JAMA. 1994;271:684-689.

27. Orlowski JP and Wateska L. The effects of pharmaceutical firm enticements on physician prescribing patterns. Chest. 1992; 102:270-273.

28. Avorn J, Chen M, Hartley R. Scientific versus commercial sources of influence on the prescribing behavior of physicians. Am J Med. 1982;73:4-8.

29. Chew, LD, et al. A Physician Survey of the Effect of Drug Sample Availability on Physicians' Behavior. J Gen Int Med. 2000;15: 478-483.

30. Caudill, TS, Johnson, MS, Rich EC, McKinney, WP. Physicians, pharmaceutical sales representatives, and the cost of prescribing. Arch of Fam Med. 1996;5:201-206.

31. Mendelsohn R. How to raise a healthy child in spite of your doctor. New York: Random House, Incorporated,1987.

32. Lam CL; Catarivas MG; Lauder IJ .Fam Pract, 1995;12(2): 171-5.

33. Boyer-Chammard A, Taylor TH, Anton-Culver H. Survival differences in breast cancer among racial/ethnic groups: a population-based study. Cancer Detect Prev 1999;23(6):463-73.

34. Mack TM, Hamilton AS, Press MF, Diep A, Rappaport EB. Heritable breast cancer in twins. Br J Cancer. 2002;87:294-300.

35. Haenszel W. Migrant Studies. In: Cancer epidemiology and prevention. Schottenfield, Fraumei JF eds. Philadelphia: WB Saunders, 1981.

36. Whelton PK, He J, Appel L. Treatment and Prevention of Hypertension. In: Prevention of Myocardial Infarction. Manson JE, Ridker PM, Gaziano JM, Hennekens CH ,eds. New York: Oxford University Press; 1996:154-155.

37. Barker Hypothesis Cadogan J, Eastell R, Jones N, Barker ME. Milk intake and bone mineral acquisition in adolescent girls: randomized, controlled intervention trial. Br Med J 1997;315:1255-60.

38. Rich-Edwards JW, et al. The primary prevention of coronary heart disease in women. New Engl J Med 1995;332;1758-66.

39. Michels KB, Trichopoulos D, Robins JM, Rosner BA, Manson JE, Hunter DJ, Colditz GA, Hankinson SE, Speizer FE, Willett WC. Birthweight as risk factor for breast cancer. Lancet 1996;348:1542-1546.

40. Reaven GM. Banting Lecture 1988. Role of insulin resistance in human disease. Diabetes 1988; 37:1595-1607.

41. Reaven GM. Insulin resistance: a chicken that has come to roost. Ann NY Acad Sci 2001;892:45-57.

42. Reaven GM, Lithell H, Landsberg L. Hypertension and associated metabolic abnormalities—the role of insulin resistance and the sympathoadrenal system. N Engl J Med 1996;334:374-381.

43. Zavaroni I, Mazza S, Dall'Aglio E, Gasparine P, Passeri M, Reaven GM. Prevalence of hyperinsulinaemia in patients with high blood pressure. J Int Med 1992;231:1128-1130.

44. Krentz AJ. Insulin resistance. Br Med J 1996;313:1385-1389.

45. McLaughlin T, Abbasi F, Kim HS, Lamendola C, Schaaf P, Reaven G. Relationship between insulin resistance, weight loss, and coronary heart disease risk in healthy, obese women. Metabolism 2001;50(7):795-800.

46. Carey DG. Abdominal obesity. Curr Opinio Lipidol 1998;9:35-40.

47. Turner NC, Clapham JC. Insulin resistance, impaired glucose tolerance and non-insulin dependent diabetes mellitus. Diabetes Res Clin Pract 1998; 42:91-99.

48. Boden G. Free fatty acids, a link between obesity and insulin resistance. Front Biosci 1998;3:D169-175.

49. Hansen BC. The Metabolic Syndrome X. Ann NY Acad Sci 1999;892:1-24.

50. Ford ES, Giles WH, Dietz WH. Prevalence of the Metabolic Syndrome Among US Adults. Findings from the Third National Health and Nutrition Examination Survey. JAMA 2002; 287:356-359.

51. Carr I. The far beginnings-a brief history of medicine. Hippocrates on the Web. University of Manitoba. Retrieved June 2002 from http://www.umanitoba.ca/faculties/medicine/units/history/histories/briefhis.html .

52. Walker M. Obesity, insulin resistance, and its link to non-insulin-dependent diabetes mellitus. Metabolism. 1995 Sep;44(9 Suppl 3):18-20. Review.

53. Boden G. Pathogenesis of type 2 diabetes. Insulin resistance.Endocrinol Metab Clin North Am. 2001;30(4):801-15, v. Review.

54. Paquot N, Scheen AJ, Dirlewanger M, Lefebvre PJ, Tappy L. Hepatic insulin resistance in obese non-diabetic subjects and in type 2 diabetic patients. Obes Res. 2002;10(3):129-34.

55. Bendich A, Deckelbaum R, eds. Primary and secondary preventive nutrition. Totowa (NJ): Humana Press Inc. 2001; pp 427.

56. The Merck Manual. Sixteenth Edition, Whitehouse Station, N.J.: Merck Research Laboratories,1992; pp 2477-2478.

57. The Merck Manual. Centennial (Seventeenth) Edition, Whitehouse Station, N.J.: Merck Research Laboratories, 1999; pp 2477-2478.

58. Shils ME, Olson JA, Shike M, eds. Modern nutrition in health and disease, 8th Ed. Vol.1: Philadelphia, PA: Lea & Febiger.1994; pp 444.

59. British National Formulary 37. British Medical Association and Royal Pharmaceutical Society of Great Britain, British Medical Association 1999.(Refer to the latest update available)

60. Lazarou J, Pomeranz BH, Corey PN, Incidence of adverse drug reactions in hospitalized patients: A meta-analysis of prospective studies. JAMA 1998;279:1200-1205.

61. The Merck Manual. Centennial (Seventeenth) Edition, Whitehouse Station, N.J.: Merck Research Laboratories, 1999; pp 2585-2586.

62. Hollman A. Plants in Cardiology. Br Med J 1992.

63. Dietary Supplements. U. S. Department of Health and Human Services. U.S. Food & Drug AdministrationCenter for Food Safety & Applied Nutrition. Retrieved May 2000 from http://www.cfsan.fda.gov/~dms/supplmnt.html.

64. Food and Nutrition Board, Institute of Medicine. How should the recommended dietary allowances be revised? Washington, DC: National Academy Press, 1994.

65. Ippolito P, Mathios A. Health claims in advertising and labeling: A study of the cereal market. Washington, DC: Bureau of Economics, Federal Trade Commission, 1989.

66. Food and Drug Administration. Labeling: general requirements for health claims for food. Federal Register 1993; 58:2787-2819. (Codified in Section 101.73, Title 21, Code of Federal Regulations.)

67. Food and Drug Administration. Food labeling: health claims and label statements; dietary saturated fat and cholesterol and coronary heart disease. Federal Register 1993; 58:2739-2786.

68. Food and Drug Administration. Food labeling: Health claims and label statements. Federal Register 2000;65:4252-4253.

69. Commission on dietary supplement labels. Report of the Commission on Dietary Supplement Labels. Washington, DC: Superintendent of Documents, 1997.

70. Food and Drug Administration. Regulations on statements made for dietary supplements concerning the effect of the product structure or function of the body; Final rule. Federal Register 2000;65:999-1050.

71. Milner JA. Nonnutritive components in foods as modifiers of the cancer process. In: Preventive nutrition: the comprehensive guide for health professionals. Bendich A, Deckelbaum RJ, eds. Totowa, NJ: Humana, 2001:131-154.

72. Graham HN. Green tea composition, consumption, and polyphenol chemistry. Prev Med 1992;21(3):334-50.

73. Steele Ve, Kelloff GJ, Balentine D, Boone CW, Mehta R, Bagheri D, et al. Comparative chemoprebioassays. Carcinogenesis 2000;21(1):63-7.

74. Hollman PC, Katan MB. Dietary flavonoids: intake, health effects and bioavailability. Food Chem Toxicol 1999;37(9,10):937-42.

75. Chow WH, Swanson CA, Lissowska J, Groves FD, Sobin LH, Nasierowska-Guttmejer A, et al. Risk of stomach cancer in relation to consumption of cigarettes, alcohol, tea and coffee in Warsaw, Poland. Int J Cancer 1999;81(6):871-6.

76. Mukhtar H, Katiyar SK, Agarwal R. Green tea and skin–anticarcinogenic effects. J Invest Dermatol 1994;102(1):3-7.

77. Kim DJ, Han BS, Ahn B, Hasegawa R, Shirai T, Ito N, et al. Enhancement by indole-3-carbinol of liver and thyroid gland neoplastic development in a rat medium-term multiorgan carcinogenesis model. Carcinogenesis 1997;18(2):377-81.

78. Rogers AE, Hafer LJ, Iskander YS, Yang S. Black tea and mammary gland carcinogenesis by 7,12-demethylbenz[a]anthracene in rats fed control or high fat diets. Carcinogenesis 1998; 19(7):1269-73.

79. Milner JA. Garlic: its antcarcinogenic and antitumorigenic properties. Nutr Rev 1996;54(11 Pt 2):S82-S86.

80. Shenoy NR, Choughuley AS. Inhibitory effect of diet and sulphydryl compounds on the formation of carcinogenic nitrosamines. Cancer Lett 1992;65(3):227-232.

81. Dion ME, Agler M, Milner JA. S-allyl cysteine inhibits nitrosmorpholine formation and bioactivation. Nutr Cancer 1997;28(1):1-6.

82. Milner JA. Nonnutritive components in foods as modifiers of the cancer process. In: Preventive nutrition: the comprehensive guide for health professionals. Bendich A, Deckelbaum RJ, eds. Totowa, NJ: Humana, 2001:145.

83. Elegbede JA, Maltzman TH, Verma AK, Tanner MA, Elson CE, Gould MN. Mouse skin tumor promoting activity of orange peel and d-limonene: a re-evaluation. Carcinogenesis 1986;7(12):2047-2049.

84. Underwood A, Springen K, Davis A. Cancer and Diet. Newsweek Magazine. 1998:48-54.

85. Taylor Hays J, Hurt RD, Dale LC. Smoking Cessation. In: Prevention of Myocardial Infarction. Manson JE, Ridker PM, Gaziano JM, Hennekens CH ,eds. New York: Oxford University Press; 1996:99-129.

86. Law MR, Wald NJ, Thompson SG. By how much and how quickly does reduction in serum cholesterol lower risk of ischaemic heart disease? Br Med J 1994;308:367-372.

87. HHS News. Diet and exercise dramatically delay type 2 diabetes medication. Metformin also effective. U.S. Department of Health and Human Services. For immediate release 2001 Retrieved August 2001 from http://www.nih.gov/news/pr/aug2001/niddk-08.htm.

88. Hankinson SE, Colditz GA, Manson JE, Speizer FE. eds. Healthy Women, Healthy Lives: A guide to preventing disease from the landmark Nurses' Health Study. New York: Simon & Schuster, 2001.

89. Grossman E, Messerli FH, Grodzicki T, Kowey P. Should a moratorium be placed on sublingual nifedipine capsules given for hypertensive emergencies and psuedoemergencies? JAMA. 1996;276:1328-31.

90. Schatzkin A, Lanza E, Corle D, Lance P, Iber F, Caan B, Shike M, Weissfeld J, Burt R, Cooper MR, Kikendall JW, Cahill J. Lack of effect of a low-fat, high-fiber diet on the recurrence of colorectal adenomas. Polyp Prevention Trial Study Group. N Engl J Med. 2000;342(16):1149-55.

Chapter 3

1. ADA. Position of the ADA. Nutrition Education for Health Care Professionals. J Am Diet Assoc 1998;98:343-6.

2. Nutrition in Medicine Project-University of North Carolina. KJN year. Retrieved August 2000, from http://www.med.unc.edu/nutr/nim/AboutNIM.htm.

3. Feldman EB. Educating physicians in nutrition: a view if the past, the present and the future. Am J Clin Nutr 1991:54:618-622.

4. Mann K, Putnam R. Physician's perceptions of their role in cardiovascular risk reduction. Prev Med 1989;18:45-58.

5. Perceptions of doctors and what they do. Editor's choice. Br Med J 2001;323.

6. McGinnis MJ, Ernst ND. Preventive nutrition: A historic perspective and future economic outlook. In: Bendich A, Deckelbaum R, eds. Primary and secondary preventive nutrition. Totowa (NJ): Humana Press Inc, 2001:11.

7. Jackson AA. Human nutrition in medical practice: the training of doctors. Proc Nutr Soc. 2001;60(2):257-63. Review.

8. Mennin SP, Krackov SK. Reflections on relevance, resistance, and reform in medical education. Acad Med 1998;73(9 Suppl):S60-4.

9. Roubenoff R, Roubenoff RA, Preto J, Balke CW. Malnutrition among hospitalized patients. A problem of physician awareness. Arch Intern Med 1987:147:1462-1465.

10. Greene J. After years of little variance in the way they teach students, medical schools are updating their courses. American Medical Association AMNews staff. 2000. Retrieved from http://www.ama-assn.org/sci-pubs/amnews.

11. Barzansky B, Jonas HS, Etzel SI. Educational Programs in U.S.Medical Schools 1998-1999 , JAMA. 1999;282:840-846.

12. The Committee on Nutrition in Medical Education. Nutrition Education in U.S. Medical Schools, 1985. Retrieved May 2001 from http://www.nap.edu/books/0309035872/html/R1.html.

13. James WPT. Historical perspective. In: Human nutrition and dietetics. Eight edition. Garrow JS, James WPT. Edinburgh: Churchill Livingstone, 1993; pp 1-11.

14. James WPT. Historical perspective. In: Human nutrition and dietetics. Eight edition. Garrow JS, James WPT. Edinburgh: Churchill Livingstone, 1993; pp 3.

15. James WPT. Historical perspective. In: Human nutrition and dietetics. Eight edition. Garrow JS, James WPT. Edinburgh: Churchill Livingstone, 1993; pp 2-5.

16. James WPT. Historical perspective. In: Human nutrition and dietetics. Eight edition. Garrow JS, James WPT. Edinburgh: Churchill Livingstone, 1993; pp 2-3.

17. James WPT. Historical perspective. In: Human nutrition and dietetics. Eight edition. Garrow JS, James WPT. Edinburgh: Churchill Livingstone, 1993; pp 6.

18. James WPT. Historical perspective. In: Human nutrition and dietetics. Eight edition. Garrow JS, James WPT. Edinburgh: Churchill Livingstone, 1993; pp 6-7.

19. Underwood A, Springen K, Davis A. Cancer and Diet. Newsweek Magazine. 1998; pp 48-54

20. Nutrition Education in U.S. Medical Schools (1985). Conclusions and recommendations.95-100. Committee on Nutrition in Medical Education, Food and Nutrition Board, National Research Council National Academy Press. http://www.nap.edu/catalog/597.html

21. Nutrition in Medicine Project-University of North Carolina). Retrieved August 2000 from http://www.med.unc.edu/nutr/nim/AboutNIM.htm.

22. Council on Scientific Affairs. Education for health: a role for physicians and the efficacy of health education efforts. JAMA 1990;263(13):1816-1819.

23. The Merck Manual. Sixteenth Edition, Whitehouse Station, N.J.: Merck Research Laboratories,1992; pp 2477-2478.

24. The Merck Manual. Centennial (Seventeenth) Edition, Whitehouse Station, N.J.: Merck Research Laboratories, 1999; pp 2477-2478.

25. Onish D, Brown SE, Sherwitz LW, et al.. Can lifestyle changes reverse coronary heart disease? Lancet 1990;336:129-133.

26. Rothman DJ. Medical professionalism: focusing on the real issues. N Engl J Med 2000;342:1284-6.

27. Boyd EA, Bero LA. Assessing faculty financial relationships with industry: a case study. JAMA. 2000;284:2209-14.

28. Chren MM, Landefeld CS. Physicians' behavior and their interactions with drug companies.JAMA.1994;271:684-9.

29. Korn D. Conflicts of interest in biomedical research. JAMA 2000;284:2234-7.

30. Cho MK, Shohara R, Schissel A, Rennie D. Policies on faculty conflicts of interest at U.S. universities. JAMA 2000;284:2203-8.

31. Butterworth C. The skeleton in the hospital closet. Nutrition Today 1974:4-8. Also, Butterworth C. The Skeleton in the Hospital Closet [Electronic version]. West J Med 2001;174:163.

32. Meguid MM, Campos AC, Hammond WG. Nutritional support in surgical practice: Part I. Am J Surg 1990;159(3):345-58

33. American Dietetic Association [ADA]. Position of The American Dietetic Association: Nutrition--an essential component of medical education. J Am Diet Assoc 1994;94(5):555-557.

34. Plaisted CS, Zeisel SH, Incorporating preventive nutrition into medical school curricula. In: Bendich A, Deckelbaum R, eds. Primary and secondary preventive nutrition. Totowa (NJ): Humana Press Inc. 2001:416-417.

35. Time Magazine. June 4, 2001.

36. Eisenberg D, Kessler R. Unconventional medicine in the United States: prevalence, costs and use of. N Engl J Med 1993;328:246-252.

37. Shils ME, Karp R, Stevenson N, Kuperman A, Gebhardt C. Evaluation of the quality and quantity of nutrition teaching in the curriculum. Bull N Y Acad Med 1984;60(6):591-601.

38. Plaisted CS, Zeisel SH, Incorporating preventive nutrition into medical school curricula. In: Bendich A, Deckelbaum R, eds. Primary and secondary preventive nutrition. Totowa (NJ): Humana Press Inc. 2001:416-418.

39. Young EA. Nutrition Education in US medical schools. Am J Clin Nutr 1997;65:1558.

40. Young EA, Weser E, McBride HM, Page CP, Littlefield JH. Development of core competencies in clinical nutrition. Am J Clin Nutr 1983;38(5):800-10.

41. ADA. Position of The American Dietetic Association: nutrition--essential component of medical education. J Am Diet Assoc 1987;87:642-7.

42. Association of American Medical College's Clinical Administrative Data Service. Nutrition, 1995-1996, 1996-1997, 1997-1998. Raw data. AAMC 1997.

43. Shils ME, Olson JA, Shike M, eds. Modern nutrition in health and disease, 8th Ed. Vol.1: Philadelphia, PA: Lea & Febiger.1994

44. Shils ME, Karp R, Stevenson N, Kuperman A, Gebhardt C. Evaluation of the quality and quantity of nutrition teaching in the curriculum. Bull N Y Acad Med 1984;60(6):591-601.

45. Plaisted CS, Zeisel SH. Barriers to adding nutrition to existing curricula. In: Bendich A, Deckelbaum R, eds. Primary and secondary preventive nutrition. Totowa (NJ): Humana Press Inc. 2001:417.

46. AMSA. Essentials of nutrition education in medical schools: a national consensus. American Medical Student Association's Nutrition Curriculum Project. Acad Med. 1996;71:969-71.Kent G. Nutrition education as an instrument of empowerment. Journal of Nutrition Education 1988;20:193-5.

47. Rodning CB. Sociopolitical influence upon medical education: the Medical College of Alabama (1859 to 1861) as a model. South Med J 1986;79(6):744-5.

48. Rabkin MT. A paradigm shift in academic medicine? Acad Med 1998;73:127-131.

49. Nelson E. Nutrition instruction in medical schools. JAMA 1976;236:2534.

50. National Research Council. Committee on Nutrition in Medical Education, Food and Nutrition Board: nutrition education in US medical schools. Washington, DC: National Academy Press, 1985.

51. Schollar A. Why med students miss their minimum daily requirement of nutrition education. New Physician 1989;38:16-21.

52. McLaren DS. Nutrition in medical schools: a case of mistaken identity. Am J Clin Nutr 1994;59(5):960-3.

53. Levine BS, Wigren MM, Chapman DS, Kerner JF, Bergman RL, Rivlin RS. A national survey of attitudes and practices of primary-care physicians relating to nutrition: strategies for enhancing the use of clinical nutrition in medical practice. Am J Clin Nutr 1993;57(2):115-9.

54. Young EA, Weser E, McBride HM, Page CP, Littlefield JH. Development of core competencies in clinical nutrition. Am J Clin Nutr 1983;38(5):800-10.

55. American Medical Student Association [AMSA]. Essentials of nutrition education in medical schools: a national consensus. American Medical Student Association's Nutrition Curriculum Project. Acad Med. 1996;71:969-71.

56. Mennin SP, Krackov SK. Reflections on relevance, resistance, and reform in medical education. Acad Med 1998;73(9 Suppl):S60-4.

57. Rollins LK, Lynch DC, Owen JA, Shipengrover JA, Peel ME, Chakravarthi S. Moving from policy to practice in curriculum change at the University of Virginia School of Medicine, East Carolina University School of Medicine, and SUNY-Buffalo School of Medicine. Acad Med 1999;74(1 Suppl):S104-11.

58. Hafferty FW. Beyond curriculum reform: confronting medicine's hidden curriculum. Acad Med 1998;73(4):403-7.

59. U.S. Department of Health and Human Services. Report to Congress on the appropriate Federal role in assuring access by medical students, residents and practicing physicians to adequate training in nutrition. Washington, D.C.: 1993.

60. Kushner RF. Barriers to providing nutrition counseling by physicians: a survey of primary care practitioners. Prev Med 1995;24(6):546-52.

61. Maillet JO, Young EA. Position of the American Dietetic Association: nutrition education for health care professionals. J Am Diet Assoc 1998;98(3):343-6.

62. Slavin SJ, Wilkes MS, Usatine R. Doctoring III: innovations in education in the clinical years. Acad Med 1995;70(12):1091-5.

63. Tillman HH, Woods M, Gorbach SL. Enhancing the level of nutrition education at Tufts University's Medical and Dental Schools. J Cancer Educ 1992;7(3):215-9.

64. Intersociety Professional Nutrition Education Consortium. Bringing physician nutrition specialists into the mainstream: rationale for the Intersociety Professional Nutrition Education Constortium. Am J Clin Nutr 1998;68:894-8.

65. British Nutrition Foundation. Nutrition in Medical Education. Report of the British Nutrition Task Force on Clinical Nutrition. Source 1983.

66. ADA. Position of The American Dietetic Association: nutrition--essential component of medical education. J Am Diet Assoc 1987;87:642-7.

67. Healthy People 2010.Office of Disease Prevention and Health Promotion, U.S. Department of Health and Human Services. Retrieved May, 2001 from http://www.health.gov.

68. Schulman JA. Nutrition education in medical schools: Trends and implications for health educators. Med Educ Online [serial online] 1999;4,4. Available from URL http://www.med-ed-online.org/f0000015.htm.

69. Implications for Health Educators: Addressing Barriers and Creating Solutions. Nutrition Education in U.S. Medical Schools (1985). Retrieved July 2000 from The National Academy of Sciences Web site: http://www.edunap.edu/openbook/0309035872/html/R1.html.

70. Davis CH. The report to Congress on the appropriate federal role in assuring access by medical students, residents, and practicing physicians to adequate training in nutrition. Public Health Rep 1994;109(Suppl 6):824-6.

71. Feldman EB. Networks for medical nutrition education—a review of the US experience and future prospects. Am J Clin Nutr 1995;62(3):512-7.

72. Hoffman C, Rice D, Sung H-Y. Persons with chronic conditions: their prevalence and costs. JAMA 1997;276:1473-9.

73. National Center for Health Statistics. Current estimates from the National Health Interview Survey. Washington, DC: U.S. Public Health Service, 1995.

Chapter 4

1. Eisenberg DM, Davis RB, Ettner SL, Appel S, Wilkey S, Van Rompay M, et al. Trends in alternative medicine use in the United States, 1990-1997. Results of a follow-up national survey. JAMA 1998;280:1569-75.

2. Lown B. The lost art of healing: practicing compassion in medicine. New York: Ballantine Books, 1999; pp.xi,xiv

3. Carr A. Restoring the soul of medicine. Br Med J 2001;322 [Electronic version]. Retrieved from http://Br Med J.com/cgi/content/full/322/7279/0.

4. Berman, BM. Editorials: Complementary medicine and medical education. BMJ 2001;322:121-122.

5. Dalen JE. Health Care in America: The good, the bad, the ugly. JAMA 2000;160:17.

6. Jackson C. The P-word: Why physicians don't like being called "providers" AMNews 2001.

7. Weil A. Afterword: Prescriptions for Society. In: Spontaneous Healing. New York: Ballantine Publishing Group; 1995; pp 341 ff.

8. Preamble to the Constitution of the World Health Organization as adopted by the International Health Conference, New York 1946; signed in 1946 by the representatives of 61 States (Official Records of the World Health Organization, no. 2, pp. 100) and entered into force in 1948. WHO definition of health. World Health Organization. Retrieved from http://www.who.int/about/definition/en/.

9. How to Live to 100, Newsweek Magazine, 1997.

10. Suzanne Somers' decision to forego conventional treatment criticized. Retrieved July 2001 from Thriveonline website http://test.bagus.org/news/medical/f2001_0402_somerscancer.html.

11. McClure MW. Smart Medicine for a Healthy Prostate NY: Avery Publishing Group, 2001.

12. Lown B. The lost art of healing: practicing compassion in medicine. New York: Ballantine Books, 1999; pp.xiv.

13. Astin JA. Why patients use alternative medicine: results of a national study. JAMA 1998; 279: 1548-1553.

14. White AR, Ernst E. Economic analysis of complementary medicine: a systematic review. Complement Ther Med 2000; 8: 111-118.

15. U.S. Department of Health and Human Services. Diet and exercise dramatically delay type 2 diabetes. Metformin also effective. Health Care Financ Rev 2001 Fall;23(1):181-2.

16. Ernst E. The role of complementary and alternative medicine. BMJ 2000;321:1133-1135.

17. Ernst E, White A. The BBC survey of complementary medicine use in the UK. Complement Ther Med 2000;8:32-6.

18. Fisher P, Ward A. Complementary medicine in Europe. Br Med J 1994;309:107-11.

19. Ernst E, Weihmayr T. UK and German media differ over complementary medicine. Br Med J 2000;321:707.

20. Lundberg GD, Stacey JH. Severed Trust: Why American medicine hasn't been fixed. New York, NY, Basic Books, 2000.

21. Rees L, Weil A. Integrated medicine. Br Med J 2001;322 119-20.

22. Read N, Czauderna J. Finding the time is most important [Electronic version]. Br Med J 2001;322:1484.

23. Wright SG. Soulless medicine. Br Med J 2001;322:1484.

24. Executive summary. National Center for Complementary and Alternative Medicine (NCCAM). Research Centers Program. Expert panel review. Retrieved Dec 13, 2000 from http://nccam.nih.gov/about/plans/centers/report.pdf.

25. NIH News Release. NIH Launches Large Clinical Trial on EDTA Chelation Therapy for Coronary Artery Disease. For immediate release: 2002. Retrieved April 2003 from http://nccam.nih.gov/news/2002/chelation/pressrelease.htm.

26. Zollman C, Vickers A. ABC of complementary medicine: What is complementary medicine? BMJ 1999; 319: 693-696.

27. The Merck Manual 1899. Centennial (seventeenth) edition, Whitehouse Station, N.J.: Merck Research Laboratories,1999.

28. Lown B. The lost art of healing: practicing compassion in medicine. New York: Ballantine Books, 1999; pp 121-124.

29. Plaisted CS, Zeisel SH, Incorporating preventive nutrition into medical school curricula. In: Bendich A, Deckelbaum R, eds. Primary and secondary preventive nutrition. Totowa (NJ): Humana Press Inc. 2001; pp 417.

30. What is complementary and alternative medicine(CAM)? National Center for Complementary and Alternative Medicine (NCCAM). NCCAMs Classification.Retrieved July 2002 from http://nccam.nih.gov/health/whatiscam/index.htm.

31. NIH Consensus Development Panel on Acupuncture. JAMA. 1998;280(17):1518-1524.

32. Hsu E. Innovation in Chinese Medicine. Cambridge: Cambridge University Press 2001.

33. Linde K, Melchart D. Randomized controlled trials of individualized homeopathy: A state-of-the-art review. J Altern Complement Med. 1998; 4(4):371-388.

34. Linde K, Clausius N, Ramirez G, Melchart D, Eitel F, Hedges LV, et al. Are the clinical effects of homoeopathy placebo effects? A meta-analysis of placebo-controlled trials. Lancet 1997; 350: 834-843

35. Bhattacharya B. M.D. programs in the United States with complementary and alternative medicine education opportunities: an ongoing listing. J Alternative Complementaary Med 2000; 6: 77-90.

36. Jacobs GD. Clinical applications of the relaxation response and mind-body interventions. Altern Complement Med. 2001;7 Suppl 1:S93-101.

37. Astin JA, Shapiro SL, Eisenberg DM, Forys KL. Mind-body medicine: state of the science, implications for practice. J Am Board Fam Pract 2003;16(2):131-47.

38. MacDonald R. Hypnotherapy: hype or healing? BMJ 2003;326(7396):S154.

39. Boudreaux ED, O'Hea E, Chasuk R. Spiritual role in healing. An alternative way of thinking. Prim Care 2002;29(2):439-54, viii.

40. Clarfield AM. Reflections. An old prayer for modern medicine. CMAJ 2002;167(12):1365-7.

41. McGuffin M. Herbal medicine. N Engl J Med 2003;348(15):1498-501.

42. Haller CA, Anderson IB, Kim SY, Blanc PD. An evaluation of selected herbal reference texts and comparison to published reports of adverse herbal events. Adverse Drug React Toxicol Rev. 2002;21(3):143-50.

43. Schneider J. Hospitals get alternative. Acupuncture, massage, and even herbs pop up in mainstream medical settings. US News World Rep. 2002;133(3):68, 70.

44. Study supports Atkins diet; heart association is skeptical. Heart Advis 2003;6(2):5.

45. Dean Ornish, MD: a conversation with the editor. Interview by William Clifford Roberts, MD. Am J Cardiol 2002;90(3):271-98.

46. Hamilton KK. Antioxidant supplements during cancer treatments: where do we stand? Clin J Oncol Nurs 2001;5(4):181-2.

47. Vaughan K, McConaghy N. Megavitamin and dietary treatment in schizophrenia: a randomized, controlled trial.Aust N Z J Psychiatry. 1999;33(1):84-8.

48. Gonzalez MJ, Miranda-Massari JR, Mora EM, Jimenez IZ, Matos MI, Riordan HD, Casciari JJ, Riordan NH, Rodriguez M, Guzman A. Orthomolecular oncology: a mechanistic view of intravenous ascorbate's chemotherapeutic activity. P R Health Sci J 2002;21(1):39-41.

49. Oppel L. St John's wort as treatment for depression. Can Fam Physician. 2002;48:1290; discussion 1290.

50. Cherkin DC, Deyo RA, Sherman KJ, Hart LG, Street JH, Hrbek A, Cramer E, Milliman B, Booker J, Mootz R, Barassi J, Kahn JR, Kaptchuk TJ, Eisenberg DM. Characteristics of licensed acupuncturists, chiropractors, massage therapists, and naturopathic physicians. J Am Board Fam Pract. 2002;15(5):378-90.

51. Ernst E. Prevalence of use of complementary / alternative medicine: a systematic review. Bull World Health Organ. 2000;78(2):252-7.

52. Gaumer G, Koren A, Gemmen E. Barriers to expanding primary care roles for chiropractors: The role of chiropractic as primary care gatekeeper. J Manipulative Physiol Ther. 2002;25(7):427-49.

53. Johnson SM, Kurtz ME. Perceptions of philosophic and practice differences between US osteopathic physicians and their allopathic counterparts. Soc Sci Med 2002;55(12):2141-8.

54. Kandela P. Massage. Lancet 2003;361(9365):1310.

55. Taylor AG, Galper DI, Taylor P, Rice LW, Andersen W, Irvin W, Wang XQ, Harrell FE Jr.Effects of adjunctive Swedish massage and vibration therapy on short-term postoperative outcomes: a randomized, controlled trial. J Altern Complement Med 2003;9(1):77-89.

56. Rubik B. Energy medicine and the unifying concept of information. Altern Ther Health Med. 1995;1(1):34-9.

57. Richards TL, Lappin MS, Lawrie FW, Stegbauer KC. Bioelectromagnetic applications for multiple sclerosis.Phys Med Rehabil Clin N Am. 1998;9(3):659-74.

58. Aveyard B, Sykes M, Doherty D. Therapeutic touch in dementia care. Nurs Older People. 2002;14(6):20-1.

59. Demmer C, Sauer J. Assessing complementary therapy services in a hospice program. Am J Hosp Palliat Care. 2002;19(5):306-14.

60. Nield-Anderson L, Ameling A. The empowering nature of Reiki as a complementary therapy.Holist Nurs Pract. 2000;14(3):21-9.

61. Lown B. Extraordinary healing techniques. In: The lost art of healing: practicing compassion in medicine. New York: Ballantine Books, 1999; pp.121-138.

62. Fisken R. Road to betrayal is short [Electronic version]. Br Med J 2001;322:119-120.

63. St. George D. The Center for Integrative Sciences in Complementary and Alternative Therapies (CISCAT).

64. Katz MD. Use of alternative products: where's the beef? [Electronic version]. West J Med 2000;172:95. Retrieved Jan 2001 from http://www.ewjm.com/cgi/content/full/172/2/95.

65. Food and Drug Administration (FDA). Medical Bulletin. Adverse events with ephedra and other botanical dietary supplements. 1994. Retrieved August 2001 from http://www.cfsan.fda.gov.

66. Food and Drug Administration. Regulations on statements made for dietary supplements concerning the effect of the product on the structure and function of the body; Final Rule. Federal Register 2000;65:999-1050.

67. National Federation of Spiritual Healers (NFSH), United Kingdom: Retrieved January 2001 from http://www.nfsh.org.uk.

68. The National Council Against Health Fraud. Retrieved June 2000 from http://www.ncahf.org/.

69. Quackwatch: Retrieved June 1999 from http://www.quackwatch.com/index.html.

70. Bessell TL, Anderson JN, Silagy CA, Sansom LN, Hiller JE. Surfing, self-medicating and safety: buying non-prescription and complementary medicines via the internet. Qual Saf Health Care 2003;12(2):88-92.

Chapter 5

1. Tanzi R. Decoding Darkness: The search for the genetic causes of Alzheimer's disease. 2001:30. Retrieved January 2000 from http://prevention.stanford.edu/brochure/healthcontent.html.

2. Ventura S. Peters K, Martin J, Maurer L. Births and deaths: United States, 1996. Monthly Vital Statistics Report. Hyatsville, MD: National Center for Health Statistics, 1997:32-22.

3. Flegal KM, Caroll D, Kuzmarski RJ, Johnson CL: Overweight and obesity in the United States: Prevalence and trends 1960-1994. Int J Obes Rel Metab Disord 1998;22:39-47.

4. Physical Activity and Health: A Report from the Surgeon General. U.S. Department of Health and Human Services. Public Health Service, Centers for Disease Control and Prevention. National Center for Chronic Disease Prevention and Health Promotion, 1996. Retrieved October 2001 from http://www.cdc.gov/nccdphp/sgr/contents.htm.

5. Ford ES, Giles WH, Dietz WH. Prevalence of the Metabolic Syndrome Among US Adults. Findings from the Third National Health and Nutrition Examination Survey. JAMA 2002; 287:356-359.

6. Reddy KS. Procor: Commentary: Health transition in developing countries. 1997. Retrieved December 2001 from ProCOR home page. ProCOR, Lown Cardiovascular Center, Brookline, MA. U.S.A; URL http://www.procor.org.

7. Lown B. Indian Heart Journal. Retrieved December 2001 from ProCOR, Lown Cardiovascular Center, Brookline, MA. U.S.A. http://www.procor.org/news.php.

8. WHO Statistical Information System (WHOSIS). Cause of death statistics. World Health Statistics Annual. 1997-1999.

9. King H, Aubert R, Herman W. Global burden of diabetes, 1995-2025: Prevalence, numerical estimates, and projections. Diabetes Care 1998; 21(9)1414-31.

10. Hennekens CH, Buring JE. Epidemiology in medicine. Boston: Little, Brown, 1987.

11. O'Donnell CJ, Sleight P, Manson JE. Coronary health promotion: An overview. In: Prevention of Myocardial Infarction. Manson JE, Ridker PM, Gaziano JM, Hennekens CH, eds. New York: Oxford University Press; 1996:89-98.

12. The Framingham Heart Study: The town that changed America's heart. Retrieved June 2001 from http://www.framingham.com/heart/backgrnd.htm.

13. Framingham heart study: 50 years of research success. Last accessed April 2003. http://www.nhlbi.nih.gov/about/framingham/index.html. Framingham heart study.

14. McGinnis JM, Foege WH. Actual causes of death in the United States. JAMA 1993;270:2207-12.

15. Gotto AM, Farmer JA. Risk factors for coronary artery disease. In: Braunwald E. Heart disease, 4th ed. Philadelphia: WB Saunders, 1992:1125-60.

16. Gaziano JM, Manson JE, Ridker PM. Primary and secondary prevention of coronary heart disease. In: Braunwald E, Zipes DP, Libby P. Heart disease, A textbook of cardiovascular medicine. 6th ed. Philadelphia: WB Saunders, 2001:1056.

17. Manson JE, Ridker PM, Gaziano JM, Hennekens CH ,eds. Prevention of Myocardial Infarction. New York: Oxford University Press; 1996.

18. Bendich A, Deckelbaum RJ, eds. Preventive nutrition: the comprehensive guide for health professionals. Totowa, NJ: Humana, 2001.

19. Eriksson KF, Lindgärde F. Prevention of type 2 (non-insulin-dependent) diabetes mellitus by diet and physical exercise. Diabetologia 1991;34:891-8.

20. Bendich A, Deckelbaum RJ, eds. Primary and secondary preventive nutrition. Totowa (NJ): Humana Press Inc. 2001.

21. Behavioral Risk Factor Surveillance System. National Center for Chronic Disease Prevention and Health Promotion. Retrieved June 200 from http://www.cdc.gov/scientific.htm.

22. From the Centers for Disease Control and Prevention. Prevalence of current cigarette smoking among adults and changes in prevalence of current and some day smoking—United States, 1996-2001. JAMA 2003;289(18):2355-6.

23. Annual smoking-attributable mortality, years of potential life lost, and economic costs— United States, 1995-1999. Morbidity and Mortality Weekly Report (MMWR). 2002;51(14):300-3.

24. Peto R, Lopez AD, Boreham J, Thun M, Heath C Jr, Doll R. Mortality from smoking worldwide. Br Med Bull. 1996;52(1):12-21.

25. Tobacco or Health: A Global Status Report Country Profiles by Region, 1997. World Health Organization Tobacco Control Program. Visit: http://www.cdc.gov/tobacco/who/whofirst.htm.

26. Eriksen MP, LeMaistre CA, Newell GR. Health hazards of passive smoking. Annu Rev Public Health. 1988;9:47-70. Review.

27. U.S. Department of Health and Human Services. The Surgeon General's call to action to prevent and decrease overweight and obesity. [Rockville, MD]: U.S. Department of Health and Human Services, Public Health Service, Office of the Surgeon General; [2001]. Available from: US GPO, Washington. http://www.surgeongeneral.gov/library.

28. National Center for Health Statistics, Centers for Disease Control and Prevention. CDC. Prevalence of overweight and obesity among adults: United States, 1999. [Hyattsville (MD)]: NCHS [cited 2001]. Retrieved September 2000 from: www.cdc.gov/nchs/products/pubs/pubd/hestats/obese/obse99.htm.

29. U.S. Surgeon General. The Surgeon General's report on nutrition and health. U.S. Department of Health and Human Services, 1998.

30. Physical Activity and Health: A Report of the Surgeon General. Washington, DC, U.S. Department of Health and Human Services, Centers for Disease Control and Prevention, 1996.

31. Helmrich SP, Ragland DR, Leung RW, Paffenbarger RS. Physical activity and reduced occurrence of non-insulin-dependent diabetes mellitus. N Engl J Med 1991;325:147-52.

32. Kannel WB, Belanger A, D'Agostino R, Israel I. Physical activity and physical demand on the job and risk of cardiovascular disease and death: the Framingham Study. AM Heart J 1986;112:820-5.

33. CDC. Participation in school physical education and selected dietary patterns among high school students: United States, 1991. Morbidity and Mortality Weekly Report (MMWR) 1992b;41:597-601,607.

34. CDC. Public health focus: physical activity and the prevention of coronary heart disease. Morbidity and Mortality Weekly Report (MMWR) 1993;42:669-72.

35. What We Eat in America. The continuing survey of food intakes by individuals (CSFII) and the diet and health knowledge survey (DHKS), 1994-96. Food Surveys Research Group. Beltsville Human Nutrition Research Center. United States Department of Agriculture (USDA). http://www.barc.usda.gov/bhnrc/foodsurvey/home.htm.

36. Dwyer J, Picciano MF, Raiten DJ; Members of the Steering Committee; National Health and Nutrition Examination Survey. Estimation of usual intakes: What We Eat in America-NHANES. J Nutr. 2003;133(2):609S-23S. Review.

37. Personal Consumption Expenditures Table, 1999, Bureau of Economic Analysis, U.S. Department of Commerce.

38. van Dam RM, Rimm EB, Willett WC, Stampfer MJ, Hu FB. Dietary patterns and risk for type 2 diabetes mellitus in U.S. men. Ann Int Med 2002;136(3):201-209.

39. Kida K, Ito T, Yang SW, Tanphaichitr V. Effects of western diet on risk factors of chronic diseases in Asia. In: Bendich A, Deckelbaum R, eds. Primary and secondary preventive nutrition. Totowa (NJ): Humana Press Inc. 2001; pp 435-436.

40. National Center for Chronic Disease Prevention and Health Promotion Nutrition and Physical Activity. Retrieved March 2002 from http://www.cdc.gov/nccdphp/dnpa/obesity/index.htm

41. Jacobson MF. Ph.D. Liquid Candy—How Soft Drinks are Harming Americans' Health http://www.cspinet.org/sodapop/liquid_candy.htm

42. U.S. Dept. Agr. Nationwide Food Consumption Survey, 1977-78; Continuing Survey of Food Intakes by Individual, 1987-88, 1994-96.

43. U.S. Department of Agriculture, 1965 and 1977-78 USDA Nationwide Food Consumption Surveys, and 1989-1991 and 1994-1995 Continuing Survey of Food Intakes by Individuals. Beltsville Human Nutrition Research Center Bldg. 308, Rm 223, BARC-East Beltsville, MD 20705. Retrieved January 2001 from http://www.barc.usda.gov.

44. Manson JE, Ridker PM, Gaziano JM, Hennekens CH, eds. Prevention of Myocardial Infarction. New York: Oxford University Press; 1996. Appendix A:534-535.

45. Prentice A. Calcium in pregnancy and lactation. Annu Rev Nutr 2000;20:249-72.

46. Prentice, A., Jarjou, L.M.A., Cole, T.J., Stirling, D.M., et al: Calcium requirements of lactating Gambian mothers: effects of a calcium supplement on breast-milk calcium concentration, maternal bone mineral content and urinary calcium excretion. Am J Clin Nutr, 62:58-67, 1995.

47. Allen LH. Women's dietary calcium requirements are not increased by pregnancy or lactation. Am J Clin Nutr 1998;67(4):591-2.

48. Antonov AN. Children born during the siege of Leningrad in 1942. J Paediatr 1947; 30: 250-259.

49. Goldberg GR. Nutrition in pregnancy: the facts and fallacies. Nurs Stand 2003;22-28;17(19):39-42

50. FAO/WHO/UNU Expert Consultation 1985 Energy and protein requirements. Technical Report Series 724. World Health Organization, Geneva.

51. Committee on Medical Aspects of Food Policy (COMA) 1991.

52. Heinig MJ, Nommsen LA, Dewey KG. Lactation and postpartum weight loss. FASEB Journal 1990;4:362A.

53. Roth G, quoted In: Better Homes & Gardens Food for Health and Healing. Ortho Books, 1999.

54. Willcox BJ, Willcox C, Suzuki M. The Okinawa Program: How the world's longest-lived people achieve everlasting health--and how you can too. New York: Three Rivers Press, 2001. pp 49, 86-87.

55. Southgate DAT, Johnson I. Food processing. In: Human nutrition and dietetics. Garrow JS, James WPT eds.. Eight edition. Edinburgh. Churchill Livingstone, 1993:335-348.

56. Karmas E, Harris RS. Nutritional evaluation of food processing, 3rd edition. New York: Van Nostrand Reinhold, 1988.

57. Joint WHO/FAO Expert Report on Diet, Nutrition and the Prevention of Chronic Disease. Executive Summary 2003. Department of Noncommunicable Disease Prevention and Health Promotion. Retrieved March 2003 from http://www.who.int/hpr/nutrition/expertconsultationge.htm.

58. Karmas E, Harris RS. Nutritional evaluation of food processing, 3rd edn. New York: Van Nostrand Reinhold, 1988.

59. Mattes R. D., Donnelly D. Relative contributions of dietary sodium sources. J Am Coll Nutr 1991;10:383-393.

60. Severi S, Bedogni G, Manzieri AM, Poli M, Battistini N. Effects of cooking and storage methods on the micronutrient content of foods. Eur J Cancer Prev. 1997;6 Suppl 1:S21-4. Review.

61. Franz MJ, Maryniuk MD. Position of the American Dietetic Association: Use of nutritive and non-nutritive sweeteners. J Am Dietetic Assn 1993; 93:816-821.

62. Morton ID. Physical, chemistry and biological changes related to different time-temperature combinations. In: Hoyem T, Kvale O (eds) Physical, chemical and biological changes in foods caused by thermal processing. Applied Science, London 1977 :135-51.

63. Reddy MB, Love M. The impact of food processing on the nutritional quality of vitamins and minerals. Adv Exp Med Biol. 1999;459:99-106. Review.

64. United States Department of Agriculture (USDA), Nutrient Data Laboratory, Agricultural Research Service. Available at http://www.nal.usda.gov/fnic/foodcomp/

65. Dwyer J, Picciano MF, Raiten DJ. Food and dietary supplement databases for What We Eat in America-NHANES Supplement: Future Directions for What We Eat in America-NHANES: The Integrated CSFII-NHANES. J Nutr. 2003;133(2):624S-34S.

66. Southgate DAT, Johnson I. Food processing. In: Human nutrition and dietetics. Garrow JS, James WPT eds. Eight Edition. Edinburgh. Churchill Livingstone, 1993:341.

67. Walker R. Food Toxicity. In: Human nutrition and dietetics. Garrow JS, James WPT eds. Eight Edition. Edinburgh. Churchill Livingstone, 1993; pp 355.

68. Hargraves WA. Mutagens in cooked foods. In Nutritional Toxicology. Vol.2. Hathcock JN, eds. Orlando, FL, Academic Press 1987.

69. National Academy of Sciences. The health effects of nitrate, nitrite and N-nitroso compounds. Washington. D. C. National Academy Press, 1981.

70. Risch HA, Jain M, Choi N, Fodor JG, Pfeiffer CJ, Howe GR, et al. Dietary factors and the incidence of cancer of the stomach. Am J Epidemiol 1985;122:947-59.

71. Buiatti E, Palli D, Bianchi S, DeCarli A, Amadori D, Avellini C, et al. A case-control study of gastric cancer and diet in Italy III. Risk patterns by histologic type. Int J Cancer 1991;48:369-74.

72. Gonzales CA, Riboli E, Badosa J, Batiste E, Cardona T, Pita S, et al. Nutritional factors and gastric cancer in Spain. Am J Epidemiol 1994;139:466-73.

73. American Heart Association. Heart and stroke facts; 1994 statistical supplement. Dallas: American Heart Association, 1993.

74. Gurr MI. Role of fats in food and nutrition. London: Elsevier Applied Science Publishers, 1992.

75. Goldman L. Cholesterol reduction. In: Prevention of Myocardial Infarction. Manson JE, Ridker PM, Gaziano JM, Hennekens CH, eds. New York Oxford University Press; 1996; pp 154-171.

76. Gaziano JM, Manson JE, Ridker PM. Primary and secondary prevention of coronary heart disease. In: Braunwald E, Zipes DP, Libby P. Heart disease, A textbook of cardiovascular medicine. 6th ed. Philadelphia: WB Saunders, 2001; pp 1048-1050.

77. Gurr M. Fats. In: Human nutrition and dietetics. Eight edition. Edinburgh. Churchill Livingstone, 1993; pp 77-102.

78. Mann J. Diseases of the heart and circulation: the role of dietary factors in aetiology and management. In: Human nutrition and dietetics. Eight edition. Edinburgh. Churchill Livingstone, 1993; pp 619-650.

79. Feldman EB. Nutrition and diet in the management of management of hyperlipidemia and atherosclerosis. In: Shils ME, Olson JA, Shike M, eds. Modern nutrition in health and disease, 8th Edition Vol.1: Philadelphia, PA: Lea & Febiger.1994; pp 1298-1316.

80. Ackman R, Hooper D. Linolenic acid artifacts from the deodorization of oils. J Am Oil Chem Soc 1974;51:42-9.

81. Manson JE, Ridker PM, Gaziano JM, Hennekens CH, eds. Prevention of Myocardial Infarction. New York: Oxford University Press; 1996. Appendix A. pp 536-537.

82. Values were based on the results of the 1989 -1991 CSFII of the USDA, and the TFA composition data was adapted from Nutrient Data Bank Bulletin Board (USDA).

83. Position Paper on trans-fatty acid. ASCN/AIN Task force on trans-fatty acids. American Society for Clinical Nutrition and American Institute of Nutrition. Am J Clin Nutr 1996; 245-260.

84. Vermunt SHF, Mensink. Health effects of trans-fatty acids. In: Bendich A, Deckelbaum R, eds. Primary and secondary preventive nutrition. Totowa (NJ): Humana Press Inc. 2001; pp 435-436.

85. Keys A, Anderson JT, Grande F. Serum cholesterol response to changes in diet—particularly saturated fatty acids in the diet. Metabolism 1965;14:747-58.

86. Ascherio A, Katan MB, Zock PL, et al. Trans fatty acids and coronary heart disease. N Engl J Med 340:1994-1998,1999.

87. Sundram K, Ismail A, Hayes KC, Jeyamalar R, PathmanathanR. Trans (elaidic) fatty acids adversely affect the lipoprotein profile relative to specific saturated fatty acids in humans. J Nutr 1997;127:514s-20s.

88. Willett WC, Stampfer MJ, Colditz GA, et al. Intake of trans fatty acids and risk of coronary heart disease among women. Lancet 1993;341:581-5.

89. Litin L, Sacks F. Trans-fatty acid content of common foods [letter]. N Engl J Med 1993;329(26):1969 -70.

90. Tracey E. Removing Trans Fats From Foods Could Save Lives, FDA Says. Quotations from Kathleen Koehler, FDA epidemiologist, Ph.D. WebMD Medical News Archive, Web, MD 2000. http://my.webmd.com/content/article/36/1728_58208.

91. McLaren DS, Loveridge N, Duthie G, Bolton-Smith C. Fat-soluble vitamins. In: Human nutrition and dietetics. Eight edition. Edinburgh. Churchill Livingstone, 1993; pp 208-210.

92. Erasmus U. Fats that heal, fats that kill. Burnaby BC Canada: Alive Books, 1993; pp 235-248.

93. Blackburn GL, Kater G, Mascioli EA, Kowalchuk M, Babayan VK, Bistrian BR. A reevaluation of coconut oil's effect on serum cholesterol and atherogenesis. J Phil Med Assoc 1989;65:144-152.

94. Bell SJ, Mascioli EA, Bistrian BR, Babayan VK, Blackburn GL. Alternative lipid sources for enteral and parenteral nutrition: Long and medium-chain triglycerides, and fish oils. J Am Diet Assoc 1991;91:74-78.

95. Mattson FH, Grundy SM. Comparison of the effects of dietary saturated, monosaturated, and polyunsaturated fatty acids on plasma lipids and lipoproteins in man. J Lipid Res 1985;26:194-202.

96. Hegsted DM, Ausman LM, Johnson JA, Dallal GE. Dietary fat and serum lipids: an evaluation of the experimental data. Am J Clin Nutr 1993;57:75-83.

97. Hayes KC. Specific dietary fatty acids in predicting plasma cholesterol. Am J Clin Nutr 1993;57:230-1.

98. Quotation attributed to Blackburn GL (Harvard) in Cajanus (Caribbean Quarterly), 1988.

99. De Roos N, Schouten EG, Katan MB. Consumption of a solid fat rich in lauric acid results in a more favorable serum lipid profile in healthy men and women than consumption of a solid fat rich in trans-fatty acids. Journal of Nutrition. 2001;131:242-5.

100. Transmissible spongiform encephalopathies, hypotheses and food safety: an overview.Sci Total Environ. 1998;217(1-2):71-82.

101. Willett WC. Introduction. In: Eat, drink, and be healthy. New York: Simon & Schuster, 2001; pp 19.

102. Garlick PJ, Reeds PJ. Proteins. In: Human nutrition and dietetics. Eight edition. Garrow JS, James WPT. Edinburgh: Churchill Livingstone, 1993; pp 56-76.

103. Hoffman, Joseph F. "Russell Henry Chittenden," The Physiologist 30(4) (1987): 81-82.

104. Rubner: Schädigung der deutschen Volkskraft durch die feindliche Blockade, Denkschrift des Reichsgesundheitsamtes, Berlin, 1919. (German)

105. Southgate DAT. Meat, fish, eggs, and novel proteins. In: Human nutrition and dietetics. Garrow JS, James WPT eds. Eight Edition. Edinburgh. Churchill Livingstone, 1993:305-316.

106. Nordin BEC, Need AG, Morris HA, Horowitz M. The nature and significance of the relationship between urinary sodium and urinary calcium in women. J Nutr 1993;123:1615-22.

107. Nordin BEC, Need AG, Morris HA, Horowitz M. Sodium, calcium and osteoporosis. In: Burckhardt P, Heaney RP, eds. Nutritional aspects of osteoporosis. New York: Raven Press, 1991; pp 279-95.

108. Cooper C, Campion G, Melton LJ 3rd. Hip fractures in the elderly: a world-wide projection. Osteoporos Int. 1992;2(6):285-9 .

109. Matkovic V, Illich JZ, Andon B, et al. Urinary calcium, sodium, and bone mass of young females. Am J Clin Nutr 1995;62:417-25.

110. de Deckere EA, korver O, Verchuren PM, Katan MB. Health aspects of fish and n-3 polyunsaturated fatty acids from plant and marine origin. Eur J Clin Nutr 1998;52:749-53.

111. Paul AA, Southgate DAT. McCance and Widdowson's The composition of food. 4th ed. London: Her Majesty's Stationery Office (HMSO), 1978.

112. Bao DQ, Mori TA, Burke V, Puddey IB, Beilen LJ. Effects of dietary fish and weight reduction on ambulatory blood pressure in overweight hypertensives. Hypertension 1998;32:710-7.

113. Mozaffarian D, Lemaitre RN, Kuller LH, Burke GL, Tracy RP, Siscovick DS. Cardiac benefits of fish consumption may depend on the type of fish meal consumed: the Cardiovascular Health Study. Circulation. 2003;107(10):1372-7.

114. Yoshizawa K, Rimm EB, Morris JS, Spate VL, Hsieh CC, Spiegelman D, Stampfer MJ, Willett WC. Mercury and the risk of coronary heart disease in men. N Engl J Med. 2002 28;347(22):1755-60.

115. Guallar E, Sanz-Gallardo MI, van't Veer P, Bode P, Aro A, Gomez-Aracena J, Kark JD, Riemersma RA, Martin-Moreno JM, Kok FJ. Mercury, fish oils, and the risk of myocardial infarction. N Engl J Med. 2002;347(22):1747-54.

116. Southgate DAT. Meat, fish, eggs, and novel proteins. In: Human nutrition and dietetics. Garrow JS, James WPT eds. Eight edition. Edinburgh. Churchill Livingstone, 1993; pp 311-313.

117. National Cholesterol Education Program 1985. National Heart, Lung, and Blood Institute. National Institutes of Health. http://www.nhlbi.nih.gov/about/ncep/index.htm.

118. Willett WC. Calcium: no emergency. In: Eat, drink and be healthy. New York: Simon & Schuster, 2001; pp 138-151.

119. Colditz GA, et al. The Nurses' Health Study: 20-year Contribution to the understanding of health among women. Journal of Women's Health 1997;6:49-61.

120. Melton LJ 3rd. Hip fractures: a worldwide problem today and tomorrow. Bone. 1993;14 Suppl 1:S1-8. Review.

121. Pereda CA, Eastell R. Calcium requirements during treatment of osteoporosis in women. In: Bendich A, Deckelbaum R, eds. Primary and secondary preventive nutrition. Totowa (NJ): Humana Press Inc. 2001; pp 307-321.

122. Heaney RP. Osteoporosis: minerals, vitamins, and other micronutrients. In: Preventive nutrition: the comprehensive guide for health professionals. Bendich A, Deckelbaum RJ, eds. Totowa, NJ: Humana, 2001; pp 271-291.

123. Gullberg B, Johnell O, Kanis JA. World-wide projections for hip fracture. Osteoporos Int.1997;7(5):407-13.

124. Lau EM, Cooper C. The epidemiology of osteoporosis. The oriental perspective in a world context. Clin Orthop. 1996;(323):65-74. Review.

125. Fujita T. Osteoporosis in Japan: factors contributing to the low incidence of hip fracture. Adv Nutr Res. 1994;9:89-99. Review.

126. Reid IR, Ames RW, Evans MC, Gamble GD, Sharpe SJ. Effect of calcium supplementation on bone loss in postmenopausal women. N Engl J Med 1993;328:460-4.

127. Cadogan J, Eastell R, Jones N, Barker ME. Milk intake and bone mineral acquisition in adolescent girls: randomized, controlled intervention trial. Br Med J 1997;315:1255-60.

128. Anderson JJ. Plant-based diets and bone health: nutritional implications. Am J Clin Nutr. 1999;70(3 Suppl):539S-542S. Review.

129. Southgate DAT. Milk and milk products; fats and oils. In: Human nutrition and dietetics. Garrow JS, James WPT eds. Eight Edition. Edinburgh. Churchill Livingstone, 1993; pp 317-324.

130. Neil Sherman. Health Scout Reporter. Giuliani has cow over milk ad. NYC mayor's prostate cancer used to knock milk, 2000.

131. Giovannucci E. Calcium and milk and prostate cancer: a review of the evidence. Minireviews. The Prostate Journal 1999;1(1):1-7.

132. G, Bjelke E, Heuch I, Vollset SE. Milk consumption and cancer incidence: a Norwegian prospective study. Br J Cancer 1990;61:454-9.

133. Giovannucci E. Calcium and Fructose Intake in Relation to Risk of Prostate Cancer. Cancer Research 58 (1998):442-7.

134. Giovannucci E, Kantoff P, Spiegelman D, Loughlin KR, Wishnow KI, Corless C,McDermott A, Willet WC, Talcott JA. The epidemic of prostate cancer and the medical literature: a causal association? Prostate Cancer Prostatic Dis. 1998;1(3):148-153.

135. Giovannucci E, Kantoff P, Spiegelman D, Loughlin KR, Wishnow KI, Corless C,McDermott A, Willet WC, Talcott JA. The epidemic of prostate cancer and the medical literature: a causal association? Prostate Cancer Prostatic Dis. 1998;1(3):148-153.

136. Chan JM, Giovannucci EL. Dairy products, calcium, and vitamin D and risk of prostate cancer. Epidemiol Rev. 2001;23(1):87-92. Review. No abstract available.

137. Chan JM, Stampfer MJ, Ma J, Gann PH, Gaziano JM, Giovannucci EL. Dairy products, calcium, and prostate cancer risk in the Physicians' Health Study.Am J Clin Nutr. 2001;74(4):549-54.

138. Whelton PK, He J, Appel L. Treatment and Prevention of Hypertension. In: Prevention of Myocardial Infarction. Manson JE, Ridker PM, Gaziano JM, Hennekens CH ,eds. New York Oxford University Press; 1996; pp 154-155.

139. He J, Klag MJ, Whelton PK, et at. Migration, blood pressure pattern, and hypertension: the Yi Migrant Study. Am J Epidemiol 1991;134:1085-101.

140. Shils ME. Magnesium. In: Shils ME, Olson JA, Shike M, eds. Modern nutrition in health and disease, 8th Edition Vol.1: Philadelphia, PA: Lea & Febiger.1994; pp 164-84.

141. Correa P, Fontham E, Pickle LW, Chen V, Lyn Y, Haenszel W. Dietary determinants of gastric cancer in south Louisiana inhabitants. J Natl Cancer Inst 1985;75:645-54.

142. Lu J-B, Qin Y-M. Correlation between high salt intake and mortality rates for esophageal and gastric cancers in Henan province, China. Int J Epidemiol 1987;16:171-6.

143. Sierra R, Chinnock A, Ohshima H, Pignatelli B, Malaveille C, Gamboa C, et al. In vivo nitrosoproline formation and other risk factors in Costa Rican children from high- and low-risk areas for cancer. Cancer Epid Biomarkers Prev 1993; 122:947-959.

144. Sato T, Fukuyama T, Suzuki H. Studies of the causation of gastric cancer. The relation between gastric cancer mortality and salted food intake in several places in Japan. Bull Inst Publ Health (Japan) 1959; 8:187-198.

145. Lee J-K, Park B-Y, Yoo K-Y, Ahn Y-O. Dietary factors and stomach cancer: a case-control study in Korea. Int J Epidemiol 1995;24:33-41.

146. Lands WEM. Alcohol: the balancing act. In: Bendich A, Deckelbaum R, eds. Primary and secondary preventive nutrition. Totowa (NJ): Humana Press Inc. 2001; pp 375-595.

147. Fuchs CS, et al. Alcohol consumption and mortality among women. N Engl J Med 1995;332:1245-50.

148. Camargo CA, Hennekens CH, Gaziano JM, Glynn RJ, Manson JE, Stampfer MJ. Prospective study of alcohol consumption and mortality in U.S. male Physicians. Arch Int Med 1997;157:79-85.

149. Rimm EB, et al. Prospective study of alcohol consumption and risk of coronary disease in men. Lancet 1991;338:464-8.

150. Reichman ME, et al. Effects of alcohol consumption on plasma and urinary hormone concentrations in premenopausal women. J Natl Cancer Inst 1993;85:722-7.

151. Boffetta P, Garfinke L. Alcohol drinking and mortality among men enrolled in a American Cancer Society prospective study. Epidemiology 1990;1:342-8.

152. Kabat GC, Ng SK, Wynder EL. Tobacco, alcohol intake and diet in relation to adenocarcinoma of the esophagus and gastric cardia. Cancer Causes Contr 1993;4:123-32.

153. Brown LM, Silverman DT, Pottern LM, Schoenberg JB, Greenberg RS, Swanson GM, et al. Adenocarcinoma of the esophagus and esophagogastric junction in white men in the United States: alcohol, tobacco and socioeconomic factors. Cancer Causes Control 1994;5:333-40.

154. Gammon MD, Schoenberg JB, Ahsan H, Risch HA, Vaughan TL, Chow WH, et al. Tobacco, alcohol, and socioeconomic status and adenocarcinomas of the esophagus and gastric cardia. J Natl Cancer Inst 1997;89:1277-84.

155. Marmot MG, Elliot P, Shipley MJ, Dyer AR, Ueshima H, Beevers DG, et al. Alcohol and blood pressure: the INTERSALT study. Br Med J 1994; 308:1263-1267.

156. Maclure M. A demonstration of deductive meta-analysis: Ethanol intake and risk of myocardial infarction. Epidemiol Rev 1994;15;328-51.

157. Rosenqvist M. Alcohol and cardiac arrhythmias. Alcoholism Clin Exp Res 198;22:318S-322S.

158. Murray CJL, Lopez AD. Global mortality, disability, and the contribution of risk factors: Global Burden of Disease Study. Lancet 1997; 349:1436-1442.

159. Hoey J, Montvernay C, Lambert R. Wine and tobacco risk factors for stomach cancer in France. Am J Epidemiol 1981;113:668-74.

160. Feinman L, Leiber CS. Alcoholism. Clin Exp Res, 1988;12:2-6.

161. Renaud S, de Lorgeril M. Wine, alcohol, platelets, and the French paradox for coronary disease. Lancet 1992;339:1523-6.

162. Lands WEM. Alcohol: the balancing act. In: Bendich A, Deckelbaum R, eds. Primary and secondary preventive nutrition. Totowa (NJ): Humana Press Inc. 2001; pp 389.

163. Potter JD. The epidemiology of diet and cancer: Evidence of human maladaptation. In: Moon TE, Micozzi MS, eds. Nutrition and Cancer Prevention. Investigating the Role of Macronutrients. New York: Marcel Dekker 1992:55-84.

164. Kennedy E, Bowman SA, Lino M, Gerrior SA, Basiotis PP. Diet quality of Americans. Healthy eating index. Retrieved January 2002 from http://www.ers.usda.gov/publications/aib750/aib750.pdf.

165. Jospipura KJ, et al. Fruit and Vegetable Intake in Relation to Risk of Ischemic Stroke. JAMA 282 1999:1233-9.

166. Ness AR, Poles JW. Fruits and vegetables and cardiovascular diseases. A review.Int J Epidemiol 1997;26:1-13.

167. Serdula MK, Coates RJ, Byers T, Simoes E, Mokdad AH, Subar AF. Fruit and vegetable intake among adults in 16 states: results of a brief telephone survey. Am J Public Health 1995;85:236-9.

168. Temple NJ. Fruits, vegetables and cancer prevention trials. J Natl Cancer Inst 1999;91(13):1164.

169. Garcia-Closas R, Gonzalez CA, Agudo A, Riboli E. Intake of specific carotenoids an flavonoids and the risk of gastric cancer in Spain. Cancer Causes Control 1999;10(1):71-5.

170. Steinmetz KA, Potter JD. Vegetables, fruit and cancer. II. Mechanisms. Cancer Causes Control 1991;2:427-42.

171. Weisburger JH. Mechanisms of action of antioxidants as exemplified in vegetables, tomatoes and tea. Food Chemical Toxicol 1999;37(9,10):943.

172. American Heart Association. MyHeartWatch. http://www.onelife.americanheart.org/

173. Coronary Heart Disease Risk Charts. The Coronary Risk Prediction Charts 1998 Heart supplement Joint British recommendations on prevention of coronary heart disease in clinical practice, prepared by David Wood, Paul Durrington, Neil Poulter, Gordon McInnes, Alan Rees and Richard Wray on behalf of the British Cardiac Society, British Hyperlipidaemia Association, British Hypertension Society and Diabetes UK. Retrieved August 2000 from http://www.diabetes.org.uk/infocentre/inform/heart.htm.

174. Joint British Societies CHD Risk Charts. Joint British Societies Coronary Risk Prediction Chart http://www.hyp.ac.uk/bhsinfo/riskview.htm

175. Camus JP. Gout, diabetes, hyperlipidemia: a metabolic trisyndrome. Rev Rhum Mal Osteoartic 1966;33:10-14 (in French).

176. Reaven GM. Banting Lecture 1988. Role of insulin resistance in human disease. Diabetes 1988;37:1595-1607.

177. Reaven GM, Abbasi F, Bernhart S, et al. Insulin resistance, dietary cholesterol, and cholesterol concentration in postmenopausal women. Metabolism 2001;50(5):594-597.

178. Reaven GM. Insulin resistance: a chicken that has come to roost. Ann NY Acad Sci 2001;892:45-57.

179. Reaven GM, Lithell H, Landsberg L. Hypertension and associated metabolic abnormalities—the role of insulin resistance and the sympathoadrenal system. N Engl J Med 1996;334:374-381.

180. Reaven G, Segal K, Hauptman J, Boldrin M, Lucas C. Effect of orlistat assisted weight loss in decreasing coronary heart disease risk in patients with syndrome X. Am J Cardiol 2001,87;827-831.

181. Facchini FS, Hua N, Abbasi F, Reaven GM. Insulin resistance as a predictor of age-related diseases. J Clin Endocrinol Metab 2001;86(8):3574-3578.

182. Zavaroni I, Mazza S, Dall'Aglio E, Gasparine P, Passeri M, Reaven GM. Prevalence of hyperinsulinaemia in patients with high blood pressure. J Int Med 1992;231:1128-1130.

183. McLaughlin T, Abbasi F, Kim HS, Lamendola C, Schaaf P, Reaven G. Relationship between insulin resistance, weight loss, and coronary heart disease risk in healthy, obese women. Metabolism 2001;50(7):795-800.

184. McLaughlin T, Abbasi F, Kim HS, Lamendola C, Schaaf P, Reaven G. Relationship between insulin resistance, weight loss, and coronary heart disease risk in healthy, obese women. Metabolism 2001;50(7):795-800.

185. Modan M, Halkin H. Hyperinsulinemia or increased sympathetic drive as links for obesity and hypertension. Diabetes Care 1991;14:470-87.

186. Wellborn TA, Wearne K. Coronary heart disease incidence and cardiovascular mortality in Busselton with reference to glucose and insulin concentrations. Diabetes Care 1979;2:154-60.

187. Ryan AS, Nicklas BJ, Berman DM. Hormone replacement therapy, insulin sensitivity, and abdominal obesity in postmenopausal women. Diabetes Care 2002;25(1):127-133.

188. Valantine H, Rickenbacker P, Kemna M, et al. Metabolic abnormalities characteristic of dysmetabolic syndrome predict the development of transplant coronary artery disease: a prospective study. Circulation 2001;103(17):2144-2152.

189. Ford ES, Giles WH, Dietz WH. Prevalence of the Metabolic Syndrome Among US Adults. Findings from the Third National Health and Nutrition Examination Survey. JAMA 2002; 287:356-359.

190. Hansen BC. The Metabolic Syndrome X. Ann NY Acad Sci 1999;892:1-24.

191. Isomaa B, Henricsson M, Almgren P, Tuomi T, Taskinen M-R, Groop L. The metabolic syndrome influences the risk of chronic complications in patients with type II diabetes. Diabetologia 2001;44:1148-1154.

192. Krentz AJ. Insulin resistance. Br Med J 1996;313:1385-1389.

193. Vega GL. Obesity, the metabolic syndrome, and cardiovascular disease. Am Heart J 2001;142:1108-1116.

194. Ferrannini E, Natali A, Bell P, et al. Insulin resistance and hypersecretion in obesity. J Clin Invest 1997;100:1166-1173.

195. 1999 World Health Organization-International Society of Hypertension Guidelines for the Management of Hypertension. Guidelines Subcommittee. J Hypertens 1999;17:151-183.

196. Grundy SM. Hypertriglyceridemia, atherogenic dyslipidemia, and the metabolic syndrome. Am J Cardiol 1998;81(4A):18B-25B.

197. Ginsberg HN, Huang LS. The insulin resistance syndrome: impact on lipoprotein metabolism and atherothrombosis. J Cardiovasc Risk 2000;7:325-331.

198. Brunzell JD, Hokanson JE. Dyslipidemia of central obesity and insulin resistance. Diabetes Care 1999;22(suppl 3):C10-13.

199. Ornish D, Brown SE, Sherwitz LW. Can lifestyle changes reverse coronary heart disease? Lancet 1990;336:129-33.

200. Ornish D, Scherwitz LW, Billings JH, et al. Intensive lifestyle changes for reversal of coronary heart disease. JAMA 1998;280:2001-7.

201. Ornish D, Brown SE, Billings JH, et al.. Can lifestyle changes reverse coronary artherosclerosis? Four-year results of the Lifestyle Heart Trial. Circulation 1993;88:I-385.

202. Tsevat J, Weinstein MC, Williams LW, Tosteson AN, Goldman, L. Expected gains in life expectancy from various coronary heart disease risk factor modifications. Circulation 1991;83,no.4;1194- 201.

203. Gaziano JM, Manson JE, Ridker PM. Primary and secondary prevention of coronary heart disease. In: Braunwald E, Zipes DP, Libby P. Heart disease, A textbook of cardiovascular medicine. 6th edition Philadelphia: WB Saunders, 2001; pp 1056.

204. Strong WB, Kelder SH. Pediatric preventive cardiology. In: Prevention of Myocardial Infarction. Manson JE, Ridker PM, Gaziano JM, Hennekens CH, eds. New York: Oxford University Press; 1996:353.

Chapter 6

1. CDC. Healthy aging: Preventing disease and improving quality of life among older Americans. National Center for Chronic Disease Prevention and Health Promotion, 2001:1.

2. Lown B. The lost art of healing: practicing compassion in medicine. New York: Ballantine Books, 1999; pp 234.

3. Vaillant GE, Mukamal K. Successful aging. Am J Psychiatry 2001;158(6):839-47

4. Vaillant GE. Surprising guideposts to a happier life from the landmark Harvard Study of Adult Development. Boston: Little Brown; 2002.

5. Quick S, Hesseldenz P, Hayhoe C, Bastin S, Flashman RH. Aging Gracefully [Electronic version], University of Kentucky. Retrieved February 2001 from http://www.ca.uky.edu/fcs/aging>.

6. Geriatric medicine: demography and healthcare. The Merck Manual. Sixteenth edition, Whitehouse Station, N.J.: Merck Research Laboratories, 1992. The Merck Manual. Centennial (seventeenth) edition, Whitehouse Station, N.J.: Merck Research Laboratories,1999; pp 240-241.

7. Strong WB, Kelder SH. Pediatric preventive cardiology. In: Prevention of Myocardial Infarction. Manson JE, Ridker PM, Gaziano JM, Hennekens CH ,eds. New York: Oxford University Press; 1996; pp 353.

8. Psalm 90:10. Holy Bible, New International Version 1978, Committee on Bible Translation.

9. Selected physiologic age-related changes in body function and composition. The Merck Manual. Centennial (Seventeenth) Edition, Whitehouse Station, N.J.: Merck Research Laboratories, 1999; pp 2504 (table).

10. Geriatric medicine: health care delivery nursing home care. The Merck Manual. Centennial (Seventeenth) Edition, Whitehouse Station, N.J.: Merck Research Laboratories, 1999; pp 2503-2505.

11. Trends in Health and Aging. National Center for Health Statistics. United States Department of Health and Human Services. Centers for Disease Control and Prevention. Atlanta, GA. Retrieved June 2001 from http://www.cdc.gov/.

12. Emmanuel EJ, Ash A, Yu W, Gazelle G. Managed care, hospice use, site of death, and medical expenditures in the last year of life. Arch Int Med 2002;162(15):1722-1728.

13. Ecclesiastes 12: 1b-3b. New International Version 1978, Committee on Bible Translation.

14. Troen BR. The biology of aging. Mt Sinai J Med 2003 ;70(1):3-22

15. Weindruch RH, Walford RL. The Retardation of Aging and Disease by Dietary Restriction. Springfield, I: Charles C Thomas, 1988.

16. Schneider EL. Theories of aging a perspective. In: Warner HR, Butler RN, Sprott RL, Schneider EL. Modern biological theories of aging. New York: Raven Press, 1987; pp 1-3.

17. Haylick L. The aging process: current theories. Drug-Nutrient Interac 1985;4:13-33.

18. Emerit I and Chance B, eds. Free radicals and aging. Basel, Switzerland: Birkhauser Verlag, 1992;398-410.

19. Manton KG. Dynamic paradigms for human mortality and aging. J Gerontol A Biol Sci Med Sci 1999;54(6):B247-54.

20. Mangel M. Complex adaptive systems, aging and longevity. J Theor Biol 2000; 213(4):559-71.

21. Ozawa T. In: Understanding the process of aging. Cadenas E, Packer L (eds). Marcel Dekker. New York:1999; pp 265-292.

22. Harman D. Aging: prospects for further increases in the functional life span. Age 1994;17:119-146.

23. Pauling L. Vitamin C and the common cold. San Francisco: Freeman WH, 1970.

24. Pauling L. Vitamin C and the common cold and the flu. San Francisco: Freeman WH, 1970.

25. Hogg N. Free radicals in disease. Semin Reprod Endocrinol 1998;16(4):241-8.

26. Thomas JA. Oxidative stress, oxidant defense, and dietary constituents. In Modern nutrition in health and disease, 8th edition Lea & Febiger, Phil.,1994; pp 501-512.

27. Droge W. Free radicals in the physiological control of cell function. Physiol Rev 2002 ;82(1):47-95.

28. Challem J. Some good things to say about free radicals (editorial). Townsend letter for doctors & patients 1995:104-5.

29. Packer JE, Slater TF, Wilson RL. Direct observation of a free radical interaction between vitamin E and vitamin C. Nature 1979;278:737-8.

30. Niki E, Saito T, Kamiya Y. The role of vitamin C as an antioxidant. Chem Lett 1983;631-2

31. Luxford C, Dean RT, Davies MJ. Radicals derived from histone hydroperoxides damage nucleobases in RNA and DNA. Chem Res Toxicol 2000;13(7):665-72

32. Begley S, Hager M. Fountain of Youth. Newsweek magazine 1990.

33. Constainescu A, Han D, Packer L. Vitamin E recycling in human erythrocyte membranes. J Biol Chem 1993;268:10906-13.

34. Frei B. Reactive oxygen species and antioxidant vitamins: mechanisms of action. Am J Med 1994;97(3A):5S-14S.

35. Steinbrecher UP, Parthasarathy S, Leake DS, et al. Modification of low density lipoprotein endothelial cells involves lipid peroxidation and degradation of low density lipoprotein phospholipids. Proc Natl Acad Sci USA 1984;81:3883-7.

36. Carr AC, Zhu BZ, Frei B. Potential antiatherogenic mechanisms of ascorbate (vitamin C) and alpha-tocopherol (vitamin E). Circ Res 2000;87(5):349-54

37. Bogden JD, Louria DB. Micronutrients and immunity in older people. In: Preventive nutrition: the comprehensive guide for health professionals. Bendich A, Deckelbaum RJ, eds. Totowa, NJ: Humana, 2001; pp134-136.

38. Aronson M. Involution of the thymus revisited: Immunological trade-offs as an adaptation to aging. Mech Ageing Dev 1993;72:49-55.

39. Schwab R, Weksler ME. Cell biology of the impaired proliferation of T cells from elderly humans. In: Goidl EA, ed. Aging and the Immune Response. New York: Marcel Dekker, 1987:67-80.

40. Weksler ME. The senescence of the immune system. Hosp Pract 1981:53-64.

41. Watkins PJ. The diabetic foot. BMJ 2003;326(7396):977-9

42. Boike AM, Hall JO. A practical guide for examining and treating the diabetic foot.

43. Cleve Clin J Med. 2002;69(4):342-8. Review.

44. Senior C. Assessment of infection in diabetic foot ulcers. J Wound Care. 2000;9(7):313-7.

45. Beisel WR. Nutrition and infection. In: Linder MC, ed. Nutritional biochemistry and metabolism. New York: Elsevier, 1985:364-94.

46. Goodwin JS, Garry PJ. Relationships between megadose vitamin supplementation and immunological function in a healthy elderly population. Clin Exp Immunol 1983;51:647-53.

47. Chandra RK. Nutrition and immunology. Contemp Nutr 1986;11:1-4.

48. McMurray DN. Cell-mediated immunity in nutritional deficiency. Prog Food Nutr Sci 1984;8:193-228.
49. James SJ, Makinodan T. Nutritional intervention during immunologic aging: past and present. In: Armbrecht HJ, Prendergast JM, Coe RM, eds. Nutritional Intervention in the Aging Process. New York: Spinger-Verlag, 1984:209-27.
50. Beisel WR. Single nutrient and immunity. Am J Clin Nutr 1982;35:417-68.
51. Bendich A. Antioxidant micronutrients and immune response. Ann NY Acad Sci 1990;587:168-180.
52. Makinodan T. Patterns of age-related immunologic changes. Nutr Rev 1995;53:S27-S34.
53. Hodis HN, Mack WJ, Sevanian. Antioxidant vitamins and atherosclerosis. In: Primary and secondary preventive nutrition. Bendich A, Deckelbaum RJ, eds. Totowa, NJ: Humana, 2001; pp 91-116.
54. Mashima R, Witting PK, Stocker R. Oxidants and antioxidants in atherosclerosis. Curr Opin Lipidol 2001;12(4):411-8
55. Gaziano JM, Manson JM, Hennekens CH. Dietary antioxidants and cardiovascular disease: Epidemiologic studies and clinical intervention trials. In: Frei B, ed. Natural antioxidants and human disease, Academic Press, 1994.
56. Gaziano JM, Manson JE, Buring JE, Hennekens CH. Dietary antioxidants in cardiovascular disease. Ann of NY Acad Sci 1992;249-59.
57. Manson JE, Stampfer MJ, Willet WC, et al. A prospective study of antioxidant vitamins and incidence of CHD in women. Circulation 1991;84:Suppl II.
58. Kok FJ, de Bruijn AM, Vermeeren R, et al. Serum selenium, vitamin antioxidants and cardiovascular mortality: a 9 year follow-up study in the Netherlands. Am J Clin Nutr 1987;45:462-8.
59. Harrison D, Griendling KK, Landmesser U, Hornig B, Drexler H. Role of oxidative stress in atherosclerosis. Am J Cardiol. 2003;91(3A):7A-11A. Review.
60. Modan M, Or J, Karasik A, et al. Hyperinsulinemia, sex, and risk of atherosclerotic cardiovascular disease. Circulation 1991;84:1165-75.
61. Takemura G, Onodera T, Millard RW, Ashraf M. Demonstration of hydroxyl radical and its role in hydrogen peroxide-induced myocardial injury: hydroxyl radical dependent and independent mechanisms. Free Radic Biol Med. 1993;15(1):13-25.
62. Consensus Conference. Lowering blood cholesterol to prevent heart disease. JAMA 1985;253:2080-6.
63. Leren P. The effect of plasma cholesterol lowering diet in male survivors of myocardial infarction: a controlled clinical trial. Acta Med Scand Suppl 1966;466:1-92.
64. Henriksen T, Evensen SA, Carlander B. Injury to human endothelial cells in culture induced by low-density lipoproteins. Scan J Clin Lab Invest 1979;39:361-8.
65. Brown MS, Goldstein JL. Receptor mediated pathway for cholesterol homeostasis. Science 1986;232;34-47.
66. Morel DW, DiCorelto PE, Chisholm GM. Endothelial and smooth muscle cells alter low density lipoprotein in vitro by free radical oxidation. Arteriosclerosis 1984;4:356-64.
67. Grundy SM. Cholesterol and coronary heart disease, a new era. JAMA 1986;256:2849-58.
68. Pathobiological Determinants of Atherosclerosis in Youth (PDAY) Research Group. Natural history of aortic and coronary atherosclerotic lesions in youth: findings from the PDAY Study. Atheroscler Thromb 1993;13:1291-8.
69. Goldstein JL, Ho YK, Basu SK, Brown MS. Binding site on macrophages that mediates uptake and degradation of acetylated low-density lipoprotein, producing massive cholesterol deposition. Proc Natl Acad Sci USA 1979;76:333-7.
70. Lipid Reseach Clinics Program. The Lipid Research Clinics Coronary Primary Prevention Trial results: I. Reduction in incidence of coronary heart disease. JAMA 1984;251:351-64.
71. Steinberg D and Workshop Participants. Antioxidants in the prevention of human atherosclerosis: summary proceedings of a National Heart, Lung, and Blood Institute Workshop: 1991. Bethesda MD. Circulation 1992;85:2337-47.

72. Tackett RL, Zumbro GL, Rubin JW, Zhao L. Increased superoxide production in vasculature of African-Americans impairs endothelial mediated relaxation. Circulation 1997;96(8):375-1. Suppl.

73. Plotnick G, Corretti MC, Vogel RA. Effect of antioxidant vitamins on the transient impairment of endothelium-dependent brachial artery vasoactivity following a single high-fat meal. JAMA 1997;278(20):1682-1686.

74. Criqui MH, Ringel BL. Does diet or alcohol explain the French paradox? Lancet 1994; 1719-23.

75. Grønbach M. et al. Mortality associated with moderate intakes of wine, beer, or spirit. British Medical Journal, volume 310, 1995, pp 1165-1169.

76. Shah PK, Schwartz I, McCarthy D, Saldana MJ, Villaran C. Sildenafil in the Treatment of Erectile Dysfunction. N Engl J Med 1998; 339:699-702, 1998.

77. NIH Consensus Conference: Impotence. NIH Consensus Development Panel on Impotence. JAMA 270:83-87, 1993.

78. Mumarriz R, Quingwei RY, Goldstein I: Blunt trauma: The pathophysiology of hemodynamic injury leading to erectile dysfunction. J of Urology 153:1831, 1995.

79. Shabsigh R. Cigarette smoking and other vascular risk factors in vasculogenic impotence, Urology 38:277, 1991.

80. Feldman HA et al. Impotence and its medical and psychological correlates: results of Massachusetts male aging study. J of Urology 151:54-61, 1994.

81. Schein M et al. The frequency of sexual problems among family practice patients. Family Practice Research Journal 7:122, 1988.

82. FitzGerald GA, Oates JA, Nowak J. Cigarette smoking and hemostatic function. AM Heart J 1988;115:267-71.

83. Murray JJ, Nowak J, Oates JA, Fitzgerald GA. Platelet-vessel wall interactions in individuals who smoke cigarettes. Adv Exp Med Biol 1990;273:189-98.

84. Ernst E, Koenig W. Smoking and blood rheology. Adv Exp Med Biol 1990;273:295-300.

85. Allen DR, Browse NL, Rutt DL. Effects of cigarette smoke, carbon monoxide and nicotine on the uptake of fibrinogen by the canine arterial wall. Atherosclerosis 1989;77:83-8.

86. Zhu B & WW Parmley. Hemodynamic and vascular effects of active and passive smoking. American Heart Journal 1995;130:1270-75.

87. Darr D, Dunston S, Faust H, et al. Effectiveness of antioxidants (vitamin C and E) with and without sunscreens as topical photoprotectants. Aca Derm Venerol 1996;76:264-8.

88. Kligman AM. Current status of topical tretinoin in the treatment of photoaged skin. Drugs and Aging 1992;2:7-13.

89. Bernstein Ef, Brown DB, Urbach F, et al. Ultraviolet radiation activates the human elastin promoter in transgenic mice: A novel approach to in vitro model of cutaneous photoaging. J Investig Dermatolog1995;105:269-73.

90. Ziboh VA, Chapikins RS. Biologic significance of polyunsaturated fatty acids in the skin. Arch Dermatol 1987;123:1686-90.

91. Alster T, Tanzi E. Hypertrophic scars and keloids : etiology and management. Am J Clin Dermatol. 2003;4(4):235-43.

92. Weeks DJ, James J. Secrets of the superyoung: the scientific reasons some people look ten years younger than they really are—and how you can, too. Berkley Publishing Group; Reissue edition, 1999.

93. Osler W. Lecture on angina pectoris and allied states. New York: Appleton, 1897.

94. Kaplan JR, Manuck SB, Williams JK, Strawn W. Psychological influences on atherosclerosis: evidence for effects and mechanisms in non-human primates. In: Blascovich J, Katkin ES, eds. Cardiovascular reactivity to psychological stress and disease. Washington, DC: American Psychological Association, 1993.

95. Jacobs S, Friedman R, Mittleman M, et al. for the MI Onset Investigators. 9-fold increased risk of myocardial infarction following psychological stress as assessed by a case –control study. Circulation 1992; 86(suppl I) I: 198.

96. Karasek RA, Theorell T, Schartz JE, et al. Job characteristics in relation to the prevalence of myocardial infarction in the U.S. Health Examination Survey (HES) and the Health and Nutrition Examination Survey (HANES). Am J Public Health 1988; 78:910-18.

97. Lown B, Temte JV, Reich P, et al. Basis for recurring ventricular fibrillation in the absence of coronary heart disease and its management. N Eng J Med 1976;294:623-9.

98. Bower, B. 2001. Look on the bright side and survive longer. Science News 159 324. Retrieved December 2001 from http://www.sciencenews.org/20010526/fob2.asp.

99. Steptoe A, Magid K, Edwards S, Brydon L, Hong Y, Erusalimsky J. The influence of psychological stress and socioeconomic status on platelet activation in men.Atherosclerosis. 2003;168(1):57-63.

100. Kuper H, Marmot M. Job strain, job demands, decision latitude, and risk of coronary heart disease within the Whitehall II study. J Epidemiol Community Health. 2003;57(2):147-53.

101. Friedman M, Rosenman RH. Type-A behavior and your heart. New York: Knopf, 1974.

102. Friedman M, Ghandour G. Medical diagnosis of type A behavior. Am Heart J 1993;126:607-18.

103. Sommers LS, Hacker TW, Schneider DM, Pugno PA, Garrett JB. Descriptive study of managed-care hassles in 26 practices. West J Med 2001;174:175-179.

104. The CMA Code of Ethics. West J Med. 2001;174:5-7.

105. Dawson D, Reid K. Fatigue, alcohol and performance impairment. Nature 1997; 88:235.

106. Wu AW, Folkman S, McPhee SJ, Lo B. Do house officers learn from their mistakes? JAMA 1991;265:2089-94.

107. Caffeine: How little, How Much for You and Your Family? American Dietetic Association,(booklet)1998.

108. Stapleton S. 2000 Omnibus Sleep in America Poll. AMNews 2001.

109. Segelken R. Maas: National (sleep) debt is killing Americans, hurting economy. Cornell Chronicle. Vol. 29, Number 18, 1998. http://www.news.cornell.edu/Chronicle/98/1.22.98/Chron.html.

110. Spiegel K, Leproult R, Van Cauter E. Impact of sleep debt on metabolic and endocrine function. Lancet 1999;354(9188):1435-1439.

111. Nutrition and physical activity. Recommended strategies to prevent chronic diseases and obesity. National Center for Chronic Disease Prevention and Health Promotion. Center for Disease Control and Prevention (CD). Retrieved May 2002 from http://www.cdc.gov/nccdphp/dnpa/obesity/recommendations.htm/.

112. Keeler TE, Hu TW, Keith A, Manning R, Marciniak MD, Ong M, Sung HY. The benefits of switching smoking cessation drugs to over-the-counter status. Health Econ. 2002;11(5):389-402.

113. Fagerstrom K. The epidemiology of smoking: health consequences and benefits of cessation. Drugs. 2002;62 Suppl 2:1-9.

114. Montalto NJ. Recommendations for the treatment of nicotine dependency. J Am Osteopath Assoc. 2002;102(6):342-8.

115. Taylor DH Jr, Hasselblad V, Henley SJ, Thun MJ, Sloan FA. Benefits of smoking cessation for longevity. Am J Public Health. 2002;92(6):990-6.

116. Ornish D. An Inquiry into Access to Complementary and Alternative Medicine in Government-Funded Programs. Washington, DC. Committee on Government Reform, Congress of the United States, House of Representatives 1999.

117. Bendich A, Deckelbaum R, eds. Primary and secondary preventive nutrition. Totowa (NJ): Humana Press Inc, 2001; pp 6-10.

118. Preventive nutrition: the comprehensive guide for health professionals. Bendich A, Deckelbaum RJ, eds. Totowa, NJ: Humana, 2001; pp 134-136.

119. Mayne ST.Antioxidant nutrients and chronic disease: use of biomarkers of exposure and oxidative stress status in epidemiologic research.J Nutr. 2003;133 Suppl 3:933S-940S. Review.

120. Sinatra ST, DeMarco J.Free radicals, oxidative stress, oxidized low density lipoprotein (LDL), and the heart: antioxidants and other strategies to limit cardiovascular damage. Conn Med. 1995;59(10):579-88. Review.

121. Diplock AT.Antioxidant nutrients and disease prevention: an overview. Am J Clin Nutr. 1991;53(1 Suppl):189S-193S. Review.

122. McDermott JH. Antioxidant nutrients: current dietary recommendations and research update.J Am Pharm Assoc (Wash). 2000;40(6):785-99. Review.

123. Willett WC. What you can believe about the diet. In: Eat, drink and be healthy. New York: Simon & Schuster, 2001; pp 27-34.

124. Forestalling frailty. The average woman can now expect live into her 80s. Whether she enjoys her later years may depend on avoiding a common, though not inevitable, consequence of aging. Harv Womens Health Watch. 2003;10(7):2-3.

125. Larson EB. Exercise, functional decline and frailty. J Am Geriatr Soc. 1991;39(6):635-6. Review.

126. Butler RN. Fighting frailty. Prescription for healthier aging includes exercise,nutrition, safety, and research.Geriatrics. 2000;55(2):20.

127. Allison M, Keller C. Physical activity in the elderly: benefits and intervention strategies.Nurse Pract. 1997;22(8):53-4, 56, 58 passim. Review.

128. Evans WJ. Exercise training guidelines for the elderly.Med Sci Sports Exerc. 1999;31(1):12-7.

129. Evans WJ, Campbell WW. Exercise, ageing, and protein metabolism. Diabetes Nutr Metab. 2000;13(2):108-12.

130. Pate RR, Pratt M, Blair SN, et al. Physical activity and public health a recommendation from the Centers for Disease Control and Prevention and the American College of Sports Medicine. JAMA 1995;273:402-7.

131. Fiatarone MA, O'Neill EF, Doyle N, Clements KM, Roberts SB, Kehayias JJ, Lipsitz LA, Evans WJ. The Boston FICSIT study: the effects of resistance training and nutritional supplementation on physical frailty in the oldest old. J Am Geriatr Soc. 1993;41(3):333-7.

132. Fiatarone MA, O'Neill EF, Ryan ND, Clements KM, Solares GR, Nelson ME, Roberts SB, Kehayias JJ, Lipsitz LA, Evans WJ. Exercise training and nutritional supplementation for physical frailty in very elderly people. N Engl J Med. 1994;330(25):1769-75.

133. Pescatello LS, Murphy D. Lower intensity physical activity is advantageous for fat distribution and blood glucose among viscerally obese older adults. Med Sci Sports Exerc 1998;30:1408-13.

134. Tanasescu M, Leitzmann MF, Rimm EB, Willett WC, Stampfer MJ, Hu FB. Exercise type and intensity in relation to coronary heart disease in men. JAMA 2002;288(16):1994-2000.

135. Chou KL, Chi I. Successful aging among the young-old, old-old, and oldest-old Chinese. Int J Aging Hum Dev. 2002;54(1):1-14.

136. Bird CE, Fremont AM. Gender, time use, and health. J Health Soc Behav. 1991;32(2)114-129.

137. Dilenschneider RL. The Critical 2nd phase of your professional life: Keys to Success from age 40 and beyond. Citadel Press, 1992.

138. Murrell SA, Meeks S. Psychological, economic, and social mediators of the education-health relationship in older adults. J Aging Health. 2002;14(4):527-50.

139. Wilcox BJ., Wilcox C, Suzuki M. The Okinawa Program: How the world's longest-lived people achieve everlasting health—and how you can too. New York: Three Rivers Press, 2001.

140. Vaillant GE, Western RJ. Healthy aging among inner-city men. Int Psychogeriatr. 2001;13(4):425-37.

141. Vaillant GE, Meyer SE, Mukamal K, Soldz S. Are social supports in late midlife a cause or a result of successful physical ageing? Psychol Med. 1998;28(5):1159-68.

142. Cui XJ, Vaillant GE. Antecedents and consequences of negative life events in adulthood: a longitudinal study.Am J Psychiatry. 1996 ;153(1):21-6.

143. Shu BC, Huang C, Chen BC.Factors related to self-concept of elderly residing in a retirement center.J Nurs Res. 2003;11(1):1-8.

144. Balick MJ, Lee R. The power of community. Altern Ther Health Med. 2003;9(1):100-3..

145. Deeg DJ, van Zonneveld RJ, van der Maas PJ, Habbema JD. Medical and social predictors of longevity in the elderly: total predictive value and interdependence. Soc Sci Med. 1989;29(11):1271-80.

146. Roos NP, Havens B. Predictors of successful aging: a twelve-year study of Manitoba elderly. Am J Public Health. 1991 ;81(1):63-8.

147. Soc Sci Med. 1989;29(11):1271-80. Achat H, Kawachi I, Spiro A 3rd, DeMolles DA, Sparrow D. Optimism and depression as predictors of physical and mental health functioning: the Normative Aging Study. Ann Behav Med. 2000 Spring;22(2):127-30.

148. Leonard WM 2nd. Successful aging: an elaboration of social and psychological factors. Int J Aging Hum Dev. 1981-82;14(3):223-32.

149. Vaillant GE, Meyer SE, Mukamal K, Soldz S. Are social supports in late midlife a cause or a result of successful physical ageing? Psychol Med. 1998;28(5):1159-68.

150. Strawbridge WJ, Cohen RD, Shema SJ, Kaplan GA. Successful aging: predictors and associated activities. Am J Epidemiol. 1996;144(2):135-41.

151. Koenig HG, Hays JC, George LK, Blazer DG, Larson DB, Landerman LR. Modeling the cross-sectional relationships between religion, physical health,social support, and depressive symptoms. Am J Geriatr Psychiatry. 1997 Spring;5(2):131-44.

152. Canova F, Siega Battel G, Carlini A, Rausa G, Rocco S. The problem of the aged person living alone: a methodological proposal for a pilot project of the aged person's and university student's cohabitation Ann Ig. 2002;14(5):427-34. Italian.

153. Blazer DG. Social support and mortality in an elderly community population. Am J Epidemiol. 1982;115(5):684-94.

Chapter 7

1. Khan MA. Evaluation of food selection patterns and preferences. CRC Critical Reviews: Food Science and Nutrition 1981;15(99)129-53.

2. Narayan KMV, Bowman BA, Engelgau ME. Prevention of type 2 diabetes. Br Med J 2001;323:63-64.

3. Guthrie C. Letters. Br Med J 2001;323:997.

4. Tuomilehto J, Lindstorm J, Eriksson JG, Valle TT, Hamalainein H, Ilanne-Parikka, et al. Prevention of type 2 diabetes by changes in lifestyle among subjects with impaired glucose tolerance. The Finnish Diabetes Prevention Study Group. N Engl J Med 2001;345(9):696-697

5. Bhopal R. South Asian children are more insulin resistant than white children. Epidemic of cardiovascular disease in South Asians. Br Med J 2002;324:625-6.

6.   Swinburn B, Egger G. Letters. Br Med J 2001;323:997.

7. Genesis 25:29-34. New International Version 1978, Committee on Bible Translation.

8. Maslow AH. Motivation and Personality. New York: Harper & Row, 1970.

9. Fieldhouse P. Food and Nutrition, Customs and Culture. London: Chapman & Hall, 1986:25.

10. Turner-McGrievy B, Airwise news report. Retrieved May 2001 from http://news.airwise.com/index.html.

11. Williams BJ. Evolution and Human Origins: an Introduction to Physical Anthropology. New York: Harper, 1973.

12. Fieldhouse P. Food and Nutrition, Customs and Culture. London: Chapman & Hall, 1986:5.

13. Fieldhouse P. Nutrition and Education of the School Child. World Rev Nutr & Diet, 1982;40:83-112

14. National Consumer Council. Your food: whose choice? HMSO, London: pp.72-94.

15. Lucas B. Normal nutrition from infancy through adolescence. In Queen PM, Lang CE, eds. Handbook of pediatric nutrition. Gaithersburg, MD: Aspen publishers,1993; pp 145-70.

16. Rosenbaum M. Marketing to schools. The Guardian (UK), 1993.

17. Sheperd R. Factors influencing food preferences and choice. Handbook of the Psychophysiology of Human Eating. Sheperd R, Wiley, eds. 1989:3-24.

18. Ward, Reale, Levinson. Children's perceptions, explanations and judgments of television advertising: a further exploration. Television and Social Behavior, Washington DC: U.S. Government Printing Office, 972:4.

19. Greenberg B, Fazal S, Wober M. Children's Views on Advertising. Independent Broadcasting Authority, 1986.

20. "60 Minutes" CBS cable television (U.S.A.), 2002.

21. Nestle M. Food Politics: How the food industry influences nutrition and health. University of California Press 2002.

22. American Diabetes Association, Type 2 Diabetes in Children and Adolescents, Pediatrics, Volume 105, No. 3, Retrieved March, 2000 from www.diabetes.org/ada/type2kids.asp.

23. Fagot-Campagna, Anne, MD, Ph.D. et al., Type 2 Diabetes Among North American Children and Adolescents: An epidemiologic review and a public health perspective, Journal of Pediatrics 2000, Volume 136, Number 5, Pg 664-672.

24. Dundee & Newcastle. Proceedings of the Nutrition Society: OCA Spring 2001:2A.

25. Dundee & Newcastle. Proceedings of the Nutrition Society: OCA Spring 2001:3A.

26. Lucas B. Normal nutrition from infancy through adolescence. In Queen PM, Lang CE, eds. Handbook of pediatric nutrition. Gaithersburg, MD: Aspen publishers, 1993; pp145-170.

27. Contento IR, Michaela JL, Williams SS. Adolescent food choice criteria: role of weight and dieting status. Appetite 1995;25:51-76.

28. Strong WB, Kelder SH. Pediatric preventive cardiology. In: Prevention of Myocardial Infarction. Manson JE, Ridker PM, Gaziano JM, Hennekens CH, eds. New York: Oxford University Press; 1996; pp 353.

29. Young LR, Nestle M. The Contribution of expanding portion sizes to the U.S. obesity epidemic: Am J of Public Health 2002;2:246-49.

30. Nielsen SJ, Popkin BM. Patterns and trends in food portion sizes, 1977-1998.JAMA. 2003;289(4):450-3.

31. Young LR. Portion sizes in the American food supply: Issues and implications [dissertation]. New York, NY: New York University, 2000.

32. Understanding the Food choices of low income families. U.S. Department of Agriculture Food and Nutrition Service; 1997. Retrieved October 1999 from http://www.fns.usda.gov/oane/menu/published/nutritioneducation/Files/NUTRI.PDF

33. Ministry of Agriculture, Fisheries and Food. Household food consumption and expenditure 1990. Annual Report of the National Food Survey Committee, Her Majesty's Stationery Office (HMSO), 1990.

34. Proceedings of the Nutrition Society Vol. 60 Meeting of 2001:177A.

35. Leather S. Less Money, Less Choice: Poverty and Diet in the UK Today. In: National Consumer Council (ed.), Your Food: Whose Choice?, London HMSO, 1992; pp 72-94.

36. Forbes AL. National Nutrition Policy, Food Labeling, and Health Claims. In: Modern nutrition in health and disease. Shils ME, Olson JA, Shike M, eds. 8th Ed. Vol.1: Philadelphia, PA: Lea & Febiger;1994; pp 1637.

37. Dietary Guidelines for Americans. USDA home and garden bulletin No. 232. 3rd ed. Washington, DC. Government Printing Office (1990-272-930), 1990.

38. Willett WC. Introduction. In: Eat, drink and be healthy. New York: Simon & Schuster, 2001; pp 15-22.

39. Willett WC. Introduction. In: Eat, drink and be healthy. New York: Simon & Schuster, 2001; pp 138.

40. Nelson ME. 2001. Strong Women Eat Well: Nutritional Strategies for a Healthy Body and Mind. New York: G. P. Putnam's Sons.

41. McGinnis MJ, Ernst ND. Preventive nutrition: A historic perspective and future economic outlook. In: Bendich A, Deckelbaum R, eds. Primary and secondary preventive nutrition. Totowa (NJ): Humana Press Inc, 2001; pp 6-10.

42. Leather S. (In: National Consumer Council (ed.), Your Food: Whose Choice?, London HMSO, 1992:56-57.

43. Food Commission. Sweet Persuasion. The Food Magazine 1990; pp 4.

44. Zuckerman P, Gianinno L. Measuring children's response to television advertising. Television advertising and children. Esserman J, ed. 1987.

45. Ward, Reale and Levinson. Children's perceptions, explanations and judgments of television advertising; a further exploration. Television and Social Behavior, U.S. Government Printing Office, Washington DC, 1972:4.

46. Van Duyn MAS, Kristal AR, Dodd K, Campbell. Association of awareness, intrapersonal and interpersonal factors, and stage of dietary change with fruit and vegetable consumption: A national survey. Am J Health Promot 2001; 16(2):69-78).

47. Trudeau E, Kristal AR, Li S et al. Demographic and psychosocial predictors of fruit and vegetable intakes differ: implications for dietary interventions. J Am Diet Assoc 1998;98(12):1412-1419.

48. Pescatello LS, Murphy D, Vollono J, Lynch E. The cardiovascular health impact of an incentive worksite health promotion program. Am J Health Promot 2001;16(1):16-20.

49. Proceedings from the Nutrition Society Vol 60; autumn 2001:158A.

50. Genesis 41:46-57. New International Version 1978, Committee on Bible Translation.

51. Southgate DAT, Johnson I. Food processing. In: Human nutrition and dietetics. Garrow JS, James WPT eds. Eight edition. Edinburgh. Churchill Livingstone, 1993:335-348.

52. Campden Food Preservation Research Association (1987) Briefing paper -11. Food Processing. The British Nutrition Foundation 1993.

53. Karmas E, Harris RS. Nutritional evaluation of food processing, 3rd edn. New York: Van Nostrand Reinhold, 1988.

54. Symposium on 'Nutritional Effects of New Processing Technologies': New Procession Technologies: an overview. Grahame W. Gould; pp 87-90.

55. What We Eat in America. The continuing survey of food intakes by individuals (CSFII) and the diet and health knowledge survey (DHKS), 1994-96. Food Surveys Research Group. Beltsville Human Nutrition Research Center. United States Department of Agriculture (USDA); http://www.barc.usda.gov/bhnrc/foodsurvey/home.htm.

56. Personal Consumption Expenditures Table, 1999, Bureau of Economic Analysis, U.S. Department of Commerce.

57. The Contextual Effect of the Local Food Environment on Residents' Diets: The Atherosclerosis Risk in Communities (ARIC) Study 2002, Vol 92, No. 11. American Journal of Public Health 1761-1768.

58. Loria CM, Obarzanek M, Ernst ND. Choose and prepare foods with less salt: Dietary advice for all Americans. Journal of Nutrition. 2001;131:536S-551S.

59. Dietary Guidelines Advisory Committee Report of the Dietary Guidelines Advisory Committee on the Dietary Guidelines for Americans 1990:1990 U.S. Department of Agriculture Washington, DC.

60. Mattes R. D., Donnelly D. Relative contributions of dietary sodium sources. J Am Coll Nutr 1991;10:383-393.

61. Hoffman C. J. Does the sodium level in drinking water affect blood pressure levels?. J Am Diet Assoc 1988;88:1432-1435.

62. Fregly M. J. Estimates of sodium and potassium intake. Ann Intern Med 1983;98:792-799.

63. Franz MJ, Maryniuk MD. Position of the American Dietetic Association: Use of nutritive and non-nutritive sweetenes. J Am Dietetic Assn 1993; 93:816-821.

64. Karmas E, Harris RS. Nutritional evaluation of food processing, 3rd edn. New York: Van Nostrand Reinhold, 1988.

65. Morton ID. Physical, chemistry and biological changes related to different time-temperature combinations. In: Hoyem T, Kvale O (eds) Physical, chemical and biological changes in foods caused by thermal processing. Applied Science, London 1977; pp 135-51.

66. Severi S, Bedogni G, Manzieri AM, Poli M, Battistini N. Effects of cooking and storage methods on the micronutrient content of foods. Eur J Cancer Prev. 1997;6 Suppl 1:S21-4. Review.

67. Fillion L, Henry CJ. Nutrient losses and gains during frying: a review. Int J Food Sci Nutr. 1998;49(2):157-68. Review.

68. Nursal B, Yucecan S.Vitamin C losses in some frozen vegetables due to various cooking methods. Nahrung. 2000;44(6):451-3.

69. Reddy MB, Love M. The impact of food processing on the nutritional quality of vitamins and minerals. Adv Exp Med Biol. 1999;459:99-106. Review.

70. Rumm-Kreuter D, Demmel I. Comparison of vitamin losses in vegetables due to various cooking methods. J Nutr Sci Vitaminol (Tokyo). 1990;36 Suppl 1:S7-14; discussion S14-5. Review.

71. Effect of Storage, Cooking, Freezing, Frozen Storage, Canning and Canned Storage on the Vitamin C content of garden peas (on a dry weight basis). Campden Food Preservation Research Association (1987). Modified from: Briefing paper -11. Food Processing. The British Nutrition Foundation 1993; pp 8-9.

72. Effect of Storage, Cooking, Freezing, Frozen Storage, and Frying the Vitamin C content of old potatoes (on a dry weight basis). Source: Campden Food Preservation Research Association (1987). Modified from: Briefing paper -11. Food Processing. The British Nutrition Foundation 1993; pp 10.

73. Tanphaichitr V. Thiamin. In Modern nutrition in health and disease, 8th ed. Lea & Febiger, Phil.,1994; pp 359-365.

74. Gann PH, Ma J, Giovannucci E, Willett W, Sacks FM, Hennekens CH, Stampfer MJ. Lower prostate cancer risk in men with elevated plasma lycopene levels: results of a prospective analysis. Cancer Res. 1999;59(6):1225-30.

75. Hallberg L, Rossander L. Effect of soy protein on nonheme iron absorption in man. Am J Clin Nutr. 1982;36(3):514-20.

76. Macfarlane BJ, van der Riet WB, Bothwell TH, Baynes RD, Siegenberg D, Schmidt U, Tal A, Taylor JR, Mayet F. Effect of traditional oriental soy products on iron absorption. Am J Clin Nutr. 1990;51(5):873-80.

77. Hurrell RF, Juillerat MA, Reddy MB, Lynch SR, Dassenko SA, Cook JD. Soy protein, phytate, and iron absorption in humans. Am J Clin Nutr. 1992;56(3):573-8.

78. Food Fortification: Technology and Quality Control. (FAO Food and Nutrition Paper - 60). Report of an FAO technical meeting. Rome, Italy, 1995. Food and Agriculture Organization of the United Nations Rome, 1996. Retrieved January 2001 from http://www.fao.org/docrep/W2840E/W2840E00.htm

79. Bauernfeind JC. Nutrification of foods. In Modern nutrition in health and disease, 8th ed. Lea & Febiger, Phil.,1994; pp 1579-1592.

80. Severi S, Bedogni G, Zoboli GP, Manzieri AM, Poli M, Gatti G, Battistini N. Effects of home-based food preparation practices on the micronutrient content of foods. Eur J Cancer Prev. 1998;7(4):331-5.

81. Yadav SK, Sehgal S. Effect of home processing on ascorbic acid and beta-carotene content of spinach (Spinacia oleracia) and amaranth (Amaranthus tricolor) leaves. Plant Foods Hum Nutr. 1995;47(2):125-31

82. Hargraves WA. Mutagens in cooked foods. In Nutritional Toxicology. Vol. 2. Hathcock J, ed. Orlando, FL, Academic Press, 1987.

83. Sugimura T, Wakabayashi K, Nagao M, et al. Heterocyclic amines in food. In Food Toxicology: A Perspective on the Relative Risks. Taylor SL, Scanlan RA, eds. New York, Marcel Dekker, 1989.

84. Andrews, et al. Food preservation using ionizing radiation. Rev Environ Contam Toxicol, 1998;154(1):1-53.

85. Ohlsson T, Bengtsson N. Microwave technology and foods. Adv Food Nutr Res. 2001;43:65-140. Review.

86. Alfrey AC. Aluminum intoxication. New England Journal of Medicine 1984, 310:1113-1115.

87. Martyn C N et al (1989). Geographical relation between Alzheimer's disease and aluminum in drinking water. Lancet 1990, 59-62.

88. Tareke E, Rydberg P, Karlsson P, Eriksson S, Törnqvist M. Analysis of Acrylamide, a Carcinogen Formed in Heated Foodstuffs. J Agric Food Chem 2002;50 (17):4998-5006.

89. Hornick SB. Factors affecting the nutritional quality of crops. AM J Alternative Ag,1992;7(1-2).

90. Transmissible spongiform encephalopathies, hypotheses and food safety: an overview.Sci Total Environ. 1998;217(1-2):71-82.

91. Smith G, Charlton R. New-variant Creutzfeldt-Jacob disease. Br J Gen Pract. 2000;50(457):611-2.

92. Smith BL. Organic foods vs. supermarket foods: J Applied Nutr,1993;45(1):35-39.

93. Baker BP, Benbrook CM, Groth E 3rd, Lutz Benbrook K. Pesticide residues in conventional, integrated pest management (IPM)-grown andorganic foods: insights from three US data sets. Food Addit Contam. 2002;19(5):427-46.

94. The National Organic Program. Last retrieved July 2002 from http://www.ams.usda.gov/nop/.

95. Asami DK, Hong YJ, Barrett DM, Mitchell AE. Comparison of the Total Phenolic and Ascorbic Acid Content of Freeze-Dried and Air-Dried Marionberry, Strawberry, and Corn Grown Using Conventional, Organic, and Sustainable Agricultural Practices. J Agric Food Chem;2003; 51(5):1237-1241.

96. Whitman DB. Genetically Modified Foods: Harmful or Helpful? Cambridge Scientific Abstracts, Hot topics series 2000; http://www.csa.com/hottopics/gmfood/overview.html

97. Martens MA. Safety evaluation of genetically modified foods. Int Arch Occup Environ Health. 2000;73 Suppl:S14-8. Review.

98. Rowland IR. Genetically modified foods, science, consumers and the media. Proc Nutr Soc. 2002;61(1):25-9.

99. Normile D. Agricultural biotechnology. Monsanto donates its share of golden rice. Science. 2000;289(5481):843-5.

100. Shouse B. Genetically modified food. TV drama sparks scientific backlash. Science. 2002;296(5575):1948-9.

101. Murphy, D. 1996. How clean is "Too Clean?" Meat Marketing and Technology (12):50-52.

102. The Royal Institute of Public Health. Are We Too Clean? A Question of Immunity Balance. Courses and symposia, 2002. Retrieved September 2002 from http://www.riphh.org.uk/symposia.html.

103. Larson L. Hygiene of the skin: when is clean too clean? Emerging Infectious Disease 2001; Vol 7 No 2:225-230. http://www.cdc.gov/ncidod/eid/vol7no2/larson.htm.

104. Rulis AM. Safety assurance margins for food additives currently in use. Regul Toxicol Pharmacol. 1987;7(2):160-8. Review.

105. Nutrition Labeling and Education Act (NLEA, 1990) which led to the mandatory requirement of specified food labels on most foods with the exception of fresh meat, poultry, fish and produce (fruits & vegetables). 166-167.

106. Nutrition Labeling and Education Act of 1990. Public Law 101- 535, 1990,104 Stat. 2353, 21 USC, 301 note,321, 337, 343, 343 notes, 343-1, 343-1 note, 345, 371.

107. The Surgeon General's Report on Nutrition and Health (1988). U.S. Department of Health and Human Services, Public Health Service, DHHS (PHS) Publ. No. 88-50210. Superintendent of Documents, Stock No. 017-001-00465-1. Washington, DC, Government Printing Office, 1988.

108. Food and Drug Administration. Food labeling: public health messages on food labels and labeling: notice of proposed rulemaking. 52 Federal Register 28843, 1987.

109. Food and Drug Administration. Food labeling: general provisions; nutrition labeling; nutrient content claims; health claims; ingredient labeling; state and local requirements; and exemptions; proposed rules. 56 Federal Register 60366, 1991.

110. Food and Drug Administration. Food labeling: mandatory status of nutrition labeling and nutrient content revision; proposed rule. 55 Federal Register 29487, 1990.

111. Food and Drug Administration. Food labeling: nutrient content claims, general principles, petitions, definition of terms; proposed rule. 56 Federal Register 60421, 1991.
112. Centers for Disease Control and Prevention. Recommendations for the use of folic acid to reduce the number of cases of spina bifida and other neural tube defects. Morbidity and Mortality Weekly Report (MMWR) 1992;41(RR-14).
113. Food and Drug Administration. Food labeling: health claims; dietary lipids and cancer; proposed rule. 56 Federal Register 60764, 1991.
114. Food and Drug Administration. Food labeling: health claims and label statements; antioxidant vitamins and cancer. Federal Register 1993;58:2622-2660.(Codified in Section 101.78, Title 21, Code of Federal Regulations).
115. Food and Drug Administration. Food labeling: health claims and label statements; sodium and hypertension. Federal Register 1993;58:2820-2849.(Codified in Section 101.74, Title 21, Code of Federal Regulations).
116. Food and Drug Administration. Food labeling: definitions of the terms cholesterol free, low cholesterol, and reduced cholesterol; tentative final rule. 55 Federal Register 29456, 1990.
117. Food and Drug Administration. Food labeling: "Cholesterol free", "low cholesterol", and "percent fat free" claims; proposed rule. 56 Federal Register 60507, 1991.
118. Dickinson A. Health Claims for foods and dietary supplements in the United States and Japan. In: Bendich A, Deckelbaum R, eds. Primary and secondary preventive nutrition. Totowa (NJ): Humana Press Inc, 2001; pp 397-411.
119. Shils ME, Olson JA, Shike M, eds. Modern nutrition in health and disease, 8th Ed. Vol.1: Philadelphia, PA: Lea & Febiger.1994:1650.
120. National Consumer Council. Your food: whose choice? HMSO, London; pp 61-62
121. Willett WC. What you can believe about the diet. In: Eat, drink and be healthy. New York: Simon & Schuster, 2001; pp 98-99.
122. Food and Drug Administration. Labeling: general requirements for health claims for food. Federal Register 1993; 58:2478-2536. (Codified in Section101.14, Title 21, Code of Federal Regulations).

Chapter 8

1. Powell A. Diabetes onset affected by diet. Harvard University Gazette 2002:9. Also retrieved from http://www.news.harvard.edu/gazette/2002/02.07/09-diabetes.html.
2. Jospipura KJ, et al. Frui and Vegetable Intake in Relation to Risk of Ischemic Stroke. JAMA 282 1999:1233-9.
3. Ness AR, Poles JW. Fruits and vegetables and cardiovascular diseases. A review. Int J Epidemiol 1997;26:1-13.
4. Cohen JH, Kristal AR, Stanford JL. Fruit and vegetable intakes and prostate cancer risk. J Natl Cancer Inst 1977;58:825-32.
5. Temple NJ. Fruits, vegetables and cancer prevention trials. J Natl Cancer Inst 1999;91(13):1164.
6. Garcia-Closas R, Gonzalez CA, Agudo A, Riboli E. Intake of specific carotenoids an flavonoids and the risk of gastric cancer in Spain. Cancer Causes Control 1999;10(1):71-5.
7. van Dam RM, Rimm EB, Willett WC, Stampfer MJ, Hu FB. Dietary patterns and risk for type 2 diabetes mellitus in U.S. men. Ann Int Med 2002;136(3):201-209.
8. De Roos N, Schouten EG, Katan MB. Consumption of a solid fat rich in lauric acid results in a more favorable serum lipid profile in healthy men and women than consumption of a solid fat rich in trans-fatty acids. Journal of Nutrition. 2001;131:242-5.
9. Molteni A, Brizio-Molteni L, Persky V. In vitro hormonal effects of soybean isoflavones. J Nutr 1995;125:751S-6S.
10. Messina MJ. Legumes and soybeans: overview of their nutritional profiles and health effects. Am J Clin Nutr 1999;70(3 suppl):439S-450S.

11. Kim H. Peterson TG, Barnes S. Mechanisms of action of the soy isoflavone genistein: emerging role for its via transforming growth factor beta signaling pathways. Am J Clin Nutr 1998; 68(6 Suppl)1418S-1425S.

12. Crowell PL. Prevention and therapy of cancer by dietary monoterpenes. J Nutr 1999;129(3):775S-8S.

13. Elegbede JA, Maltzman TH, Verma AK, Tanner MA, Elson CE, Gould MN. Mouse skin tumor promoting activity of orange peel and d-limonene: a reevaluation. Carcinogenesis 1986;7(12):2047-49.

14. Appel LJ, Morre TJ, Obarzanek E, et al. A clinical trial of the effects of dietary patterns on blood pressure. DASH Collaborative Research Group. N Eng J Med 1997;336:1117-24.

15. Potischman N, Swanson CA, Coates RJ, Gammon MD, Brogan DR, Curtin J, et al. Intake of food groups and associated micronutrients in relaion to risk of early-stage breast cancer. Int J Cancer 1999;82(3):315-21.

16. Canivenc-Lavier MC, Bentejac M, Miller ML, Leclerc J, Siess MH, Latruffe N, et al. Differential effects of nonhydroxylated flavonoids as inducers of cytochrome P450 1A and 2B isozymes in rat liver. Toxicol Appl Pharmacol 1996;136(2):348-53.

17. Van Duuren BL, Goldschmidt BM, Cocarcinogenic and tumor-promoting agents in tobacco carcinogenesis. J Natl Cancer Inst 1976;56(6):1237-42.

18. Milner JA. Nonnutritive components in foods as modifiers of the cancer process. In: Preventive nutrition: the comprehensive guide for health professionals. Bendich A, Deckelbaum RJ, eds. Totowa, NJ: Humana, 2001; pp 134-136.

19. Gaziano JM, Manson JE, Ridker PM. Primary and secondary prevention of coronary heart disease. In: Braunwald E, Zipes DP, Libby P. Heart disease, A textbook of cardiovascular medicine. 6th ed. Philadelphia: WB Saunders, 2001; pp 1056.

20. Niebauer J, Hambrecht R, Mauburger C, et al. Impact of intensive physical exercise and low-fat diet on collateral vessel formation in stable angina pectoris and angiographically concerned coronary artery disease. Am J Cardiol 1995;76:771-5.

21. Ascherio A, Katan MB, Zock PL, et al. Trans fatty acids and coronary heart disease. N Engl J Med 340:1994-1998,1999.

22. Yusuf S, Dagenais G, Pogue J, et al: Vitamin E supplementation and cardiovascular events in high-risk patients. The Heart Outcomes Prevention Evaluation Study Investigators. N Engl J Med 342:154-160,2000.

23. Dietary supplementation with n-3 polyunsaturated fatty acids and vitamin E after myocardial infarction: Gruppo Italiano per lo Studio della Sopravvivenza nell'Infarto miocardio. Lancet 1999;354:447-55.

24. Bauernfeind J. Tocopherols in foods: In: Vitamin E—a Comprehensive Treatise. Ed. Machlin. New York: Marcel Dekker, 1980.

25. Farrell PA, Roberts RJ. Vitamin E. In Modern nutrition in health and disease, 8th ed. Philadelphia, PA: Lea & Febiger, 1994:326-358.

26. Morrison, E. Y. S. A., H. Thompson, et al. (1991). Extraction of an hyperglycemic principle from the annatto (Bixa orellana): A medicinal plant in the West Indies. Tropical and Geographical Medicine 43(1-2): 184-188.

27. Stephens NG, Parsons A, Schofield PM, et al. Randomized controlled trial of vitamin E in patients with coronary artery disease: Cambridge heart antioxidant heart study (CHAOS). Lancet 347:781, 1996.

28. Rapola JM, Virtamo J, Ripatti S, et al. Randomized trial of alpha-tocopherol and beta-carotene supplements on incidence of major coronary events in men with previous myocardial infarction. Lancet 349:1715,1997.

29. Gersh BJ, Braunwald E, Bonow RO. Chronic coronary heart disease. In: Braunwald E, Zipes DP, Libby P. Heart disease, A textbook of cardiovascular medicine. 6th ed. Philadelphia: WB Saunders, 2001; pp 1284.

30. Willet WC. Nutritional Epidemiology, Second Edition. New York: Oxford University Press; 1998.

31. Willett WC. What you can believe about the diet. In: Eat, drink and be healthy. New York: Simon & Schuster, 2001; pp 27-34.

32. Willett WC, Stampfer MJ. Total energy intake: implications for epidemiologic analyses. Am J Epidemiol 1986;124:17-27.

33. Bendich A, Deckelbaum RJ. Preventive nutrition throughout the life cycle. In: Bendich A, Deckelbaum R, eds. Primary and secondary preventive nutrition. Totowa (NJ): Humana Press Inc. 2001; pp 427-441.

34. Keys A. Seven Countries: a multivariate analysis of death and coronary heart disease. Cambridge, Massachusetts: Harvard University Press; 1980.

35. Keys A, Menotti A, Karvonen MJ, et al. The diet and 15-year death rate in the seven countries study. Am J Epidemiol 1986;124:903-15.

36. Verschuren WM, Jacobs DR, Bloemberg BP, et al. Serum total cholesterol and long-term coronary heart disease mortality in different cultures: twenty-five year follow-up of the seven countries study. JAMA 1995;274:131-6.

37. The Framingham Heart Study: The town that changed America's heart. Retrieved June 2001 from http://www.framingham.com/heart/backgrnd.htm.

38. Framingham heart study: 50 years of research success. Last accessed April 2003. http://www.nhlbi.nih.gov/about/framingham/index.html. Framingham heart study Bibliography: http://www.nhlbi.nih.gov/about/framingham/bib-menu.htm

39. de Lorgeril,M. et al. "Mediterranean Alpha-linolenic Acid-rich Diet in Secondary Prevention of Coronary Heart Disease." Lancet 1994;343:1454-59.

40. Leaf A. Dietary prevention of coronary heart disease: the Lyon diet heart study. Circulation 1999, 99(6) p733-5.

41. Gruppo Italiano per lo Studio della Sopravvienza nell'Infarto Miocardico. "Dietary supplementation with n-3 polyunsaturated fatty acids and vitamin E after Myocardial infarction: Results of the GISSI-Prevenzione trial." Lancet 354(1999): 447- 455.

42. Leelagul P, Tanphaichitr V. Current status on diet-related chronic diseases in Thailand. Intern Med 1995;11:28-33.

43. Statistics and Information Department, Minister's Secrearia, Ministry of Health and Welfare of Japan. Vital Statistics of Japan, 1993.

44. National Statistics Office, Republic of Korea. Annual Report of Case of Death Statistics, 1994.

45. Willett WC. Potential benefits of preventive nutrition strategies: lessons for the United States. In: Bendich A, Deckelbaum R, eds. Primary and secondary preventive nutrition. Totowa (NJ): Humana Press Inc. 2001; pp 450.

46. Kida K, Ito T, Yang SW, Tanphaichitr V. Effects of western diet on risk factors of chronic diseases in Asia. In: Bendich A, Deckelbaum R, eds. Primary and secondary preventive nutrition. Totowa (NJ): Humana Press Inc. 2001; pp 435-436.

47. Block G, Patterson BH, Subar AF. Fruit, vegetables, and cancer prevention: a review of the epidemiological evidence. Nutr Cancer 1992;18:1-29.

48. Steinmetz KA, Potter JD. Vegetables, fruit, and cancer. I. Epidemiology. Cancer Causes Control 1991;2:325-57

49. Steinmetz KA, Potter JD. Vegetables, fruit, and cancer. II. Mechanisms. Cancer Causes Control 1991;2:427-42.

50. Verhoeven DTH, Goldbohm RA, Van Poppel G, et al. Epidemiological studies on brassica vegetables and cancer risk. Cancer Epidemiological biomarkers Prev 1996;5:733-748.

51. Willett WC, Trichopoulos D. Nutrition and cancer: a summary of the evidence. Cancer Causes Control 1996;7:178-180.

52. Bertram JS, Dolonel LN, Meyskens FL. Rationale and strategies for chemprevention of cancer in human. Cancer Res 1987;47:3012-3031.

53. Moon TE, Micozzi MS. Nutrition and and Cancer Prevention: Investigating the Role of Micronutrients. New York: Marcel Dekker, 1988.

54. Diplock AT. Antioxidant nutrients and disease prevention: an overview. Am J Clin Nutr 1991;53(Suppl.):189-193.

55. Greaves KA, Wilson MD, Rudel LL, et al. Consumption of soy protein reduces cholesterol absorption compared to casein protein alone or supplemented with an isoflavone extract or conjugated equine estrogen in ovariectomized cynomolgus monkeys. J Nutr 2000;130(4): 820-6.

56. Baum JA, Teng H, Erdman JW, et al. Long-term intake of soy protein improves blood lipid profiles and increases mononuclear cell low-density-lipoprotein receptor messenger RNA in hypercholesterolemic, postmenopausal women. Am J Clin Nutr, 1998;68(3):545-51.

57. Ho SC, Woo JL, Leung SS, et al. Intake of soy products is associated with better plasma lipid profiles in the Hong Kong Chinese population. J Nutr, 2000;130(10):2590-3.

58. Milner JA. Nonnutritive components in foods as modifiers of the cancer process. In: Preventive nutrition: the comprehensive guide for health professionals. Bendich A, Deckelbaum RJ, eds. Totowa, NJ: Humana, 2001; pp 131-154.

59. Higdon JV, Frei B. Tea catechins and polyphenols: health effects, metabolism, and antioxidant functions. Crit Rev Food Sci Nutr. 2003;43(1):89-143.

60. Leung LK, Su Y, Chen R, Zhang Z, Huang Y, Chen ZY. Theaflavins in black tea and catechins in green tea are equally effective antioxidants.J Nutr. 2001;131(9):2248-51.

61. Leenen R, Roodenburg AJ, Tijburg LB, Wiseman SA. A single dose of tea with or without milk increases plasma antioxidant activity in humans. Eur J Clin Nutr. 2000;54(1):87-92.

62. Appel LJ, Morre TJ, Obarzanek E, et al. A clinical trial of the effects of dietary patterns on blood pressure. DASH Collaborative Research Group. N Eng J Med 1997;336:1117-24.

63. Sacks FM, Svetkey LP, Vollmer WM, et al for the DASH-Sodium Collaborative Research Group. Effects on blood pressure of reduced dietary sodium and the Dietary Approaches to Stop Hypertension (DASH) diet. N Engl J Med. 2001;344:3-10.

64. Hankinson SE, Colditz GA, Manson JE, Speizer FE. eds. Healthy women, healthy lives: A guide to preventing disease from the landmark Nurses' Health Study. New York: Simon & Schuster, 2001.

65. Colditz GA, et al. The Nurses' Health Study: 20-year contribution to the understanding of health among women. Journal of Women's Health 1997;6:49-61.

66. Van Dam RM, Rimm EB, Willett WC, Stampfer MJ, Hu FB. Dietary patterns and risk for type 2 diabetes in U.S. men. Ann Int Med 2002;136(3):201-9.

67. Ornish D, Brown SE, Sherwitz LW. Can lifestyle changes reverse coronary heart disease? Lancet 1990;336:129-33.

68. Ornish D, Scherwitz LW, Billings JH, et al. Intensive lifestyle changes for reversal of coronary heart disease. JAMA 1998;280:2001-7.

69. Ornish D. An Inquiry into access to complementary and alternative medicine in Government-funded programs. Washington, DC. Committee on government reform, Congress of the United States, House of Representatives 1999.

70. Kato H, Tillotson J, Nichamen MZ, et al. Epidemiologic studies of coronary heart disease and stroke in Japanese men living in Japan, Hawaii and California: serum lipids and diet. Am J Epidemiol 1973;97:372-85.

71. Robertson TL, Kato H, Rhoads GG, et al. Epidemiologic studies of coronary heart disease and stroke in Japanese men living in Japan, Hawaii and California: Incidence of myocardial infarction and death from coronary heart disease. Am J Cardiol 1977;39:239-43.

72. Willett WC. Migrant studies and secular trends. In: Prevention of Myocardial Infarction. Manson JE, Ridker PM, Gaziano JM, Hennekens CH, eds. New York: Oxford University Press; 1996; pp 353.

73. Oldways Preservation & Exchange Trust. Boston, MA. Retrieved December 2001 from http://www.oldwayspt.org/html/p_med.htm.

74. Harmon N, Trichopoulou A. The Mediterranean Diet Cookbook. New York: Bantam Doubleday Dell Pub.;1994.

75. The Omega Diet: The Lifesaving Nutritional Program Based on the Diet of the Island of Crete by Artemis P. Simopoulos, Jo Robinson. New York. HarperCollins; 1999.

76. The Omega Diet by Artemis Simopoulos, MD and Jo Robinson. HarperCollins Publishers: New York;1999.

77. Simopoulos AP. Omega-3 fatty acids in health and disease and in growth and development. Am J Clin Nutr 1991;54:438-63.

78. de Lorgeril M, Salen P, Martin JL, Monjaud I, Delaye J, Mamelle N, "Mediterranean diet, traditional risk factors, and the rate of cardiovascular complications after myocardial infarction: Final report of the Lyon Diet Heart Study," Circulation. 1999;99:779-785.

79. Kris-Etherton P, Eckel RH, Howard BV, et al. AHA Science Advisory: Lyon Diet Heart Study. Benefits of a Mediterranean-style, National Cholesterol Education Program/American Heart Association Step I Dietary Pattern on Cardiovascular Disease. Circulation 2001;103:1823-5.

80. Voelker R. Mediterranean Diet after MI. JAMA 2000;284:2919-2926.

81. Anderson W. Rapid Alerts: Advice to Industry - Contamination of olive pomace oil. Retrieved December 2001 from http://www.fsai.ie/rapid_alerts/alerts/advice_pomace_contamination.htm

82. United States standards for grades of olive oil. www.ams.usda.gov/standards/oliveoil.pdf

83. Ang CYW, Health implications of ingredients in Asian diets. Session 27, Developing technologies on functional ingredients for improving the health benefits of Asian foods. Annual Meeting and Food Expo - Anaheim, California. Retrieved June , 2002 from http://ift.confex.com/ift/2002/techprogram/paper_9712.htm.

84. Yamori Y, Miura A, Taira K. Implications from and for food cultures for cardiovascular diseases: Japanese food, particularly Okinawan diets. Asia Pac J Clin Nutr. 2001;10(2):144-5. Review.

85. Kurzer MS, Xu X. Dietary phytoestrogens. Annu Rev Nutr. 1997;17:353-81. Review. Fourth International Symposium on the Role of Soy in Preventing and Treating Chronic Disease. San Diego, California, USA. November 4-7, 2001. Proceedings and abstracts. J Nutr. 2002 Mar;132(3):545S-619S.

86. Kris-Etherton PM, Hecker KD, Bonanome A, Coval SM, Binkoski AE, Hilpert KF, Griel AE, Etherton TD. Bioactive compounds in foods: their role in the prevention of cardiovascular disease and cancer. Am J Med. 2002 30;113 Suppl 9B:71S-88S. Review.

87. Tham DM, Gardner CD, and Haskell WL. Clinical Review 97: Potential health benefits of dietary phytoestrogens: a review of the clinical, epidemiological, and mechanistic evidence. J Clin Endocrinology Metabol. 1998;83(7):2223-35.

88. Barnes S, Boersma B, Patel R, Kirk M, Darley-Usmar VM, Kim H, Xu J. Isoflavonoids and chronic disease: mechanisms of action. Biofactors. 2000;12(1-4):209-15. Review.

89. Lee HP, Gourley L, Duffy SW, Esteve J, Lee J, Day NE. Dietary effects on breast-cancer risk in Singapore. Lancet 1991;337:1197-1200.

90. Severson RK. Normura AMY, Grove JS. Stemmermann GN. A prospective study of demographics, diet, and prostate cancer among men of Japanese ancestry in Hawaii. Cancer Res 1989;49:1857-60.

91. Goodman MT, Hankin JH, Wilkens LR, Lyu L-C, McDuffie K, Lui LQ, Kolonel LN. Diet, body size, physical activity, and the risk of endometrial cancer. Cancer Res 1997;57:5077-85.

92. Yuan JM, et al. Diet and breast cancer in Shanghai and Tianjin, China. Br J Cancer 1995;71:1353-8.

93. Anderson JW, Smith BM, Washnock CS. Cardiovascular and renal benefits of dry bean and soybean intake. Am J Clin Nutr. 1999 Sep;70(3 Suppl):464S-474S. Review.

94. Goodman MT, Hankin JH, Wilkens LR, Kolonel LN. Dietary phytoestrogens and the risk of endometrial cancer. Am J Clin Nutr 1998;68(Suppl.):1524S-30S.

95. Hollman PC, Katan MB. Dietary flavanoids: intake, health effects and bioavailability. Food Chem Toxicol 1999;37(9,10):937-42.

96. Moyad MA. Soy, disease prevention, and prostate cancer. Semin Urol Oncol. 1999;17(2):97-102. Review.

97. Washburn S, Burke GL, and Morgan T, et al. Effect of soy protein supplementation on serum lipoproteins, blood pressure, and menopausal symptoms in perimenopausal women. Menopause. Spring 1999;6(1):7-13.

98. Anderson JW, Johnstone, BM, and Cook-Newell ME. Meta-analysis of the effects of soy protein intake on serum lipids. N Engl J Med 1995;333(5):276-82.

99. Albertazzi P, Pansini F, and Bonaccorsi G, et al.. The effect of dietary soy supplementation on hot flushes. Obstetrics & Gynecology 1998;91(1):6-11.

100. Fournier DB, Erdman JW Jr, Gordon GB. Soy and cancer prevention. In: Bendich A, Deckelbaum R, eds. Primary and secondary preventive nutrition. Totowa (NJ): Humana Press Inc. 2001; pp 51.

101. Lock M, Kaufert P. Menopause, local biologies, and cultures of aging. Am J Human Biol 2001;13(4):494-504.

102. Satia JA, Patterson RE, Kristal AR, Hislop TG, Pineda M. A household food inventory for North American Chinese. Public Health Nutr 2001;4(2):241-7.

103. Goddard MS, Young G, Marcus R. The effect of amylose content on insulin and glucose responses to ingested rice. Am J Clin Nutr 1984;39(3):388-92.

104. Hagop EG, Younis SA, Shahatha HA. Proteins and amino acids of some local varieties of rice seeds (Oryza Sativa L.). Plant Foods Hum Nutr 1990;40(4):309-15.

105. Tufts University Health & Nutrition Letter 2001.

106. Burkitt D. Related disease—related cause? Lancet 1969;2:1229-1231.

107. Trowell H. Non-infected disease in Africa. Edward Arnold, ed. London: 1960:217-22.

108. Liu S, et al. A Prospective Study of Dietary Glycemic Load, Carbohydrate Intake and Risk of Coronary Heart Disease in U.S. Women. Am J Clin Nutr 2000;71:1455-61.

109. Salmeron J, et al. Dietary Fiber, Glycemic Load, and Risk of Non-Insulin-Dependent Diabetes Mellitus in Women. JAMA 1997;277:472-7.

110. National Research Council (US), Committee on Diet and Health. Diet and Health. Implications for Reducing Chronic Disease Risk. National Academy Press, US, 1989.

111. Jacobs DR Jr, et al. Whole-grain intake and cancer: An expanded review and meta-analysis. Nutrition and Cancer 1998;30:85-89.

112. Jang M et al. Cancer chemopreventive activity of resveratrol, a natural product derived from grapes Science. 1997;275:218-220.

113. Martin W. The combined role of atheroma, cholesterol, platelets, the endothelium and fibrin in heart attacks and strokes. Med Hypoth 1984;15:305-22.

114. Renaud S, de Lorgeril M.Wine, alcohol, platelets, and the French paradox for coronary heart disease. Lancet 1992;339:1523-26.

115. Goldberg DM et al. Beyond alcohol: Beverage consumption and cardiovascular mortality. Clin Chim Acta 1995;237:155-87.

116. Goldberg DM. Does wine work? Clin Chem 1995;41:14-16.

117. Hertog MG et al. Dietary antioxidant flavonoids and risk of coronary heart disease: the Zutphen Elderly study. Lancet 1993;342:1007-11.

118. Mediterranean epidemiological evidence on tomatoes and the prevention of digestive-tract cancers. Proc Soc Exp Biol Med 1998;218:125-28.

119. Mills PK, et al. Cohort study of diet, lifestyle, and prostate cancer in Adventist men. Cancer 1989;64:598-604.

120. Agarwal S, et al. 1998. Tomato lycopene and low density lipoprotein oxidation: a human dietary intervention study. Lipids 33:981-84.

121. Gionvannucci E. Tomatoes, tomato-based products, lycopene, and cancer: review of the epidemiological literature. J Natl Cancer Inst 1999;91(4): 317–331.

122. Giovannucci E and Clinton SK. Tomatoes, lycopene, and prostate cancer. Proc Soc Exp Biol 1998;218: 129–139.

123. Stahl W, et al. Carotenoid mixtures protect multilamellar liposomes against oxidative damage: synergistic effects of lycopene and lutein. FEBS Lett 1998;427:305-8.

124. Mangels, A.R., J.M. Holden, G.R. Beecher, M.R. Forman, and E. Lanza. (1993). Carotenoid content of fruits and vegetables: an evaluation of analytic data. J. Am. Diet. Assoc., 93:284-296.

125. Milner JA. Nonnutritive components in foods as modifiers of the cancer process. In: Preventive nutrition: the comprehensive guide for health professionals. Bendich A, Deckelbaum RJ, eds. Totowa, NJ: Humana, 2001; pp 134-139.

126. Maskalyk J. Grapefruit juice: potential drug interactions. Can Med Assoc J 2002;167(3):279-280.

127. Curhan GC, Willett WC, Speizer FC, Stampfer MJ. Beverage use and risk for kidney stones in women. J Urol 1999;162(2):635-636.

128. Plotnick G, et al.Vitamins C and E temporarily block some harmful effects of high-fat meal. JAMA. 1997;278:1682-1686.

129. Seddon JM et al. NIH eye disease case-control study JAMA. 1994; 272: 1413-1420.

130. Diets high in carotenoids may lower risk of macular degeneration. Medical Sciences Bulletin 1995.

131. Shils ME. Magnesium. In: Shils ME, Olson JA, Shike M, eds. Modern nutrition in health and disease, 8th Ed. Vol.1: Philadelphia, PA: Lea & Febiger.1994; pp 164-84.

132. Beecher CW. Cancer preventive properties of varieties of Brassica oleracea: a review. Am J Clin utr 1994;59:1166S-1170S.

133. Joseph JA, Shukitt-Hale B, Denisova NA, Prior RL, Cao G, Martin A, Taglialatela G, Bickford PC. Long-term dietary strawberry, spinach, or vitamin E supplementation retards the onset of age-related neuronal signal transduction and cognitive behavioral deficits. J Neurosci 1998;18:8047-55.

134. Plant Pigments Paint a Rainbow of Antioxidants. Agricultural Research 1996:4-8.

135. USDA Agriculture Research Magazine 1999. United States Department of Agriculture (USDA). http://www.usda.gov/.

136. Mei X, Lin X, Liu J, Lin XY, Song PJ, Hu JF, et al. The blocking effect of garlic on the formation of N-nitrosoproline in humans. Acta Nutr Sin 1989;11:141-5.

137. Lin X-Y, Liu JZ, Milner JA. Dietary garlic suppresses DNA adducts caused by N-nitroso compounds. Carcinogenesis 1994;15:349-52.

138. National Research Council (US), Committee on Diet and Health. Diet and Health. Implications for Reducing Chronic Disease Risk. National Academy Press, US, 1989.

139. Frier HI, Greene HL. Obesity and chronic disease. In: Bendich A, Deckelbaum R, eds. Primary and secondary preventive nutrition. Totowa (NJ): Humana Press Inc. 2001; pp 416.

140. Flegal KM, Caroll D, Kuzmarski RJ, Johnson CL: Overweight and obesity in the United States: Prevalence and trends 1960-1994. Int J Obes Rel Metab Disord 1998;22:39-47.

141. Flancbaum L, Choban PS. Surgical implications of obesity. Annu Rev Med 1998;49:215-34.

142. Abdel-Moneim RI. The hazards of surgery in the obese. Int Surg 1985;70(2):101-3.

143. Jannsen I, Katzmarzyk PT, Ross P. Body mass index, waist circumference, and health risk. Evidence in support of current National Institutes of Health guidelines. Arch Int Med 2002; 162:2074-2079.

144. Metropolitan Life Insurance Co. New weight standards for men and women 1959; New York: Statistics Bulletin.

145. Garrow JS. Obesity. In: Human Nutrition and Dietetics. 9th Edition. Edinburgh. Churchill Livingstone 1993; pp. 465-6.

146. Rose GA, Blackburn H (1982). Cardiovascular survey methods. WHO Monograph Series no.58. Geneva: WHO.

147. Hartz AJ, Rupley DC, Rimm AA. The association of girth measurements with disease in 32,856 women. Am J Epidemiol 1984; 119:71-80.

148. Vague J. The degree of masculine differentiation of obesity: A factor determining predisposition to diabetes, atherosclerosis, gout and uric-calculous disease. Am J Clin Nutr 1956; 4:20-34.

149. Bjorntorp P. Classification of obese patients and complications related to the distribution of surplus fat. Am J Clin Nutr 1987:45S:1120-1125.

150. Hsieh SD, Yoshinaga H. Abdominal fat distribution and coronary heart disease risk factors in men-waist/height ratio as a simple and useful predictor. Int J Obesity 1995:19:585-589.

151. Han TS, van Leer EM, Seidell JC, Lean MEJ. Waist circumference action levels in the identification of cardiovascular risk factors: Prevalence study in a random sample. Br Med J 1995; 311:1401-1405.

152. Roche AF. Anthropometric methods: New and old, what they tell us. Int J Obesity 1984; 8:509-523.

153. Willett WC. Anthropometric measures and body composition. In: Nutritional Epidemiology 1998. 2nd Edition. New York. Oxford University Press; pp 244-272.

154. Gallagher D, Visser M, Sepulveda D. How useful is a body mass index for comparison of body fatness across age, sex, and ethnic groups? Am J Epidemiol 1996; 143:228-239.

155. Ornish D. Eat More, Weigh Less: Dr. Dean Ornish's Life Choice Program for Losing Weight Safely while Eating Abundantly. New York: Harper Paperbacks, 1993.

156. Shintani T.The Hawaii Diet. New York: Pocket Books, 1999.

157. Dwyer JT, Rippe JM. (eds.) Lifestyle Nutrition. Malden, MA: Blackwell Science, Inc.,2001:130-131.

158. Bren L. Losing weight: more than counting calories. FDA Consum 2002;36(1):18-25.

159. Willet WC. Eat, drink and be healthy. The Harvard Medical School guide to healthy eating. New York: Simon & Schuster 2001; pp 80.

160. Nelson ME. 2001. Strong Women Eat Well: Nutritional Strategies for a Healthy Body and Mind. New York: G. P. Putnam's Sons.

Chapter 9

1. Physical Activity and Cardiovascular Health. NIH Consensus Statement 1995;13(3):1-33

2. Physical activity and health: A Report of the Surgeon General. Washington, DC: U.S. Department of Health and Human Services, Centers for Disease Control and Prevention, 1996.

3. Charleton G. Pets benefit from weight loss programs. Texas A&M University College of Veterinary Medicine's Veterinary Teaching Hospital in College Station, Texas. Retrieved March 2002 from http://www.tamu.edu/univrel/aggiedaily/news/stories/archive/102595-1.html.

4. Colditz GA. Economic costs of obesity and inactivity. Medicine and Science in Sports and Exercise 1999;31(Suppl 11):S663–S667.

5. Pratt M, Macera CA, Wang G. Higher direct medical costs associated with physical inactivity. The Physician and Sports Medicine 2000;28(10):63–70.

6. U.S. Department of Health and Human Services. The Surgeon General's call to action to prevent and decrease overweight and obesity. Washington: U.S. Department of Health and Human Services, Public Health Services, Office of the Surgeon General; 2001. Available from U.S. GPO, Washington or online at http://www.surgeongeneral.gov/topics/obesity/default.htm.

7. Estimated percentage of adults with sedentary lifesytyle by race and sex.-U.S. 1991-1992. Chronic Disease in Minority Populations, Centers for Disease and Prevention, 1994.

8. National Center for Health Statistics. 1998. National Health Interview Survey (NHIS) Public Use Data Release. NHIS Survey Description. Centers for Disease Control and Prevention. U.S. Department of Health and Human Services. 2000. ftp://ftp.cdc.gov/pub/Health_Statistics/NCHS/Dataset_Documentation/NHIS/1998/srvydesc.pdf.

9. Schoenborn CA, Barnes PM. Leisure-time physical activity among adults: United States, 1997-1998: Advance Data from Vital and Health Statistics. Atlanta: CDC. No.325 2002

10. Pescatello LS. Exercising for health: The merits of lifestyle physical activity. West J Med 2001;174:114-118.

11. Dunn AL, Andersen RE, Jakicic JM. Lifestyle physical activity interventions history, short- and long-term effects, and recommendations. Am J Prev Med 1998;15:398-412.

12. American College of Sports Medicine Position Stand. The recommended quantity and quality of exercise for developing and maintaining cardiorespiratory and muscular fitness, and flexibility in adults. Med Sci Sports Exerc 1998;30:975-991.

13. Pescatello LS, Costanzo D, Murphy D. Low-intensity physical activity benefits blood lipids and lipoproteins in older adults living at home. Aging 2000;29:433-439.

14. Pescatello LS, Murphy D. Lower intensity physical activity is advantageous for fat distribution and blood glucose among viscerally obese older adults. Med Sci Sports Exerc 1998;30:1408-13.

15. Weiler AM, Faghri PD, Pescatello LS, Aiudi B, Camaione DN. The effectiveness of a behavior modification lifestyle physical activity program among worksite employees. Med Sci Sports Exerc 2000;32:S141.

16. Andersen RE, Wadden TA, Bartlett SJ, Zemel B, Verde TJ, Franckowiak SC. Effects of lifestyle activity vs structured aerobic exercise in obese women. JAMA 1999;281: 335-340.

17. Dunn AL, Marcus BH, Kampert JB, Garcia ME, Kohl HW III, Blair SN. Comparison of lifestyle and structured interventions to increase physical activity and cardiorespiratory fitness a randomized trial. JAMA 1999;281:327-334.

18. Hakim AA, Curb JD, Petrovitch H, et al. Effects of walking on coronary heart disease in elderly men: the Honolulu Heart Program. Circulation 1999;100:9-13.

19. Mayer-Davis EJ, D'Agostino R, Karter AJ, et al. Intensity and amount of physical activity in relation to insulin sensitivity the insulin resistance atherosclerosis study. JAMA 1998;279: 669-674.

20. Pescatello LS. Exercise prescription and management for cardiometabolic health. ACSM's Health Fitness J 1999;3:15-21.

21. Gaziano JM, Manson JE, Ridker PM. Primary and secondary prevention of coronary heart disease. In: Braunwald E, Zipes DP, Libby P. Heart disease, A textbook of cardiovascular medicine. 6th ed. Philadelphia: WB Saunders, 2001; pp 1054.

22. Carvalho JJM, Baruzzi RG, Howard PF, et al. Blood pressure in four remote populations in INTERSALT Study. Hypertension 1989;14:238-46.

23. Paffenbarger RS Jr., I-Min Lee. Exercise and Fitness. In: Prevention of Myocardial Infarction. Manson JE, Ridker PM, Gaziano JM, Hennekens CH, eds. New York: Oxford University Press; 1996; pp 193.

24. Stefanick ML. Exercise and weight loss. In: Clinical Trials in Cardiovascular Disease: A Companion Guide to Braunwald's Heart Disease, ed. Hennekens CH. Philadelphia: WB Saunders, 1999; pp 375-391.

25. Stefanick ML, Mackey S. Sheehan M. et al. Effects of diet and exercise in men an postmenopausal women with low levels of HDL cholesterol and high levels of LDL cholesterol. N Engl J Med 339:12-20, 1998.

26. Mayer-Davis EJ, D'Agostino R Jr, Karter AJ, et al: Intensity and amount of physical activity in relation to insulin sensitivity: The Insulin Resistance Atherosclerosis Study. JAMA 279:669-674, 1998.

27. Halbert JA, Silagy CA, Finucaine P, et al. The effectiveness of exercise training in lowering blood pressure: A meta-analysis of randomized controlled trials of 4 weeks or longer. J Hum Hypertens 11:641-649, 1997.

28. Franklin BA, McCullough PA, Timmis GC: Exercise. In: Clinical Trials in Cardiovascular Disease: A Companion Guide to Braunwald's Heart Disease, ed. Hennekens CH. Philadelphia: WB Saunders, 1999; pp 278-295.

29. Pollock ML, Franklin BA, Balady GJ, et al: AHA Science Advisory Resistance exercise in individuals with and without cardiovascular disease: Benefits, rationale, safety, and prescription: An advisory from the Committee on Exercise, Rehabilitation, and Prevention, Council on Clinical Cardiology, American Heart Association; position paper endorsed by the American College of Sports Medicine. Circulation 101: 828-833, 2000.

30. Morris JN, Heady JA, Raffle PAB, et al. Coronary heart disease and physical activity of work. Lancet 1953; 329:1677-83.

31. Kahn HA. The relationship of reported coronary heart disease mortality to physical activity of work. Am J Public Health 1963; 53:11058-67.

32. Paffenbarger RS Jr., Hale WE. Work activity and coronary heart mortality. N Engl J Med 1975;292:545-50.

33. Paffenbarger RS Jr., Wing AL, Hyde RT. Physical activity as an index of heart attack risk in college alumni. Am J Epidemiol 1978;108:161-75.

34. Morris JN, Everitt MG, Pollard R, et al. Vigorous exercise in leisure-time: protection against coronary heart disease. Lancet 1980;2:1207-10.

35. Lee IM, Paffenbarger RS Jr. Physical activity and stroke incidence. The Harvard Alumni Health Study. Stroke 1988;29:2049-54.

36. Blair SN, Kohl HW III, Paffenbarger RS Jr., et al. Physical fitness and all-cause mortality: a prospective study of healthy men and women. JAMA 1989;262:2395-401.

37. Physical Activity and Cardiovascular Health. NIH Consensus Statement 1995;13(3):1-33.

38. Weeks DJ, James J. Secrets of the superyoung: The scientific reasons why some people look ten years younger than they really are—and how you can too. New York: Villard Books (Random House), 1998.

39. Heitler S. The power of two: secrets to a strong and loving marriage. Oakland, CA: New Harbinger Publications, 1997.

40. Southwestern Library. Exercise and your sex life. UT Southwestern library. Retrieved August 2002 from http://www3.utsouthwestern.edu/library/consumer/sexlife.htm.

41. Leon AS, Connett J, Jacobs DR Jr, Rauramaa R. Leisure-time physical activity levels and risk of coronary heart disease and death: the Multiple Risk Factor Intervention Trial. JAMA 1987;258:2388-95

42. Manson JE, Hu FB, Rich-Edwards JW, et al. A prospective study of walking compared with vigorous exercise in the prevention of coronary heart disease in women. N Engl J Med 1999;341:650-8.

43. Ornish D. Dr. Dean Ornish's program for reversing heart disease. New York: Ballantine Books, 1990.

44. Missed opportunities in preventive counseling for cardiovascular disease—United States, 1995. Morbidity and Mortality Weekly Report (MMWR) 1998;47:91-5.

45. Centers for Disease Control and Prevention (2000) Fact Sheet: Youth Risk Behavior Trends. Adolescent and School Health web site. Updated 6–9-2000. Retrieved June 2000 from. http://www.cdd.gov/nccdphp/dash/yrbs/trend.htm.

46. Pratt M., Macera C. A., Blanton C. Levels of physical activity and inactivity in children and adults in the United States: current evidence and research issues. Med. Sci. Sports Exerc. 1999;31:S526-S533.

47. Centers for Disease Control and Prevention (2000) Youth risk surveillance summary— United States, 1999. In: CDC Surveillance Summaries, Morb. Mortal. Wkly. Rep. 49: 1–96.

48. Trudeau F., Laurencelle L., Tremblay J., Rajic M., Shephard R. J. Daily primary school physical education: effects on physical activity during adult life. Med. Sci. Sports Exerc. 1999;31:111-117.

49. Troiano RP, Macera CA, Ballard-Barbash R. Be Physically Active Each Day. How Can We Know? Journal of Nutrition. 2001;131:451S-460S.

50. Kraus WE, Houmard JA, Duscha BD, Knetzger KJ, Wharton MB, McCartney JS, Bales CW, Henes S, Samsa GP, Otvos JD, Kulkarni KR, Slentz CA. Effects of the amount and intensity of exercise on plasma lipoproteins. N Engl J Med 2002;347(19):1483-92.

51. Kelley GA, Kelley KS, Tran ZV. The effects of exercise on resting blood pressure in children and adolescents: a meta-analysis of randomized controlled trials. Prev Cardiol 2003 Winter;6(1):8-16.

52. Franklin BA, Swain DP, Shephard RJ. New insights in the prescription of exercise for coronary patients. J Cardiovasc Nurs 2003;18(2):116-23.

53. Mullooly C. Cardiovascular fitness and type 2 diabetes. Curr Diab Rep 2002;2(5):441-7.

54. Fitts RH. Effects of regular exercise training on skeletal muscle contractile function. Am J Phys Med Rehabil 2003;82(4):320-31.

55. Chau DL, Edelman SV, Chandran M. Osteoporosis and diabetes. Curr Diab Rep 2003;3(1):37-42.

56. LaStayo PC, Ewy GA, Pierotti DD, Johns RK, Lindstedt S. The positive effects of negative work: increased muscle strength and decreased fall risk in a frail elderly population. J Gerontol A Biol Sci Med Sci 2003;58(5):M419-24.

57. Schmitz KH, Jensen MD, Kugler KC, Jeffery RW, Leon AS. Strength training for obesity prevention in midlife women. Int J Obes Relat Metab Disord 2003;27(3):326-33.

58. Shrier I. Flexibility versus stretching. Br J Sports Med 2001;35(5):364.

59. Nelson ME. Strong Women Stay Slim. New York: Bantam Books, 1999.

60. Proverbs 24:6. Holy Bible, New International Version 1978, Committee on Bible Translation.

61. Armen J, Smith BW. Exercise considerations in coronary artery disease, peripheral vascular disease, and diabetes mellitus. Clin Sports Med 2003;22(1):123-33, viii.

62. Tanasescu M, Leitzmann MF, Rimm EB, Willett WC, Stampfer MJ, Hu FB. Exercise type and intensity in relation to coronary heart disease in men. JAMA 2002;288(16):1994-2000.

63. Palatini P. Exercise capacity and mortality. N Engl J Med 2002;347(4):288-90; author reply 288-90.

64. Flood L, Constance A. Diabetes and exercise safety. Am J Nurs 2002;102(6):47-55.

65. Bell DS. Exercise for patients with diabetes. Benefits, risks, precautions. Postgrad Med 1992;92(1):183-4, 187-90, 195-8.

66. Young JC. Exercise prescription for individuals with metabolic disorders. Practical considerations. Sports Med 1995 ;19(1):43-54.

67. McCaffree J. Physical activity: how much is enough? J Am Diet Assoc 2003;103(2):153-4.

68. Lee IM, Sesso HD, Oguma Y, Paffenbarger RS Jr. Relative intensity of physical activity and risk of coronary heart disease. Circulation 2003;107(8):1110-6.

69. Berg AO; US Preventive Services Task Force. U.S. Preventive services task force. Behavioral counseling in primary care to promote physical activity: recommendation and rationale. Am J Nurs 2003;103(4):101-7; discussion 109.

70. How to exercise an hour a day. Three strategies will help you reach the impossible dream. Heart Advis 2003;6(3):4-5.

71. Ransdell LB, Taylor A, Oakland D, Schmidt J, Moyer-Mileur L, Shultz B. Daughters and mothers exercising together: effects of home- and community-based programs. Med Sci Sports Exerc 2003;35(2):286-96.

72. Resnicow K, Jackson A, Braithwaite R, DiIorio C, Blisset D, Rahotep S, Periasamy S. Healthy Body/Healthy Spirit: a church-based nutrition and physical activity intervention. Health Educ Res 2002;17(5):562-73

73. Warren-Findlow J, Prohaska TR, Freedman D. Challenges and opportunities in recruiting and retaining underrepresented populations into health promotion research. Gerontologist 2003;43 Spec No 1:37-46.

74. Young DR, Gittelsohn J, Charleston J, Felix-Aaron K, Appel LJ. Motivations for exercise and weight loss among African-American women: focus group results and their contribution towards program development. Ethn Health 2001;6(3-4):227-45.

75. Hu FB, Li TY, Colditz GA, Willett WC, Manson JE. Television watching and other sedentary behaviors in relation to risk of obesity and type 2 diabetes mellitus in women. JAMA 2003;289(14):1785-91.

Chapter 10

1. Joint WHO/FAO Expert Report on Diet, Nutrition and the Prevention of Chronic Disease. Executive Summary 2003. Department of Noncommunicable Disease Prevention and Health Promotion. Retrieved March 2003 from http://www.who.int/hpr/nutrition/expertconsultationge.htm.

2. Ecclesiastes 7:8. Holy Bible, New International Version 1978, Committee on Bible Translation.

3. Third National Health and Nutrition Examination Survey (NHANES III) 18 JAMA Vol.287 No.3 2002.

4. Morreale SJ, Schwartz NE. Helping Americans eat right: developing practical and actionable public nutrition education messages based on the ADA. Survey of American Dietary Habits. J Am Diet Assoc. 1995;95:305-8.

5. Pollard J, Greenwood D, Kirk S. Lifestyle Factors affecting fruit and vegetable consumption in the UK. Women's Cohort Study. Appetite 2000;37:71-9.

6. Macario E, Emmons KM, Sorensen G, et al. Factors influencing nutrition education for patients with low literally skills. J Amer Diet Assoc 1998;98:559-564.

7. Winkleby MA, Kraemer HC, Ahn DK, Varady AN. Ethnic and socioeconomic differences in cardiovascular risk factors: findings for women from the Third National Health and Nutrition Examination Survey, 1988-1994. JAMA 1998;280:356-362.

8. Morland K, Wing S, Diez Roux A. The contextual effect of the local food environment on residents' diets: the atherosclerosis risk in communities study. Am J Public Health 2002;92(11):1761-7.

9. Gates G, McDonald M. Comparison of dietary risk factors for cardiovascular disease in African-American and white women. J Am Diet Assoc 1997;97:1394-1400.

10. Glanz K. Nutrition intervention to lower the risk of cardiovascular disease: behavioral and educational considerations. In: Lifestyle Nutrition. Dwyer JT, Rippe JM. Malden, MA: Blackwell Science, 2001; pp 127-151.

11. I Samuel 17: 4ff. Holy Bible, New International Version 1978, Committee on Bible Translation.

12. Genesis 37-50. Holy Bible, New International Version 1978, Committee on Bible Translation.

13. Swindoll C. Attitude. Insight for Living. Fullerton CA. Retrieved Dec. 2000 from http://www.geocities.com/Heartland/Lake/5433/attitude.html.

14. Bandura A. Self-efficacy: The exercise of control. New York: WH Freeman, 1997.

15. Bandura A. Social foundations of thought and action: a social cognitive theory. Englewoods Cliffs, NJ: Prentice-Hall, 1986.

16. Glanz K, Rimer BK. Theory at a glance: a guide for health promotion practice. NIH Publication No. 95-3896. Bethesda, MD: National Cancer Institute, 1995.

17. Glanz K, Eriksen MP. Individual and community models for dietary behavior change. J Nutr Educ 1993;25:80-6.

18. Glanz K. Nutritional intervention: A behavioral and educational perspective. In: Ockene IS, Ockene JK, eds. Prevention of coronary heart disease. Boston: Little, Brown, 1992; pp 231-65.

19. Glanz K. Patient and public education for cholesterol reduction: A review of strategies and issues. Patient Educ Couns 1988;12:235-57.

20. Roberts HJ. The hazards of very-low-calorie dieting. Am J Clin Nutr 1985 ;41(1):171-2.

21. Rudd P. Cardiovascular risks from very low calorie diets. Compr Ther 1985;11(8):3-6.

22. Proverbs 25: 28. Holy Bible, New International Version 1978, Committee on Bible Translation.

******

Book Resources:

Books Related to Nutrition and Lifestyle

1. Adams P. 1998. Gesundheit: Bringing good health to you, the medical system, and society through physician service, complementary therapies, humor, and joy. Rochester, Vermont: Healing Arts Press.
2. Arvigo R, Balick M. 1993. Rainforest remedies: one hundred healing herbs of Belize. Twin Lakes, WI: Lotus Press.
3. Bendich A, Deckelbaum RJ. (eds.) 2001. Preventive nutrition: the comprehensive guide for health professionals, 2nd edition. Totowa, New Jersey: Humana Press.
4. Bendich A, Deckelbaum RJ. (eds.) 2001. Primary and secondary preventive nutrition. Totowa, New Jersey: Humana Press.
5. Bernstein RK. 1997. Dr. Bernstein's diabetes solution: a complete guide to achieving normal blood sugars. Boston, MA: Little, Brown and Company.
6. Better Homes and Gardens. 1999. Better homes and gardens: food for health and healing. DesMoines, Iowa: Meridith Books.
7. Braunwald E, Zipes DP, Libby P. (eds.) 2001. Heart disease: a textbook of cardiovascular Medicine, 6th edition. Philadelphia, PA: W.B. Saunders Company.
8. Challem J, Berkson B, Smith MD. 2000. Syndrome X: the complete nutritional program to prevent and reverse insulin resistance. New York: John Wiley & Sons, Inc.
9. Cooper K. 1990. Preventive medicine program: overcoming hypertension. New York: Bantam Books.
10. Dwyer JT, Rippe JM. (eds.) 2001. Lifestyle nutrition. Malden, MA: Blackwell Science, Inc.
11. Filedhouse P. 1986. Food and nutrition: customs and culture. London: Chapman & Hall.
12. Garrow JS, Jame WPT. (eds.) 1993. Human nutrition and dietetics, 9th edition. London: Churchill Livingstone.
13. Gibson DM. Harling M, Kaplan B. (eds.) 1987. Studies of homeopathic remedies. Bucks, England: Beaconsfield Publishers Ltd.
14. Graboys TB, Blatt CM. 1997. Angina pectoris: management strategies, 2nd edition. Caddo, Ok: Professional Communications, Inc.
15. Griffith HW. 1998. Complete guide to vitamins, minerals and supplements. Tucson, Arizona: Fisher Books.
16. Hankinson SE, Colditz GA, Manson JE, Speizer FE. (eds.) 2001. Healthy women, healthy lives: a guide to preventing disease from the landmark nurses' health study. New York: Simon & Schuster Source.
17. Herbert V, Subak-Sharpe GJ. (eds.) 1995. Total nutrition: the only guide you'll ever need. New York: St. Martin's Griffith.
18. Hollman A. 1992. Plants in cardiology. Tavistock Square, London: British Medical Journal.
19. Krall L, Beaser R. 1989. Joslin diabetes manual, 12th edition. Malvern, PA: Lea & Febiger.
20. Lown B. 1999. The lost art of healing: practicing compassion in medicine. New York: Ballantine Books.
21. Maggi A, Boucher J. 2000. What you can do to prevent diabetes: simple changes to improve your life. New York: John Wiley & Sons, Inc.
22. National Consumer Council. 1992. Your food: whose choice. London: HMSO Publications.
23. Natow AB, Heslin J. 1996. The cholesterol counter, 4th edition. New York: Pocket Books.
24. Nelson ME. 2001. Strong women eat well: nutritional strategies for a healthy body and mind. New York: G. P. Putnam's Sons.

25. Nicolici D. 1972. The original diet, 6th edition. Auburn, Australia: Religious Liberty Publishing Association.
26. Ornish D. 1990. Dr. Dean Ornish's program for reversing heart disease: The only system scientifically proven to reverse heart disease. New York: Ballantine Books.
27. Ornish D. 1993. Eat more, weigh less: Dr. Dean Ornish's life choice program for losing weight safely while eating abundantly. New York: Harper Paperbacks.
28. Owen D. 1976. In sickness and in health: the politics of medicine. London: Quartet Books, Ltd.
29. Schwarzbein D, Deville N. 1999. The Schwarzbein principle: the truth about losing weight, being healthy and feeling younger. Deerfield Beach, FL: Health Communications, Inc.
30. Shintani T. 1999. The Hawaii diet. New York: Pocket Books.
31. Swifton D. (ed.) 1995. The PDR family guide to nutrition and health. Montvale, New Jersey: Medical Economics.
32. Texas Heart Institute. 1996. The Texas Heart Institute heart owner's handbook. New York: John Wiley & Sons.
33. Weil A. 2000. Eating well for optimum health: the essential guide to food, diet, and nutrition. New York: Alfred A. Knopf.
34. Weil A. 1995. Spontaneous healing: how to discover and embrace your body's natural ability to maintain and heal itself. New York: Ballantine Books.
35. Whitaker J. 2001. Reversing diabetes. New York: Warner Books.
36. White EG. 1976. Counsels on diet and foods. Washington, DC: Review and Herald Publishing Association.
37. Willett WC. 2001. Eat, drink, and be healthy: the Harvard Medical School guide to healthy eating. New York: Simon & Schuster.
38. Willett WC. 1998. Nutritional epidemiology. New York: Oxford University Press.

******

General Index

A

AbioCor artificial heart, 109
advertising
    children and food choices, 262
    direct, 80
    direct-to-consumer (DTC)
        marketing, 81
    dishonesty in direct drug marketing,
        80
    drug ads and the medicalization of
        trivial ailments, 82
    media and drug choices, 81
    overmedicated society and, 79
    "pester power", 81
    prescription ads, 80
aging
    accelerated or premature, 216
    accelerators, 233, 241
    aged (old), 211
    aging skin
        photo-aging, 232
        race and, 232
        sun exposure accelerates, 232
        wrinkles, 231
    as a risk factor, 217
    attitudes toward the elderly, 243
    begins in childhood, 215
    chronic disease in the elderly, 219
    chronological aging, 214
    chronology and biology, 215
    definitions of aging, 215
    depressing associations with, 213
    educational level, 246
    elderly and healthcare resources,
        219
    elderly population and healthcare,
        219

external images, 214
figures for U.S. population, 218
financial status, 246
five major aging accelerants, 234
functional ability and, 215
gender and, 233
gerontology, 216
healthy aging and longevity, 214
nutritional status, 246
Okinawa study, 244
    calorie restriction, 245
    formula, 244
perceptions and misconceptions,
    213
related free radical damage, 221
retirees, 244
social isolation, 245
socioeconomic status and longevity,
    246
spectrum of aging and disease, 218
stress and, 234
the mind and, 243
the process and perception, 213
theories on why we age, 220
theory of aging, 221
Western attitudes towards the
    elderly, 244
work maintains dignity, 244
agriculture, 367
    commercially grown crops, 295
    farming revolution, 115
    fertilizers, herbicides, pesticides,
        antibiotics, 294
    "food mountains and milk
        ponds,"115
    intensive farming, 295

practice of rendering, 295
alcohol
    alcohol abuse, 201
        damage to liver and cirrhois, 201
    alcoholic beverages, 201
    heavy drinking raises blood
        pressure and risk of stroke, 201
    intake and cancer, 201
    risks vs benefits, 200
    the French paradox (and a
        paradox), 200
alternative medical systems 142-148
    Ayurveda, 147
    biological-based therapies
        herbal, 149
        orthomolecular, 149
        special diet, 149
    EDTA chelation therapy, 149
    Eisenberg study, 139
    energy therapies
        bioelectromagnetic-based
            therapies, 150
        Qi-gong, 150
        reiki, 150
        therapeutic touch, 150
    homeopathic medicine, 148
    manipulative and body-based
        methods
        chiropractors, 149
        massage therapists, 150
        osteopaths, 149
    mind-body interventions
        cognitive behavioral therapies,
            148
        meditation, 148
    naturopathic medicine, 148
    traditional Oriental medicine, 146
American Aging Association (AGE),
    221
American Cancer Society, 202
American Diabetic Association
    (ADA), 126
American Heart Association (AHA),
    325
    MyHeartWatch, 203

American Medical Student
    Association (AMSA)
    nutrition curriculum project, 124
Ameri-sizing, 363
    "doggie-bag", 180
    bigger is better, 176
    fast-food nation, 175
    increase in size of various foodstuff
        as in bagels, muffins, pasta, 265
    portion control
        lack of, 265
    super sizing, 265
Anderson, Gerald, 63
antibiotics
    abuse of, 83
antioxidants, 221, 222, 322, 334, 346
    alpha lipoic acid, 232
    beta-carotene and flavanoids, 321
    Cambridge Heart Antioxidant Study
        (CHAOS), 321
    Heart Outcome Prevention
        Evaluation (HOPE), 321
    in the body, 223
    mechanisms, 223
    superoxide dismutase,catalase,
        glutathione peroxidase, 223
    synthetic, 182
    vitamin C, 95
Appert, Nicholas, 181
arthritis, 379
Association of American Medical
    Colleges (AAMC), 123
Atheroclerosis
    angioplasty, 103
Atwater, Wilbur Olin, 114

B

Bagshaw, John, 63
Bal, Dileep, 165
Barker Hypothesis, 89
Begley, Sharon, 224
behavior
    type A behavior pattern and
        personality, 235
behavior therapists, 394

Belize, 97, 267, 294, 383, 393
Bendich, Adrianne, 93
Benedict, Francis Gano, 114
Berman, Brian, 131
bioflavonoids, 95
Blackburn, George, 189
blood
    triglycerides, 102
    vessels
        and cholesterol, 226
blood lipids, 29, 184
body mass index (BMI), 353
book
    emphasis where it belongs, 56
    outlook, 54
botulism, 182
bovine spongiform encephalopathy
    (BSE)
    mad cow disease, 295-296
Bratman, Steven, 69
British Nutrition Foundation (BNF),
    125
Burkitt, Dennis, 77, 342
Butterworth, Charles, 120
    skeleton in the hospital closet, 120

C

caffeine
    how much, 239
calories
    caloric restriction, 180, 245
cancer, 48, 87, 224, 317
    benefits of physical activity, 374
    breast cancer, 88
        rates, 327
        rates in Japanese, Chinese, and
            American women, 88
        tamoxifen, 345
    carcinogens (cancer-causing), 182
    effects of green or black teas, 100
    free radicals, DNA, and, 224, 231
    genetic contribution less than
        believed, 88
    nitrosamines, 100, 327

phytochemicals cancer fighting
    activity, 347
pre-cancerous colon polyps (colon
    cancer), 104
prevention, 338
prostate, 327
    lycopene reduces risk, 286
    milk and dairy products, 197
smoking increases risk, 172
stomach
    salted foods and, 200
stomach cancer, 327
carbohydrates
    fiber and whole grains, 323
    high fiber, 323
    whole grains
        deception about, 306
carcinogens
    acrylamide, 293
    carbolines, quinolines, 291
cardiovascular diseases, 227, 323
    among African Americans, 228
    among Asians, 327
    antioxidants role in prevention of,
        321
    behavioral risk factors, 171
    benefits of physical activity, 374
    birth weight and, 89
    cardiovascular system, 227
    coronary heart disease risk charts,
        204
        American Heart Association's
            My Heart Watch, 203
        Texas Heart Institute Heart-
            Health Test, 203
    Framingham Heart Study, 168
    free radicals and, 226, 346
    get medical clearance before
        exercise, 379
    heart attack, 165, 169
    homocysteine and blood clots, 346
    impact of physical activity, 373
    Mediterranean-style diet reduces
        occurrence of heart attacks, 325

MyHeartWatch (American Heart Association), 203
omega-3 fatty acids protect against, 193
pediatric cardiologists, 215
peripheral vascular disease (arterial claudication), 226
prevention, 117
preventive cardiologists, 264
smoking and, 230
studies
    Framingham Heart Study, 168, 169
    Nurses Health Study, 102
    Physicians Health Study, 102
studies in prevention
    Alpha-Tocopherol and Beta-Carotene(ATBC), 321
    Asian diet studies, 326
    Cambridge Heart Antioxidant Study (CHAOS), 321
    DASH trial, 327
    Framingham Heart Study, 325
    GISSI-Prevenzione study, 326
    Heart Outcome Prevention Evaluation (HOPE), 321
    Keys Seven Countries Study, 323
    Lifestyle Heart Study, 328
    Lyon Diet Heart Study, 325
    Nurses' Health Study, 328, 343
    Offspring Study, 325
    Omni Study, 325
transient ischemic attack (TIA), 227
Cauter, Eve Van, 240
Centers for Disease Control (CDC), 368
cerebral arteries, 226
chest pains (angina pectoris), 226
children
    "exploiting kids, corrupting schools", 263
    American youth, food choices, 263
    food choices and, 264
    overweight, 264
    "pester power", 262

poverty and social deprivation, 264
preventive cardiologists, 264
Chittenden, Russel, 191
cholesterol
    angioplasty, 117
    animal fat contributes to high blood LDL cholesterol, 191
    atherosclerosis, 226, 229
        process of, 227
    cholesterol plaques, 184
    dietary fiber lowers LDL-cholesterol levels, 343
    dietary sources are strictly animal, 195
    HDL (high density lipoprotein), 169, 184, 185
    LDL (low density lipoprotein), 169, 184, 185
    lowering effect of soy, 338
    National Cholesterol Education Program(NCEP), 195
    oxidized LDL cholesterol, 227
    reversal of clogging, 329
citrus
    antioxidant benefits of, 318
    citrus oils, 345
    composition of and related health benefits, 318
    flavonoids (citrus bioflavonoids), 345
    grapefruit
        juice interferes with metabolism of drugs, 346
    Nurses' Health Study
        grapefruit juice and marginal increase in kidney stones, 346
    terpenes
        d-limonene, 318, 345, 361
cocaine, 97
cold sores (fever blisters), 95
collagen, 232
complementary and alternative medicine
    allopaths, 143
    alternative therapies, 144

CAM users, 135, 139
chelation therapy, 142
Cochrane collaboration, 143
complementary therapies, 144
definitions of, 143
disparaging opinions against, 134
doctors have mixed views, 150
herbal medicines increase in
    popularity, 139
holistic therapies, 144
list of CAM practices, 146
motivations for trying, 138
National Center for
    Complementary and Alternative
    Medicine (NCCAM), 142, 144
National Institutes of Health (NIH)
    classification list, 148
osteopathic manipulative medicine
    (OMM), 143
osteopaths, 143
preventive therapies, 144
types of therapies, 142
complementary and alternative
    medicine, National Institute of
    Health (NIH) classification of, 146
consumer books, 54
contraceptive pill
    Nurses' Health Study
        long term effects, 328
cooking
    aluminium toxicity and, 292
    curing, smoking, and charcoal-
        grilling
            formation of heterocyclic amines
                (HCAs), 199
    deep-fat frying and reheating of
        oils, 293
    frying
        at high temperatures, unhealthy,
            294
    health concerns over some
        methods, 291
    learning experience, 359
    quick and easy, 359
    recipes

cosmopolitan jerk chicken stir-
    fry (Dr. Bulwer's recipe), 360
reducing nutrient losses, 290
sensible culinary habits at home,
    290
smoking, grilling, charboiling, 291
steaming, 291
stir-frying, 291
coronary arteries, 226
Creutzfeld Jacob disease (CJD)
    new variant CJD (nvCJD), 295
culture
    food choices and, 261
Czauderna, Jack, 141

D

Dalen, James, 72
deaths
    causes of, in the United States, 49
Deckelbaum, Richard, 93
deoxyribonucleic acid (DNA), 224
diabetes mellitus (type II), 48, 49, 54-
    56, 90-92, 167, 315
    behavioral risk factors, 170
    behind the scene damage, 90
    birth weight and, 89
    counting calories, 357
    diabetes prevention study, 136
    diagnosis of type II diabetes, 136
    direct and indirect costs, 50
    hyperlipidemic, 165
    insulin-producing beta cells, 92
    mellitus is a metabolic disease, 92
    mellitus, type II, 92, 389
    metformin, 102
    "once diabetic, always diabetic," 136
    pre-diabetic state, 91, 216
    risk factors and deaths, 170
    root of the matter, 90
    studies
        Nurses' Health Study, 102
        Physicans' Health Study, 102
    trigerring effect, 321
    type I (juvenile onset, 264
    type II, 264, 358

World Health Organization's
    document, 71
diet, 315
    American-style diet/Western diet,
        173-203
    American diet and food processing,
        281ff
    American-style vs Japanese-style,
        177
    Best Diets for tomorrow, 315, 329-
        664
    calorie intake, 355
    calorie intake (eat more, weigh less),
        177
    clear thinking, beyond quick fixes,
        388
    cross-pollination of, 261
    daily calories from fats, 183
    daily protein requirement, 191
    dietary changes, 274
    dietary patterns, 328
    dietary supplements, 320
    disease prevention and, 324
    do the right things, 356
    eat more and weigh less, 355
    Far East, 336
        dietary practices, 336
    fruit and nut desserts, 346
    hara hachi bu, 180
    health benefits of Asian diets and
        lifestyle, 341
    helping Americans eat right, 389
    high protein intake leads to losses
        of calcium, 191
    how much meat should we eat?,
        191
    hyper-responders, 195
    knowledge and principles, 356
    lifestyle habits and risk factors, 91
    Mediterranean diet, 228
    Mediterranean style, 325, 336
        attitude, 334
        pitta bread, feta cheese, 332
    new diets, 315
    Oriental style, 177, 178

    concepts of, 337
        greens and, 339
    portions and serving sizes, 265
    pregnancy, 179
    prudent cosmopolitan
        foundation based on local
            choices, 330
        pillars of Mediterranean-styled
            and Asian styled diets, 330
        plan for a diet, 311
    reductionist approach, 321
    regimented dietary prescriptions,
        357
    restrictive diets, 355
    role in preventing diseases, 323
    super-sized portions, 265
    the whole diet, 229, 316
    traditional Mediterranean-style diet
        pyramid, 333
    vegetarian, 264
    vegetarians and high grade proteins,
        191
    Western diet 173-203, 181, 183, 323
        coleslaw, potato salad, 334
    Western diet and processed foods,
        276
    Westernization of Asian diet, 327
Dietary Approaches
    to Stop Hypertension (DASH
        study), 327
dietary behavior
    individual-personal factors, 273
Dietary Supplements and Health
    Education Act (1994), 153
diets
    food more than just for nutritional
        needs, 68
    healthy eating, virtue to vice, 70
    healthy living, 67
    sucesses, 56
    tastes are learned behaviors, 67
diseases
    adopting preventive strategies, 93
    aggressive prevention, 207
    Alzheimer's disease, 64, 87, 293

and high cholesterol, 165
atherosclerosis, 168
band-aid therapies, 90
cancer. See cancer
cardiovascular diseases. see
    cardiovascular diseases
cerebrovascular disease, 226
chronic diseases, 48
    ABCs of, 90
    common denominators, 54
    deaths due to, 48
    figures, 65
    number of Americans living
        with, 49
chronic disease statistics in the
    elderly, 219
diet and prevention, 324
herpes simplex virus, 226
historical notions, 78
hyperinsulinemia, 91, 206
hypertension (high blood pressure).
    see hypertension
lifestyle diseases, 166
mortality tables, 48
nutraceutical approach, 319
of the heart and ciruclation, 49
orthorexia nervosa, 69
osteoporosis (thinning of the
    bones), 191, 196
peptic ulcer disease
    medical therapies in 1899, 144
prevention, 56, 392
prevention-oriented model, 46, 122
stress aggravates disease, 235
the stress of disease, 141
doctors
    and stress, 237
    attitudes toward nutrition and
        prevention, 118
    basic outlook of medical school
        education, 111
    clinical skills, 111
    concerns about CAM, 152
    conflict of interest, 119

doctor-patient relationship, 111,
    253
hassle factor, 72
healers, 78
health policy and priorities, 108
helping health professionals
    become nutritionally literate, 127
Hippocratic maxim, 141
improperly prescribing morphine
    and heroin (diamorphine), 84
inadequate nutrition background in
    medical schools, 116
looking for quick results, 104
medical school curriculum, U.S.,
    111
nutrition education in medical
    schools
    trends and implications for
        health educators, 126
nutrition excluded from medicine,
    113
patient desire for better relationship
    with, 71
personal reflections, 236
plastic surgeons and dermatologists,
    214
propagate disparaging second-hand
    opinions about alternative
    therapies, 133
quick-results mentality, 102
role of complementary adjunct in
    healing process, 135
drugs
    anti-platelet drugs
        aspirin, ticlopidine, clopidogrel,
            230
    antiviral (acyclovir, penciclovir), 95,
        119
    caffeine, 97
    cocaine, 98
    composition of herbal medications,
        98
    Ephedra, 153
    erythroxylon coca, 78
    fatal side effects, 95

hashish, 78
heroin, 98
history of, 77
illegal cannabis, 99
illegal drugs, 65
improper use of morphine and
    heroin (diamorphine), 84
Indian hemp (cannabis), 77
legal drug trade, 65
medical marijuana, 98
morphine, 98
natural does not mean safer, 97
opium wars, 78
plant kingdom, 97
prescription drugs, 79
    medicare, 77
purgative
    senna, 97
St. John's wort, 153
Viagra (sildenafil citrate), 230
war on illegal drugs, 65

E

Eisenberg, David, 139
    Eisenberg study, 139
endothelium, 227
Environmental Protection Agency
    (EPA), 293
erectile dysfunction (ED), 229, 374
    Massachusetts Male Aging Study,
    230
Ernst, Edzart
    motivations for alternative
        medicine, 137
    reasons for popularity of
        complementary and alternative
        medicine (CAM), 137
exercise, 369
    aerobic exercises, 376
    and sexual activity, 373
    barriers to exercise, 382
    benefits of, 371
    definition of, 369
    establishing good habits

humans are creatures of habit,
    382
flexibility exercises, 376
get medical clearance for these
    conditions, 379, 380
get moving, 384
get professional advice, 378
habits in U.S. population '90-'98,
    369
health benefits of, 377
misconceptions about, 375
misconceptions in developing
    countries, 382
overcoming the psychological
    barriers
    demands of time, 381
personal reflections, 383
recommendations for moderate or
    vigorous exercise, 368
strengthening or resistance
    exercises, 376
success requires setting goals,
    discipline and perseverance, 394
sudden cardiac death and, 378
weight-lifting
    beginnners need medical
        clearance, 379
when to check with your doctor,
    379

F

fats
    animal fats, 183
        contribute to high blood LDL
            cholesterol, 191
    avocado (See Figure 5-7), 189
    blood cholesterol levels and, 184
    coconut oil, 187
    daily calories from, 183
    docosahexanoic acid (DHA), 193
    effects on blood lipids, 184
    eicosapentanoic acid (EPA), 193
    metabolic, 183
    monosaturated, 326
        avocados, 345

monosaturated fats (MUFAs), 183
negative effects of hydrogenated
    fats, 186
omega-3 fatty acids
    alpha-linolenic acids, 325
    docosahexanoic acid (DHA) and
        eicosapentaenoic acid (EPA),
        326
    fatty fish sources, 193
    protect against heart disease, 193
omega-6 fatty acids, 325
palm oil, 187
polyunsaturated fats (PUFAs), 183
saturated, 323
saturated fats
    (SFAs), 183, 188
    dairy fat, 197
storage (triglycerides), 183
structural, 183
total fat intake, 183
trans-fatty acids, 185, 187, 190
    content in some foods, 186
    major food sources, 185
triglycerides, 205
vegetable oils and animal fats, 185
vegetable shortenings and
    margarine, the worst, 185
Federal Trade Commission (FTC), 154
fetal programming, 89
Fiaratone, Maria, 243
fiber, 317, 323, 334
    dietary fiber, 388
        non-starch polysaccharide (NSP),
            342
        protects against a variety of
            diseases, 343
        soluble and insoluble, 342
    health benefits of whole grains, 344
    lower cases of appendicitis, 341
    lowers cholesterol
        Nurses' Health Study, 343
    roughage, 341
fish, 334
    affected by breeding cycle and
        method of preparation, 193

composition of some, 193
fatty fish, 193
fatty vs. white fish, 193
lower rates of heart disease, 193
shellfish,content of, 193
Fisken, Roger, 151
flavonoids, 119, 281, 318, 345
    anthocyanins (pigments in berries),
        347
    anticancer effects
        tangeretin and nobiletin, 345
    citrus bioflavonoids, 119
Fleming, Alexander, 79
Flexner, Abraham, 110
food, 316
    airport food, 259
    Asian styled, 337
    calorie intake, 177
    cereals
        sorghum and millet, 341
    convienence foods, 265
    cookbooks, 362
    fortification, 115
    garlic, onions, chives, leeks (allium
        species), 347
    genetically modified (GM), 298
    high grade non-meat proteins, 191
    high in sodium, 283
    high salt and pickled foods can
        promote stomach cancer, 200
    individual nutrients vs food
        sources, 321
    international dishes, 363
    maize, 298
    meat consumption, 190
    microwaved and irradiated, 292
    money spent on food, 265
    National Organic Program, (NOP),
        297
    naturally-occuring chemicals, 301
    nutrient losses and fortification, 290
    nutrients, 316
    organo-sulfur compounds (allyl
        sulfides), 347
    poisoning (botulism), 182

shopping, 358
supplements
    antioxidants, 322
tastes and preferences, 67
USDA food guide pyramid, 268
whole grains and fiber, 343
food advertising
    food and beverage industry, 264
        food politics, 263
    marketing appeal, 272
Food and Consumer Service (FCS)
    Thrifty Food Plan (TFP), 267
    U.S. Food Stamp Program, 267
Food and Drug Administration
    (FDA), 81
food choices
    and socio-economic differences,
        266
    can we legislate healthy eating?, 275
    culture and, 260
    demanding jobs, nuclear families,
        single-parent households and,
        259
    dynamics of low-income
        Americans, 267
    dynamics of socialization and
        acquisition of food habits, 260
    eating out
        buffet-style restaurants, 362
    eating out, 361
    economic access and, 257
    factors influencing adolescents, 264
    factors influencing children, 263
    factors that influence choice, 255
    family and social relationship
        effects on, 362
    fast-food culture, 257
    food and drink choices of children,
        262
    global cuisines, 362
    globalization of, 272
    human behavior and choices, 255
    impact of income, 266
    in rural communities, 267
    in schools, 262

individual issues, 273
infants and toddlers, 260
market forces, 263
more money, more choices, 265
politics and, 268
poor limited in choices, 266
promote health and prevent disease,
    274
shopping
    practical choices, 358
social and peer pressures, 262
socialization defined, 260
socioeconomic status and, 266
the developing world and, 260
the poor and, 256
the reason people chooose the
    foods they do, 253
understanding low income food
    choices, 268
urbanization and, 272
vegetarian, 258
food habits, 260
food industry
    advertisement and, 271
    children and, 263
    contribution to food preservation
        and storage, 281
    convenience-food industry
        fast foods, 181
    diary industry's "milk moustache",
        270
    government policies, 275
    impact of women in the workplace,
        277
    lobby groups, 269
    lobbyists, 275
    Monsanto, 299
    targeting children, 271
food labeling
    of food products and drugs, 154
food labels
    "fat" descriptors, 306
    deception scenario, 304
    flexi-labeling, 305

genetically modified (GM) foods, 298

health claims, 302, 308

ingredients, 305

meat, 305

Nutrition Labeling and Education Act (NLEA), 301

olive oils, 304

organics, 297

serving size, 305

the new food label, 304

food marketing

American influence, 261

food policy

changes by market forces, consumer demand and food environment, 257

establishing U.S. food policy, 269

food processing

additives and preservatives, 182

advantages of, 282

biological agents, 279

butylated hydroxytoluene (BHT), 182

bytylated hydroxyansole (BHA), 182

chemical agents, 279

disadvantages of, 282

early industrial methods, 277

fortification, 290

hidden content, 181

hidden sources of salt and sodium, 284

history, 181

impact on vitamins, 285

industrial, 278

nutritional value, 280

introduction, 275

ionizing radiation, 292

minimally processed foods, 358

newer methods, 280

nutrification, 290

physical agents, 278

sodium nitrite, 182

botulism, 182

traditional methods, 276

food safety

response to antibiotics and hormones, 192

food supply

additives, hormones, antibiotics, pesticides and fertilizers, 300

excessive food hygiene, 300

food safety and hygiene, 299

food scares, 296

food security, 301

germ warfare, 299

significant changes in, 276

Forbes, Allan, 271

fortification

of foods, 290

free radicals, 223, 228

and cellular function, 221

cardiovascular system, 226, 346

cardiovascular system and, 228

cell membrane, 224

effects, 220

effects of smoking, 231

fibrous plaque, 228

foam cells, 228

free radical stress, 222

immune systems
T-cells, 225

impact of attack on DNA, 224

nitric oxide, 221

oxidant stress (free-radical stress), 221

oxidative stress (free radical stress), 225

reactive oxygen species, 221

sources and diseases, 222

superoxide, 221

theory of aging, 221

Freeman Hospital, 85

French paradox, 70, 201

Friedman, 235

fruits and vegetables, 315, 318, 319, 323, 334

avocado, 189

berries
(blackberries,blueberries,strawber
ries, cranberries, raspberries,
gooseberries), 347
blackberries (organic vs non-
organic), 297
citrus fruits, 318, 345
colored fruit
carotenoids and flavonoids, 344
flavonoids, 345
freshly-squeezed juices vs. juices
from concentrate, 348
grapes, tomatoes, eggplant,
avocados, peppers, 26, 313, 344
green leafy vegetables, 339
green salads, 346
health aspects of some fruits and
vegetables, 344
intake, 202
papaya, canteloupe, watermelon,
346
peppers, 345
recommended levels
Five-a-Day, 202
tomatoes
lycopene, 286, 344

G

Gaynor, Mitchell, 101
gene research, 86
designer drugs, 88
genes, 86
gene-sequencing, 86
genetic effects on cancer
unfounded, 88
genetic manipulation, 298
money in the medicine, 87
gerontology. See aging
Giovannucci, Edward, 197
calcuim and milk and prostate
cancer
a review of the evidence, 197-198
GISSI-Prevenzione study, 326
Giuliani, Rudolph, 197
globalization, 363

glucose tolerance impaired, 91
glycemic index, 342
glycemic loads of foods and, 343
high vs low glycemic index, 343
glycemic load, 343
grades of consumer olive oil, 335
grapes
wine and raisins, 344
Gruman, Jessie, 51
Guthrie, Colin, 253, 256

H

Hager, Mary, 224
Harman, Denham, 221
health
another side to healing, 133
balance of good health, 308
Cardiovascular Health Awareness
Program (CHAP), 274
culture of blame, 393
defined as, 132
democratization of health
information, 122
developing world, 273
get a grip on your health, 396
globalization trends, 273
historical notions, 78
human health and healing, 132
negative triggers for, 378
optimal health, 358, 389, 392
going in for the long haul, 395
physical activity and, 370
problems from bad choices, 388
Victoria Declaration on Heart
Health, 46
women's health
Nurses' Health Study, 328
World Health Organization (WHO),
132
healthcare
acceptable medical practices, 132
approaches, 47
chronic diseases and lifestyle-based
diseases, 47
complementary medicine, 135

crisis-management approach to, 46
diagnostic overkill, 63
elderly population and healthcare
    resources, 219
excessive reliance on high
    technology care, 72
expensive medical intervention
    programs, 64
fix-it mode, 63
growing resenting under present
    systems of managed care, 132
health maintenance organizations
    (HMOs), 132
mainstream medicine, 139, 141
managed care organizations, 132
overall view, 47
patient-centered, 70
policies of reimbursement, 132
prevention model, 47
towards a global definition of
    healthcare, 71
traditional disease-based, 53
healthcare costs
    cardiovascular diseases, 49
    costliest treatments in America, 50
    U.S. expenditure, 48
healthy living
    genuine rewards, 67
    not quick fixes, 101
    proper food versus pharmaceutical
        drugs, 101
heart disease. see cardiovascular
    diseases
Heart Outcome Prevention
    Evaluation (HOPE), 321
herbal industry
    exempted from FDA regulation, 99
herbs
    composition of herbal medications,
        98
    garlic, 347
        nitrosamines, 347
    healing, 77
    spice trade, 99
Herman, William, 49

herpes simplex virus, 95
    acyclovir (Zovirax), effective and
        potentially toxic, 95
    approaches to fighting this viral
        attack (pharmaceutical or
        nutritional), 95
    preventing virus from multiplying,
        95
    sleeper-agent, 95
Hersey, Harry, 70
heterocyclic amines (HCAs),199, 291
Hippocrates, 96
Hoffman, Felix, 97
holistic medical practice, 392
Hoover, Robert, 88
Hu, Frank, 315
Human Genome Project, 88
Hypertension, 54, 83, 92
    and (DASH) dietary approaches to
        stop, 327
    and alcohol, 201
    and free radicals, 228
    classic definition of, 216
    prevention, role of environments,
        88
    processed foods and, 199
    salt (excess sodium) and, 200
hypoglycemia (low blood sugar), 379

I

impotence. See erectile dysfunction
impotence (erectile dysfunction), 374
insulin resistance syndrome. see
    metabolic syndrome
integrative medicine, 145, 146
International Obesity Task Force
    (IOTF), 351
isoflavones, 317, 318

J

Jones, Marion, 393
joy of living, 332
juices
    fruit, 281

processed fruit juices, 281
strawberry vs strawberry-flavored,
281

K

Katz, Michael, 152
Keys, Ancel, 325
Seven Country Study, 323
Koehler, Kathleen, 187
Koplan, Jeffrey, 241

L

Leaf, Alexander, 110, 325
life expectancy, 180
lifestyle
revolution in the way people live
and work, 173
lifestyle based approach, 46
lifestyle choices
Prudent Cosmopolitan Diet,
smoking cessation and increased
physical activity, 349
lifestyle diseases, 166
behavioral risk factors, 173, 174
secondary prevention
never too late, 241
six leading diseases, 170
statistics from National Center for
Health Statistics(NCHS), 48
lifestyle factors
discipline not extremism, 395
establishing good habits, 382
good changes do not occur
overnight, 394
healthy lifestyles can help you lose
weight, reduce blood pressure,
cholesterol and triglycerides, 389
Lifestyle Heart Trial, 119
lifestyle physical activity defined,
370
nutrition factors, 54
personal tastes, preferences, 394
physical inactivity (sedentary
lifestyle levels) in U.S. adults, 368

power to change, 389
self-examination, 391
set your own agenda, 392
some triggers for healthier lifestyle
and physical activity, 378
UK Women's Cohort Study, 390
useful strategies for change, 391
lifestyle patterns
amendable lifestyle changes, 170
globalization of, 166
lignocaine (lidocaine), 97
lipoprotein, 183
Lown, Bernard, 97, 135, 140
book: The Lost Art of Healing, 145
Lundberg, George, 140
severed trust, why American
medicine hasn't been fixed, 140
lycopene
reduces risk of prostate cancer, 286

M

Maas, James, 238
mad cow disease (bovine spongiform
encephalopathy (BSE), 190
Mandela, Nelson, 393
Maslow, Abraham, 258
Maslow's hierarchy
as applied to food habits, 258
McClure, Dr, 134
McCrensky Heitler, Susan, 374, 440
the power of two- secrets to a
strong and loving marriage, 374,
440
meats
composition of, 192
cured, smoked, and charcoal-grilled,
198
fatted calf, blessing, 190
high consumption contributes to
high blood LDL cholesterol
levels, 191
historical attitudes towards, 190
nitrosamines, 198
N-nitroso compounds, 198
poultry, 192, 194

seafood
    low fat protein source, 193
medical advances
    ballon angioplasty (blocked
        arteries), 112
    lithotripsy (kidney stones), 112
medical education
    ad hoc apprenticeship, 110
    focus on fixing not preventing, 108
    hospital-based training, 111
    medical has largely dismissed
        alternative health practices, 134
    overcrowded curriculum, 122
    postgraduate training, 112
    problem-based learning (PBL), 124
    residency training, 112
    SPs, OSCEs, USMLEs, CSA
        examinations, 112
    Western, 107
medical research and publication
    publish or perish, 117
medical school
    madness in the medical profession,
        236
    programs in industrialized societies,
        110
Medicare
    current system of, 65
    modernizing, 64
    political, 64
    program, 73
    the future of the U.S. system, 73
medicine
    good medicine is not just saving
        lives, 246
    herbal medicine difficult to
        standardize, 98
    legal drug trade, 65
    market driven forces dictate, 253
    of the future, 101
    preventive medicine beyond
        preventing disease, 206
    romance with high tech medicine,
        64
    traditional knowledge, 94

Mendelssohn Robert, 84
mentality
    pill-for-every ill, 316
    quick fix, 317
Merck Manual (1899), 144
metabolic syndrome (insulin resistance
    syndrome, syndrome X), 54-56, 90-
    92, 121, 176, 204-206, 216, 351, 388
    aspects of, 206
    hyperinsulinemia, 206
    hyperinsulinemia (Figure 0-3), 54
    obesity (Figure 5-9), 205
Michels, Karin Dr, 89
milk
    butter, 197
    consumption in the Far East, 339
    dairy products and, 195, 339
    designed for babies, 196
    popular misconceptions about, 339
    excess dairy fat elevates blood
        cholesterol, 196
    low fat alternatives (skimmed, semi-
        skimmed), 197
    milk of different species, 197
Milken, Mike, 258
minerals
    calcium, 196
        excess linked to prostate cancer,
            196
        osteoporosis, 191
        significant losses due to high
            protein consumption, 191
    magnesium, 200
        best sources of, 346
Motwani, Dave, 117, 119
Mukamal, Kenneth, 211

N

National Cancer Institute
    personal factors influence on food
        choice and dietary behavior, 274
National Cholesterol Education
    Program(NCEP), 195
National Federation of Spiritual
    Healers (NFSH), 154

National Institutes of Health (NIH), 373
Nebergall, Peter, 77
Nelson, Miriam, 269, 376
   strong women stay slim, 377
Nestle, Marion
   "Food politics," 263
   Surgeon General's report on
     nutrition and health in 1988, 271
nitrites, 100
nitrosamines, 198, 327
   cancer causing, 182, 347
nutrition, 53
   abandonment of nutrition
     education, 116
   and doctors, 109
   anti-nutrients
     anti-vitamins, plant estrogens,
       hallucinogens, plant phenolic
       compounds, 287
   attitudes affect choices, 390
   attitudes concerning nutrition and
     prevention, 118
   departments of diabetes and
     nutrition, 121
   diversity of views, 388
   eating right
     never too late, 242
   enteral and parenteral, 108
   food exchanges, 357
   food science, 114
   formal nutrition programs, 116
   good choices prevent, halt, and
     sometimes reverse health
     problems, 388
   good nutrition leads to optimal
     heath, 389
   heat-labile anti-nutritional factors,
     289
   helping Americans eat right, 389
   history in 1900s, 113
   integrity of our bodies, 109
   largely disregarded, 116
   lifestyle good choices, 356
   linked to infectious diseases, 113

malnutrition, 113
   communicable diseases and, 113
   of hospitalized patients, 108, 120
"medicalization" of, 321
neglect of, 113
Nutrition Curriculum Project, 124
nutrition education in U.S. medical
   schools 1985 report, 126
nutrition education takes time, 389
nutrition in medical education, UK,
   125
Nutrition in Medicine Project
   (NIM), 116
nutrition knowledge, 387
nutrition's role in medical schools,
   U.S.See Figure 3-2, 123
overconsumption of inferior-quality
   foods, 282
pay attention to the whole person,
   396
prevention agenda, 93
preventive nutrition
   primary and secondary levels, 47
principles, 357
protective foods, 114
public interest and knowledge of,
   107
re-education, 395
success of nutrition programs, 124
Surgeon General's Report on
   Nutrition and Health in 1998, 46
technology and therapeutics, 115
unbalanced nutrition and chronic
   diseases, 349
U.S. national policy, 268
vitamin and nutrition research, 114
nutrition-based therapies
   more than quick results, 104
Nutrition in Medicine (NIM) Project,
   124
Nutrition Labeling and Education Act
   (NLEA), 121, 301
nutrition-based therapies
   compared to pharmaceutical drugs,
     103

O

obesity, 53, 55, 85, 86, 87, 91, 92, 165-166, 170, 171, 173, 175-180, 204-206, 350-358
  abdominal, 176, 206
  American obesity epidemic, 265, 388
  and quality of life
    Nurses' Health Study, 351
  android vs. gynecoid obesity, 354
  battle of the bulge, 354
  birth weight and, 89
  central (abdominal/visceral) obesity
    abdominal circumference, 354
    hip circumference, 353
    waist circumference, 353
    waist-hip ratio (WHR), 354
  classification, 352
  costs of obesity, 351
  diseases linked to, 351
  excess food can shorten lifespan, 180
  exercise
    when to check with your doctor, 379
  fattening of America, 271
  genetics in obesity, 355
  genetics vs lifestyle factors, 87
  global epidemic of obesity, 255
  global obesity epidemic, 173, 350, 354
  high-calorie junk food and, 376
  infulences of modernity, megacities and automation, 367
  Japanese sumo wrestlers, 177
  lack of portion control, 265
  lifestyle problems and solutions, 354
  low calorie diets, 387
  measurements
    skinfold measurements, densititometry studies, bioelectrical impedance,deuterium

      dilution,x-ray absorption methods, 354
  medical handicaps and, 352
  metabolic syndrome, 54-55, 90-92, 204-206
  "obesogenic" environment, 256
  osteoarthritis associated with excess body weight, 351
  overconsumption, 176
  overweight, 388
    children, 264
  practical treatment for overcoming obesity, 354
  prevention, 90
  protein sparing fasting, 387
  reasons for high rate of treatment failure, 85
  sucessful approaches to its management, 356
  terms of overweight and obesity, 352
  weight for height charts, 352
  weight management, 85
obesogenic environments, 256
oils
  coconut oil
    major fatty acids in, 188
  coconut oil debate, 189
  compare vitamin E content, 320
  copra oils., 188
  how extraction affects quality, 335
  industrial manufacturing deodorization, 185, 189
  industrially prepared tropical oils, 317
  olive oil, 190, 332, 334
    grades of olive oil, 335
      pomace, 335
        aromatic hydrocarbons polycyclic (PAHs), 335
  olive,avocado, almond, cashew, and rapeseed (canola) oils and products, 183
  palm kernel oils, 189
  soy and sunflower, 325

soybean and corn oil, 183
tropical, 188
Okinawa
longevity, 180, 244-245
olive oils, 332-325
cold pressed, 305
pomace warning, 304,332,333
organic foods, 294
benefits of, 297
certified organic (USDA), 296
definitions, 296
Ornish, Dean, 119, 328
how to reverse heart disease without
drugs or surgery, 140
Osler, William, 234
outlook
of this book, 53-54

P

Pauling, Linus, 221
penicillin, 79
penile arteries (what is bad for the
heart, is bad for the brain, is bad for
the)
Viagra, 227
personal reflections, 157, 236, 308,
359, 383
misery loves company, 236
Pescatello, Linda, 369
pester power
marketing of foods to children, 262
pharmaceutical drugs
atropine (anesthesia and
cardiology), 98
compared to nutrition-based
therapies, 103
coumadin (or warfarin), 98
cozy relationship between
pharmaceutical companies and
doctors, 83
digoxin (heart failure and dropsy),
98
ergotamine (uterine
bleeding/migraine headaches), 97
give credit where due, 96

in the medical establishment, 101
interaction with food (e.g.,
grapefruit juice and Lipitor), 346
Lipitor and Zocor, 97
"money in the medicine", 79, 87
nabilone (anti-nausea), 99
nifedipine, 103
over-the-counter drug market, 79
oxycodone, 98
oxycontin controversy, 84
pharmaceutical industry most
profitable sector in U.S.
economy, 79
pharmaceutical industry revenues,
99
potentially toxic compounds, 95
prescription drug cost vs. benefit,
79
quinidine (irregular heart rhythms),
98
tamoxifen (breast cancer), 317
vast array, 94
vs. herbal drugs (turf war), 99
pharmaceutical industry, 84
physical activity, 367
and sexual activity, 373
benefits of, 371
benefits of moderate-level activity,
374
can compensate for excess food
intake, 370
cardiovascular health, 367
challenges to, 376
cumulative effect of, 374
definition of, 369
establishing good habits
humans are creatures of habit,
382
for health and longevity, 371
for optimized health and disease
prevention, 370
leads to optimal health, 389
lifestyle strategies, 381
misconceptions about, 375
moderate or vigorous exercise, 368

modern living and, 381
National Institutes of Health (NIH)
    statement on cardiovascular
    heath and physical activity,
    373
outdoor and school exercises, 376
overcoming the psychological
    barriers, 381
patterns carry symbolisms, 382
personal reflections, 383
physical education classes, 376
quick facts on U.S. adults, 368
reduction in levels of physical
    activity, 367
rejuvenates the elderly, 243
strength-training program, 243
studies on physical activity and
    health, 371
Surgeon General's report, 367
trigger factors for, 378
weight-training program, 243
physical inactivity, 170, 172
sedentary lifestyle, 173
sedentary lifestyle levels in U.S.
    adults, 368
sedentary lifestyle the norm, 368
unhealthy eating and preventable
    deaths, 368
phytochemicals
cancer fighting activity
    indole-3-carbinol and
        sulphoraphane, 347
lutein, 346
phytonutrients, 286
zeaxanthin, 346
phytoestrogen, 317
placebo effect, 96
positive benefits, 96
randomized double-blind placebo-
    controlled studies, 56
placebos
placebo medicine, 96
Plaisted, Claudia, 124
platelets, 230

polycyclic aromatic hydrocarbons
    (PAHs), 198
pyrolysis, 291
potatoes
fried potato products
    acrylamide, 293
poverty, 264
pregnancy
breastfeeding, 179
calcium intake during, 179
eating for two, false, 179
lactation, 179
outcomes in abnormal
    environments (siege of
    Leningrad), 179
proteins
lipoprotein, 186, 189
Prudent Cosmopolitan Diet
attic (supplements role), 349
ceiling (reduce Western diet), 349
first pillar (Mediterrranean-style
    diet), 349
foundation (local foods), 349
good choices and nutrition plan,
    349
second pillar (Asian-style diet), 349

Q

Quackwatch
combating health-related frauds,
    154
Quick, Sam
aging gracefully, 246

R

Read, Nick, 141
Reaven, Gerald, 54
metabolic syndrome, 205
Rees, Lesley, 138, 143
integrated medicine, 141
repetitive strain injury, 381
re-socialization, 394
restaurants, 281
rice

methods of cooking, 340
polished vs. parboiled or brown, 286
starchy, 340
sticky, 340
Rich-Edwards, Janet, 89
risk
  absolute risk, 203
  beyond risk, 206
  concept of, 167
  factors defined, 169
  factors for heart attack and stroke, 168, 169
  identifying factors for diseases, 168
  major factors (See lifestyle diseases), 170
  probability of developing diseases, 167
  risk factors controlled, 207
  risk factors for heart attack, stroke and erectile dysfunction (impotence), 229
  totality of good evidence, 168
Rosenbaum, Martin, 81
  "marketing to schools", 81
Rosenman (and type A personality), 235
Roth, George, 180
Rubner, Dr, 191

S

salt
  foods high in, 283
  ⋅ hidden sources, 284
  pickled food, 200
  sodium/potassium ratio, 199
  table salt or sodium chloride, 199
Schulman, Jessica
  trends and implications for health educators, 126
sedentary lifestyle. See physical inactivity
self efficacy, 394
sexual activity, 373

male sexual function (impotence), 229
  sexual performance, 374
sexual health, 374
Shils, Maurice, 124
skin
  aging and race, 232
  cellulite, 233
  cumulative sun exposure and, 232
  photo-aging, 232
  skin cancer, 232
  sun damage, 232
  the effects of sun, smoke, race, and sex, 232
sleep, 238
sleep deprivation
  chronic, 237
  effects on healthy young men, 241
  indicators of, 240
  medical effects of, 240
  sleepy drivers, 238
Smith, David, 63
smoking
  and the cardiovascular sytem, 231
  benefits of cessation, 241, 242
  cessation
    never too late, 241
  cessation and risk reduction, 169
  cessation leads to optimal health, 389
  cessation of, 102
  cigarette smoking and death, 172
  environmental tobacco smoke (ETS, second hand smoke), 172
  risk factor for heart disease and stroke, 169
  source of free radicals, 230
  statistics on disease and death, 172
  when a smoker quits, 242
social cognitive theory (SCT), 394
socioeconomics, 367
  adverse circumstances, 393
  broke,busted, and disgusted, 390
  economically-disadvantaged communities, 390

impact on food choices, 266
poor in America vs. poor in Belize, 266
premium placed on meat consumption, 190
principles to overcome barriers, 394
reflected in types of food consumed, 190
status and education, 390
upward social mobility, 267
sodium
dietary, 283
preservatives and flavor enhancers, 283
table salt (sodium chloride), 283
soft drinks, 176, 263, 264
Coca Cola advertising, 273
diet drinks vs water, 348
sodas, 348
soy
categories of soy foods, 339
genetically modified, 298
glycosides,phytosterols, protese inhibitors,phytic acid, isoflavone,genistein, 318
isoflavones, 317
isoflavones and cancer prevention, 338
products, 338
raw soybean, 288
soy product consumption, 327
the complex food, 317
spices
terpenes
d-limonene
anti-cancer properties, 100
citrus
peel,cardamom,coriander, thyme, mint, caraway, 100
St. George, David, 151
Stewart, Moira, 71
Steyer, Terrence, 152
stimulants
caffeinated beverages, 238
Strandal, Angeline, 133

stress, 234
academic and personal, 236
and doctors, 237
and modern living, 234
stroke, 165
sugars
excess calories, 284
high-fructose corn syrup, 284

T

Tanzi, Rudolph, 165
teas
black, oolong or green, 340
catechins, 100
epigallocatechin-3-gallate (EGCG), epigallocatechin (EGC), epicatechin-3-gallate (ECG), 327
flavonoids, 340
green and black teas against cancer, 100
green teas, 340
reduce cancer rates, 327
herbal tea industry, 100
link to lower cancer rates, 340
polyphenol, 100, 340
traditional, 100
un-oxidized, partially-oxidized and oxidized teas, 100
traditions
Hindu Ayurvedic, 77
Judeo-Christian
Mosaic theocratic rule, 77
triglycerides, 9
Trowell, Hugh, 342

U

U.S. Congress, 268
U.S. Postal Service, 154
United States Department of Agriculture(USDA), 269, 296
Food Guide Pyramid, 268, 270

V

Van Cauter, Eve, 241
Vickers, 145
  abc of complementary medicine,
    152
vitamin C
  and the common cold and the flu,
    221
vitamins
  effects of storing and cooking on
    vitamin C, 288
  folic acid
    lowers blood levels of
      homocysteine, 346
  impact of food processing, 285
  oil-soluble vitamins (A,E,K), 345
  peppers
    a rich source of, 345
  stability in varying conditions, 286
  vitamin A
    deficiency treated, 299
  vitamin B1 (thiamin), 285
  vitamin C, 226, 285, 318
    antioxidant health benefits, 232
    deficiency results in scurvy, 232
    fights viral attacks, 95
  vitamin E, 223, 319
    cell membranes and, 224
    content of viatmin E in some
      nuts, seeds, and oils, 320
    natural vs supplement, 319
    sources of, 319
  you win some, you lose some, 286

W

Weeks, David
  secrets of the superyoung, 373
  sexual activity, 233
Weil, Andrew, 138, 140, 143
  integrated medicine, 141
  prescriptions for society, 140
  spontaneous healing, 140
wheat
  milling, minerals, and vitamins, 286
Whelton, Paul, 88
Wilkes, Michael, 81
Willett, Walter, 56, 127, 196, 266, 306
  Eat, drink, and be healthy, 270
  healthy eating pyramid, 271
  Nurses' health study, 187
wine
  resveratol, 344
  with meals
    reservatol and ellagic acid, 334
work
  demands of, 377
World Health Organization (WHO),
  71
Wright, Stephen, 141

Z

Zeisel, Steven, 124
Zollmann, 145
  ABC of Complementary Medicine,
    152

******

Prudent Cosmopolitan Diet

"The Best Diets All Under One Roof"

The Prudent Cosmopolitan Diet is a simple model of healthy eating that embraces the best of the healthiest diets in the world and places them all under one roof. It serves as a framework on which to build your personal strategy to prevent disease and optimize health *(Charts IV, V, and Chapter 8)*.

It incorporates the best of those dietary patterns that are scientifically linked to the lowest rates of nutrition- and lifestyle-related diseases. This approach addresses the urgent need to tackle the modern epidemic of obesity, cardiovascular diseases, type II diabetes, and cancer *(Chart I, II, III, and Chapter 5)*.

The **Prudent Cosmopolitan Diet** is a logical prescription for eating in modern cosmopolitan societies:

- The **foundation** is the *best of American or local foods*. The upward direction of the arrow symbolizes the need to increase the intake of these foods (Chapter 8).
- The **first pillar** is a *Mediterranean-style diet* (Chapter 8). The upward direction of the arrow (chimney) recommends increased intake of these cuisines.
- The **second pillar** is an *Asian-style diet* (Chapter 5 and Chapter 8). The upward direction of this arrow (chimney) recommends increased intake of these foods.
- The **ceiling** with the downward-pointing arrow ("chandelier") represents the advice to consume less of all foods that comprise *the Western diet* (Chapter 5 and Chapter 7).
- Hidden somewhere in the **attic** is a bottle of dietary supplements with the label marked, *"Supplements…not substitutes."* These can play a role, but they are never substitutes for a healthy nutrition and lifestyle (Chapter 2, Chapter 6, and Chapter 8).
- Occupying the **entrance** is a human figure in running form to highlight the need for increased physical activity (Chapter 9).

Good Choices in Nutrition and Lifestyle

(Chart V) summarizes the "big picture:" Your Prudent Cosmopolitan Diet, smoking cessation, and increased physical activity are the 3 key players to prevent and control a broad range of nutrition and lifestyle-related diseases: obesity, cardiovascular diseases, type II diabetes and several forms of cancer.

✓ COLOR VERSIONS OF THESE CHARTS ARE AVAILABLE ON REQUEST

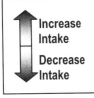

Increase Intake

Decrease Intake

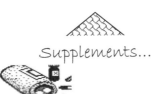

Supplements...

Not substitutes!

Worst of the

Western Diet

High Fat, Red Meats, Highly Processed Foods, Fast Foods, Soft Drinks Dairy Products

Best of

Mediterran -ean Diets

**Vegetable Salads
Virgin Olive Oils
Wine with Meals
Fruits, Nuts, Grains**

Joie de vivre

Best of

Asian Diets

**Soy Products
Green Teas
Stir frys
Greens, Fruits, Nuts, Grains**

High rice and noodle intake with less meats and fats

Best of

American, Regional or Local Diets

Fruits, Vegetables, Whole Grains, Nuts, Fish-especially fatty fish, Skinless-Boneless Poultry & occasional Lean Meats

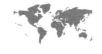 # Prudent Cosmopolitan Diet

"The Best Diets All Under One Roof"

Your Prudent Cosmopolitan Diet is a simple model of healthy eating that embraces the best o the healthiest diets in the world and places them all under one roof. It serves as a framework on which to build your personal strategy to prevent disease and optimize health.

See Chapter 8, Figure 8-3 and text "Constructing a Prudent Cosmopolitan Diet."

Your Doctor
Can't Make You
HEALTHY
Evidence-based insights into protecting your health and
preventing the major lifestyle killers of modern man

Bernard E. Bulwer, M.D.

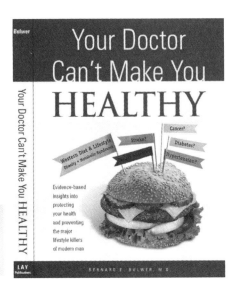

To Order Books

TOLL FREE	**ISBN 0-9725532-0-7**
Book Orders:	Paperback / 472 pages
800-247-6553	US$ 24.95; Can$34.95

Fax: 419-281-6883 **http://www.LookAfterYourHealth.net**

E MAIL ORDERS:..................	drbulwer@LookAfterYourHealth.net
	order@bookmasters.com
ONLINE ORDERS.................	http://www.LookAfterYourHealth.net
Security: PayPal© and VeriSign©	http://www.Atlasbooks.com
SPEAKING	
LECTURES etc......................	drbulwer@LookAfterYourHealth.net

Bernard E. Bulwer, M.D. c/o Bookmasters, Inc. Distribution Services Division,
30 Amberwood Parkway, Ashland, Ohio 44805; Tel: 419/281-1802; Fax: 419/281-6883

Include $3.95 shipping and handling for one book, and $1.95 for each additional book. Canadian orders must include payment in US funds, with 7% GST added. Payment must accompany orders. Allow 3 weeks for delivery.

Name:_____

Organization:_____

Address:_____

City:_____State:_____Zip:_____

Daytime telephone:_____

E-Mail:_____

Payment: □ Cheque □ Visa □ Mastercard □ AMEX □ Discover

#:_____

Name on Card:_____ Exp. Date:_____

By Telephone: (800) 247 6553
Bookmasters, Inc., Distribution Services Division, 30 Amberwood Parkway, Ashland, Ohio 44805

Also available from: **Amazon.com**   ISBN 0-9725532-0-7